Manual of
Hematology

Manual of
Hematology

Editor

Sanjeev Kumar Sharma MD DM
Director, Hemato-oncology and BMT
Incharge, Academics and Research
Department of Hemato-oncology and Bone Marrow Transplantation
BLK-MAX Superspeciality Hospital
Rajendra Place, New Delhi, India

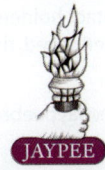

JAYPEE BROTHERS MEDICAL PUBLISHERS
The Health Sciences Publisher
New Delhi | London

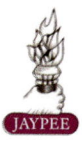

Jaypee Brothers Medical Publishers (P) Ltd

Headquarters
EMCA House, 23/23-B
Ansari Road, Daryaganj
New Delhi 110 002, India
Landline: +91-11-23272143, +91-11-23272703
+91-11-23282021, +91-11-23245672
e-mail: jaypee@jaypeebrothers.com

Corporate Office
4838/24, Ansari Road, Daryaganj
New Delhi 110 002, India
Phone: +91-11-43574357
Fax: +91-11-43574314
e-mail: jaypee@jaypeebrothers.com

Overseas Office
JP Medical Ltd.
83, Victoria Street, London
SW1H 0HW (UK)
Phone: +44-20 3170 8910
e-mail: info@jpmedpub.com

EU GPSR Authorised Representative
Logos Europe, 9 rue Nicolas Poussin
17000, La Rochelle, France
Phone: +33 (0) 6 67 93 73 78
e-mail: contact@logoseurope.eu

Website: www.jaypeebrothers.com
Website: www.jaypeedigital.com

© 2026, Jaypee Brothers Medical Publishers

The views and opinions expressed in this book are solely those of the original contributor(s)/author(s) and do not necessarily represent those of editor(s) or publisher of the book.

All rights reserved. No part of this publication may be reproduced, stored or transmitted in any form or by any means, electronic, mechanical, photocopying, recording or otherwise, without the prior permission in writing of the publishers.

All brand names and product names used in this book are trade names, service marks, trademarks or registered trademarks of their respective owners. The publisher is not associated with any product or vendor mentioned in this book.

Medical knowledge and practice change constantly. This book is designed to provide accurate, authoritative information about the subject matter in question. However, readers are advised to check the most current information available on procedures included and check information from the manufacturer of each product to be administered, to verify the recommended dose, formula, method and duration of administration, adverse effects and contraindications. It is the responsibility of the practitioner to take all appropriate safety precautions. Neither the publisher nor the author(s)/editor(s) assume any liability for any injury and/or damage to persons or property arising from or related to use of material in this book.

This book is sold on the understanding that the publisher is not engaged in providing professional medical services. If such advice or services are required, the services of a competent medical professional should be sought.

Every effort has been made where necessary to contact holders of copyright to obtain permission to reproduce copyright material. If any have been inadvertently overlooked, the publisher will be pleased to make the necessary arrangements at the first opportunity.

Inquiries for bulk sales may be solicited at: jaypee@jaypeebrothers.com

Manual of Hematology / Sanjeev Kumar Sharma

First Edition: **2026**
ISBN: 978-93-6616-024-5
Printed in India at Sterling Graphics Pvt. Ltd.

Contributors

Aastha Gupta MD DM
Additional Director and Head
Department of
Hematopathology and
Molecular Oncology
Fortis Memorial Research
Institute
Gurugram, Haryana, India

Abhishek Purohit MD DM
Additional Professor
Department of Pathology
All India Institute of Medical
Sciences
Jodhpur, Rajasthan, India

Aditi Mittal MD(Pathology)
Consultant
Department of Hematology and
Molecular Biology
Laboratory Services
BLK-MAX Superspeciality
Hospital
Rajendra Place, New Delhi, India

Anamika Bakliwal MD DM
Consultant
Department of Hemato-oncology
and Bone Marrow Transplantation
BLK-MAX Superspeciality
Hospital
Rajendra Place, New Delhi, India

Ankur Ahuja MD DM
Professor
Department of Pathology and
Hematopathology
Armed Forces Medical College
Pune, Maharashtra, India

Brig (Dr) Bhushan Asthana
MD DNB DM
Consultant
Department of
Hematopathology
Command Hospital
Lucknow, Uttar Pradesh, India

Maj (Dr) Blessy Mathew MD
Graded Specialist
Department of Pathology
Command Hospital
Pune, Maharashtra, India

Devasis Panda MD
PDF(Hematopathology) DipRCPath
Consultant
Department of
Hematopathology
Rajiv Gandhi Cancer Institute
and Research Centre
Rohini, New Delhi, India

Divya Doval MD
Senior Consultant
Department of Hemato-oncology and Bone Marrow
Transplantation
BLK-MAX Superspeciality
Hospital
Rajendra Place, New Delhi, India

Gadha K Leons MSc PhD Student
Laboratory Oncology
Dr BRA Institute Rotary Cancer
Hospital
All India Institute of Medical
Sciences
New Delhi, India

Gp Capt (Dr) Preeti Tripathi
MD DM
Professor Hematopathology
Department of Laboratory
Sciences, Army Hospital
Research and Referral
New Delhi, India

Gurleen Oberoi MD DM DNB MNAMS
Senior Consultant
Department of Hematology
Medanta – The Medicity
Gurugram, Haryana, India

Gurmeet Singh MD DM
Deputy Chief Medical Officer
Hematopathologist and
Hematologist
Jawahar Lal Nehru Hospital and
Research Centre
Bhilai, Chhattisgarh, India

Gurpreet Kaur MD
Associate Professor
Department of Pathology and
Hematopathology
Armed Forces Medical College
Pune, Maharashtra, India

Jatin Munjal MD
(Ex Senior Consultant
Hematology, NRL, Dr Lal Path
Labs)
Fellow, Department of
Hematology and Molecular
Biology, BLK-MAX
Superspeciality Hospital
Rajendra Place, New Delhi, India

Jitender Mohan Khunger MD DM
Professor and Head
Department of Hematology
Vardhman Mahavir Medical College and SafdarJung Hospital
New Delhi, India

Jyoti Bajaj Sawhney MD DM
Assistant Professor
Department of Oncopathology
Gujarat Cancer and Research Institute
Ahmedabad, Gujarat, India

Kaninnika Sanyal MD
Senior Resident
Department of Pathology
University College of Medical Sciences and Guru Teg Bahadur Hospital
Dilshad Garden, New Delhi, India

Kanwaljeet Kaur Chopra DM
Incharge Pediatric,
Department of Hemato-oncology
ESI PGIMSR
Basai Dara pur, New Delhi, India

Kriti Batni MD
Senior Resident
Department of Transfusion Medicine
Post Graduate Institute of Child Health (PGICH),
Noida, Uttar Pradesh, India

Col (Dr) Kundan Mishra MD DNB PGDHHM PGDCR MNAMS FICP DM
Professor and Head
Department of Clinical Hematology and Stem Cell Transplant
Medical Division
Command Hospital
Lucknow, Uttar Pradesh, India

Metaanksha Ahuja MBBS(Final Year)
Himalayan Institute of Medical Sciences
Dehradun, Uttarakhand, India

Mitu Dogra MD
Consultant
Department of Transfusion Medicine, BLK-MAX Superspeciality Hospital
Rajendra Place, New Delhi, India

Monica Sharma MD DM
Consultant and Associate Professor
Department of Hematology
Vardhman Mahavir Medical College and SafdarJung Hospital
New Delhi, India

Mousumi Kar MD(Pathology) DM(Hematopathology)
Associate Consultant
Department of Hematology and Molecular Biology, BLK-MAX Superspeciality Hospital
Rajendra Place, New Delhi, India

Mrinalini Kotru MD DM
Director Professor
Department of Pathology
University College of Medical Sciences and Guru Teg Bahadur Hospital
Dilshad Garden, New Delhi, India

Nagarjun Sai MD
Fellow of Hematopathology
Department of Pathology
All India Institute of Medical Sciences
Jodhpur, Rajasthan, India

Nivedita Dhingra MD DM FNB
Pediatric Hemato-oncology
Associate Director
Hematology, Hemato-oncology and Bone Marrow Transplant
Max Super Speciality Hospital
Patparganj, New Delhi, India

Prarthana MD
Senior Resident
Department of Pathology
University College of Medical Sciences and Guru Teg Bahadur Hospital
Dilshad Garden, New Delhi, India

Prashant Mane MD PDCC
Associate Consultant
Department of Histopathology and Cytopathology
BLK-MAX Hospital
Rajendra Place, New Delhi, India

Rahul Arora MD DrNB
Senior Consultant
Hematology and BMT
Department of Hematology
MAX Hospital
Nagpur, Maharashtra, India

Rajan Duggal MD DNB
PDCC Renal and Transplant Pathology
ASH-VTP Lymph Node Pathology
UICC-ICRETT Fellow
Uropathology
Director, Head
Department of Histopathology and Cytopathology
BLK-MAX Super Speciality Hospital
Rajendra Place, New Delhi, India

Col (Dr) Rama Hariharan MD DM
Senior Advisor
Department of Pathology and Hematology
Command Hospital
Lucknow, Uttar Pradesh, India

Rasika Dhawan Setia MD
Director and Head
Department of Transfusion Medicine
BLK-MAX Super Speciality Hospital
Rajendra Place, New Delhi, India

Sanjeev Kumar Gupta MD DNB MNAMS DM
Professor
Laboratory Oncology
Dr BRA Institute Rotary Cancer Hospital
All India Institute of Medical Sciences
New Delhi, India

Contributors

Sanjeev Kumar Sharma MD DM
Director, Hemato-oncology and BMT
Incharge, Academics and Research, Department of Hemato-oncology and Bone Marrow Transplantation
BLK-MAX Superspeciality Hospital
Rajendra Place, New Delhi, India

Sarjana Tiwari MD DM
Consultant Laboratory Hematology
Max Super Speciality Hospital
Patparganj, New Delhi, India

Satyam Arora MD
Additional Professor
Department of Transfusion Medicine, Post Graduate Institute of Child Health (PGICH)
Noida, Uttar Pradesh, India

Shrinidhi Nathany
MD(Pathology) Fellow (Molecular Hemato-oncology), Molecular Oncology Masters, DipRCPATH (Molecular Pathology)
Consultant
Fortis Memorial Research Institute
Gurugram, Haryana, India

Tanvi Gupta MD DNB(Pathology) PDF(Cytogenetics)
Consultant
Department of Genomics and Molecular Diagnostics
Max Superspeciality Hospital
Saket, New Delhi, India

Vandana Puri MD DNB MNAMS DM
Professor
Lady Hardinge Medical College and Associated Hospitals
Ministry of Health and Family Welfare
New Delhi, India

Vipin Khandelwal MD FNB
Consultant Pediatric
Department of Hemato-oncology and BMT Physician
Apollo Hospitals
Navi Mumbai, Maharashtra, India

Preface

Hematology is a diverse branch of medicine that covers both laboratory and clinical aspects of hematology. Both these branches have evolved significantly with newer advances further enhancing the newer concepts and developments in the field of hematology.

This book highlights the older and newer concepts in laboratory hematology in a question and answer format. This book is particularly intended for undergraduate and postgraduate students and fellows and includes the questions faced by students in the routine laboratory hematology.

The various chapters in the book have been written by experts in the field of hematopathology and clinical hematology. The topics focus mainly on the laboratory aspects of benign and malignant hematology and incorporate old and new techniques used in diagnosis and management of hematological diseases. The editor of the book, Dr Sanjeev Kumar Sharma, is a well-known author of three books: "MCQs in Hematology", "Basics of Hematopoietic Stem Cell Transplant", and "My 32 Days in BMT Ward" (in English and Hindi), and has published various articles in national and international journals.

Hopefully, this book will be of immense help to all those interested in hematology and will solve many issues faced by them on day-to-day practice.

Sanjeev Kumar Sharma

Contents

1. **Peripheral Smear** — 1
   Jyoti Bajaj Sawhney
2. **White Blood Cells** — 8
   Mrinalini Kotru, Kaninnika Sanyal, Prarthana
3. **Red Blood Cells** — 40
   Bhushan Asthana, Rama Hariharan, Blessy Mathew
4. **Basics of Complete Blood Count** — 45
   Jitender Mohan Khunger
5. **Rare Causes of Anemia** — 49
   Sanjeev Kumar Sharma, Anamika Bakliwal
6. **Thalassemias** — 53
   Gurmeet Singh
7. **Hemostasis** — 63
   Ankur Ahuja, Gurpreet Kaur, Metaanksha Ahuja
8. **Heparin-induced Thrombocytopenia** — 80
   Jatin Munjal
9. **Von Willebrand Disease** — 85
   Preeti Tripathi
10. **Hemophilia** — 95
    Kanwaljeet Kaur Chopra
11. **Thrombotic Thrombocytopenic Purpura** — 106
    Monica Sharma
12. **Thrombophilia** — 111
    Sanjeev Kumar Sharma, Anamika Bakliwal
13. **Inborn Errors of Immunity** — 114
    Vipin Khandelwal
14. **Bone Marrow Examination** — 124
    Jyoti Bajaj Sawhney
15. **Flowcytometry** — 134
    Gurleen Oberoi

16.	**Cytogenetics** *Vandana Puri, Tanvi Gupta*	**146**
17.	**Molecular Diagnostics** *Sanjeev Kumar Gupta, Gadha K Leons*	**158**
18.	**Next-generation Sequencing** *Shrinidhi Nathany*	**170**
19.	**Evaluation of Lymph Node** *Rajan Duggal*	**179**
20.	**Lymphoproliferative Disorders** *Devasis Panda, Mousumi Kar*	**188**
21.	**Myelodysplastic Neoplasm** *Aastha Gupta*	**205**
22.	**Myeloproliferative Neoplasm** *Anamika Bakliwal*	**210**
23.	**Myeloid Malignancies** *Sarjana Tiwari, Nivedita Dhingra*	**215**
24.	**Acute Promyelocytic Leukemia** *Rahul Arora*	**221**
25.	**Hodgkin Lymphoma** *Prashant Mane*	**229**
26.	**Serum Protein Electrophoresis** *Nagarjun Sai, Abhishek Purohit*	**237**
27.	**Light Chain Myeloma** *Gurleen Oberoi*	**247**
28.	**Basics of Transfusion Medicine** *Rasika Dhawan Setia, Mitu Dogra*	**269**
29.	**Blood Banking Procedures** *Kriti Batni, Satyam Arora*	**282**
30.	**CAR T-cell Therapy** *Sanjeev Kumar Sharma, Divya Doval*	**294**
31.	**Clinical Case Studies** *Kundan Mishra*	**298**
32.	**Interesting Cases in Hematology** *Aditi Mittal*	**311**

Index   **333**

1. Peripheral Smear

Jyoti Bajaj Sawhney

Q1. How should blood samples be collected?

Ans: Blood is drawn from a vein (venipuncture), usually from the inside of the elbow or the back of the hand. The phlebotomist should have hand-hygiene materials (soap and water or alcohol rub), well-fitting nonsterile gloves, single-use disposable needles, and syringes or lancing devices in sufficient numbers to ensure that each patient has a sterile needle and syringe or equivalent for each blood sampling. Clean the site with a 70% alcohol swab for 30 seconds and allow to dry completely (30 seconds). The vein should be entered swiftly at a 30° angle or less.[1]

Q2. Which anticoagulants are used in tube used for collecting blood samples?

Ans: Whole blood is collected in blood collection tubes or syringes that contain the appropriate anticoagulant to inhibit coagulation.

Routine hematology tests require a blood collection tube containing ethylenediaminetetraacetic acid (EDTA), a chelating anticoagulant. EDTA acts as a chelating agent to bind cofactor divalent cations (mainly calcium) to inhibit enzyme reactions involved in the clotting cascade specifically the conversion of prothrombin to thrombin and subsequent inhibition of the thrombolytic action on fibrinogen to fibrin necessary for clot formation. EDTA preserves the morphology of the cellular elements of blood, making it a satisfactory anticoagulant for hematologic studies. Blood collection tubes containing heparin, which stabilizes the red blood cell (RBC) membranes, are used for specialized hematology studies, such as red cell fragility tests and several specialized chemistry tests. Blood collection tubes containing sodium citrate are used for coagulation studies.[2]

Q3. What preanalytic variables should be monitored when evaluating a blood sample?

Ans: Laboratory results are dependent on the quality of the specimen analyzed. Preanalytical steps, the major source of mistakes in laboratory diagnostics, arise during patient preparation, sample collection, sample transportation, sample preparation, and sample storage. The preanalytical phase accounts for the majority of laboratory errors. It has been estimated that preanalytical errors account for more than two-thirds of all laboratory errors, while errors in the analytical phase and postanalytical phase account for one-third of all laboratory errors.[3]

The most commonly reported types of preanalytical error are:
- Missing sample and/or test request
- Wrong or missing identification
- Contamination from infusion route
- Inappropriate containers
- Hemolyzed or clotted sample
- Number of samples with insufficient volumes
- Inappropriate blood to anticoagulant ratio
- Inappropriate transport and storage conditions

Q4. **What information can be obtained from a blood smear?**

Ans: The blood film is one of the world's most widely and frequently used tests.

Blood smear examination serves three important objectives:[4]
1. It serves as a quality control tool in verifying the results generated by the automated analyzers.
2. It allows for identification of abnormal/immature/atypical cells, if present.
3. It allows for recognition of clinically significant morphologic abnormalities, which the analyzers are incapable of either flagging or detecting and identifying.

Currently available automated hematology analyzers do not generate any reportable information about the presence of many of the:
- Red cell abnormalities such as elliptocytes/ovalocytes, target cells, sickle cells, acanthocytes, echinocytes, SC crystalloids, stomatocytes, tear drop cells, rouleaux, Howell–Jolly bodies, pappenheimer bodies, basophilic stippling, and intraerythrocytic organisms
- White cell abnormalities (Auer rods, toxic granulation, toxic vacuolization, Dohle bodies, hypogranular/agranular granulocytes intraleukocytic organisms, etc.)
- Platelet abnormalities (platelet satellitosis, abnormal granulation, and hypogranulation/agranulation bizarre platelets).

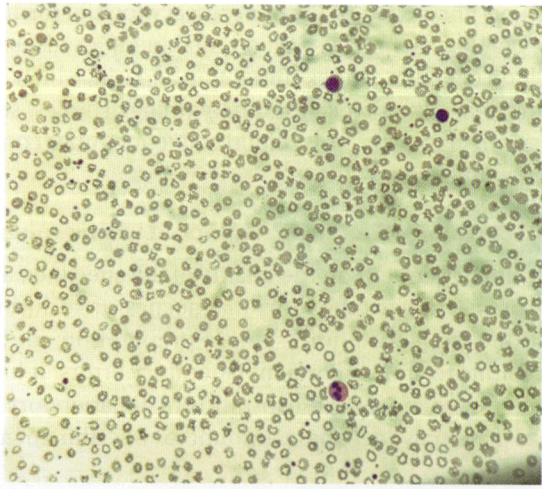

FIG. 1: Peripheral smear showing neutrophil and lymphocyte in the background of red blood cells (10×).

Q5. What are the artifacts that can affect peripheral blood smears?

Ans: An artifact on peripheral blood smear refers to "an artificial structure or tissue alteration on a prepared microscopic slide as a result of an extraneous factor". They are the major source of diagnostic confusion. The most common artifacts on the peripheral smear are caused by poor spreading techniques, slow drying in humid conditions, insufficient or delayed fixation, and fixing solutions that contain water.

Certain cell types can be damaged or ruptured easily by the blood film preparation itself. These are called smudge cells.[5] These are associated with special conditions like those with large numbers of atypical lymphocytes, chronic lymphocytic leukemia, and acute leukemia.

Slow drying causes cells to contract, whereas, water in excess of 3% in the methanol fixing solution can cause the development of artificial vacuoles. Degenerative changes, such as cytoplasmic vacuolization in monocytes and neutrophils, nuclear lobulation, or fragmentation of nucleated cells, and apoptotic changes are caused by prolonged or inadequate sample storage.

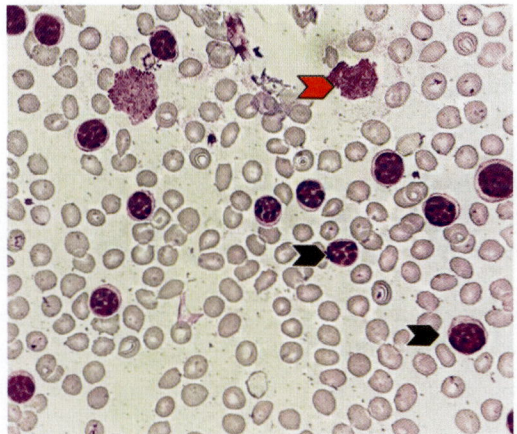

FIG. 2: Case of chronic lymphocytic leukemia: Peripheral smear (100×). Arrowhead (black)—mature lymphocytes with clumped chromatin resembling soccer ball. Arrowhead (red)—smudge cell.

Courtesy: Dr Abhishek Purohit.

Q6. What can be the false-positive and false-negative results from automated analyzers?

Ans:
- *White blood cells (WBCs)*: Causes of spurious decrease:[6]
  - Agglutination of polymorphonuclear leukocytes (PMN) (EDTA-related)
  - Agglutination of WBC other than PMN (lymphocytes, lymphoma cells, and leukemic blasts)
  - Excess amount of K3-EDTA anticoagulant
  - Coagulation within the sample
- *WBC*: Spurious increase—
  - Platelet aggregates
  - Very large platelet
  - Nucleated RBC
  - RBC resistant to lysis (newborns, abnormal Hb, chemotherapy, uremia, liver disease)

- Cryoglobulin, cryofibrinogen, and immunoglobulins
- Lipids
- Microorganisms (bacterial aggregates)
- *RBC*: Spurious decrease—
  - Cold agglutinins, warm agglutinins
  - Very small RBC
  - Cryoglobulins (↓ flow, inadequate aspiration)
  - In vitro hemolysis
  - Coagulation
- *RBC*: Spurious increase—
  - High WBC counts
  - Giant platelets
- *Hemoglobin: Spurious increase*—
  - Lipids
  - High WBC counts
  - Immunoglobulins (cryoglobulins)
  - In vitro hemolysis
  - Carboxyhemoglobin (high amount)
  - Bilirubin (>250–300 mg/L)
- *Hemoglobin*: Spurious decrease—
  - Coagulation within the sample
  - Overfilling vacuum tube
  - Venipuncture near a drip
  - Sulfhemoglobin
- *Mean corpuscular volume (MCV)*:
  - Cold agglutinins, warm agglutinins: ↑
  - High WBC counts: ↑
  - Hyperglycemia: ↑
  - K2 EDTA in excess: ↑
  - Hyper- or hyponatremia: ↑ or ↓

Conditions leading to possible interference with automated methods for reticulocyte analysis:
- *Inaccurate gating of RBCs*: Giant platelets, platelets clumps, abnormal WBCs, abnormal number of WBCs, WBC fragments, and nucleated RBCs
- *Intraerythrocytic particles*: Howell–Jolly bodies, pappenheimer bodies, basophilic stippling, Heinz bodies, sickle cells, spherocytes, hemoglobin H inclusions, *Plasmodium*, and *Babesia*
- *Others*: Cold agglutinin disease, autofluorescence of RBCs (drugs, porphyria), paraproteins, hemolysis, and diagnostic intravenous fluorescent dyes

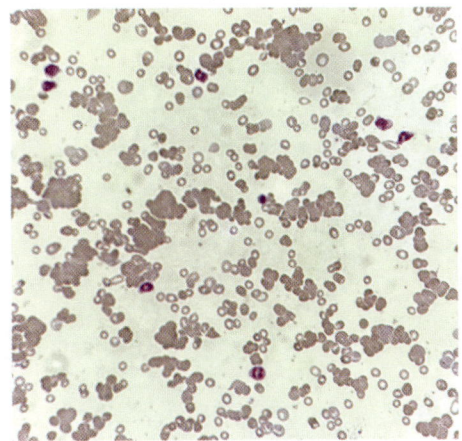

FIG. 3: Peripheral blood smear showing RBC agglutination.
Courtesy: Dr Abhishek Purohit.

Q7. What is rouleaux? What is its significance?

Ans: The RBCs in the plasma tend to form aggregates or rouleaux that appear similar to a stack of coins. Rouleaux formation is determined largely by increased levels of plasma fibrinogen and globulins. It is a reversible aggregation process. Although myeloma and macroglobulinemias are first considered by hematologists, other causes that occur more frequently include acute and chronic infections, connective tissue diseases, and chronic liver disease.[7]

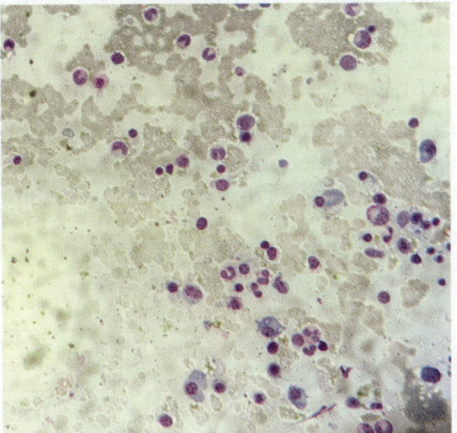

FIG. 4: Rouleaux formation in bone marrow aspirate in case of multiple myeloma with plasma cells.
Courtesy: Dr Jyoti Sawhney.

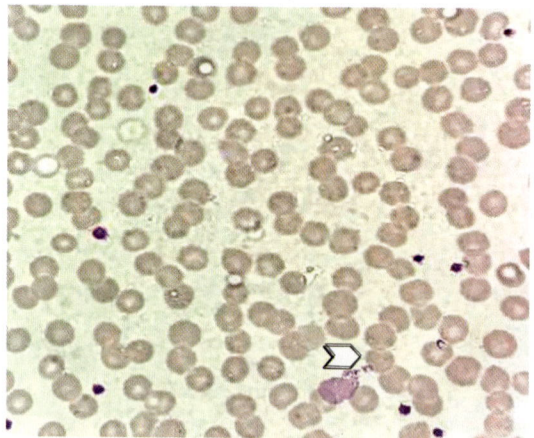

FIG. 5: Peripheral smear (100×): Rouleaux formation (arrowhead).
Courtesy: Dr Abhishek Purohit.

Q8. What are the limitations of the blood smear?

Ans: Few limitations of the peripheral smear examination are:[8]
- Experience is required to make technically adequate smears.
- There is a nonuniform distribution of WBCs over the smear, with larger leukocytes concentrated near the edges and lymphocytes scattered throughout. This can lead to erroneous estimation of total leukocyte count (TLC) and differential count.
- There is a nonuniform distribution of RBC over the smear, with small crowded RBCs at the thick edge and large flat RBCs without central pallor at the featured edge.

Q9. Which parasites can be identified on the peripheral smear?

Ans: The microscopic examination of thick and thin peripheral blood smears stained with Giemsa stain is used for detection and identification of *Plasmodium, Babesia,* and *Trypanosoma* species and filarial nematodes species (i.e., *Brugia, Mansonella,* and *Wuchereria*).[9]

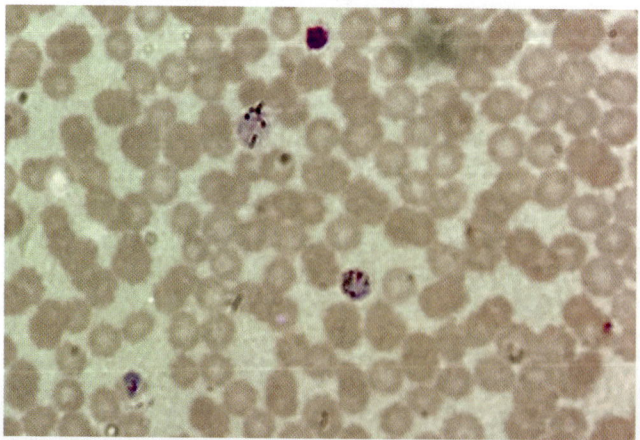

FIG. 6: *Plasmodium vivax* schizont.
Courtesy: Dr Abhishek Purohit.

Q10. **What are commonly used routine and cytochemical stains for peripheral smear?**

Ans: Romanowsky stains are used universally for routine staining of blood films.[10] The remarkable property of the Romanowsky dyes of making subtle distinctions in shades of staining, and of staining granules differentially, depends on two components: (i) azure B (trimethyl thionine) and (ii) eosin Y (tetrabromofluorescein). Among the Romanowsky stains in use, Jenner is the simplest and Giemsa is the most complex. Leishman stain, which occupies an intermediate position, is widely used in the routine staining of blood films, although the results are better obtained by combining May–Grünwald–Giemsa, Jenner–Giemsa, and azure B–eosin Y methods. Cytochemical stains are special stains used for staining peripheral blood and bone marrow smears that help in classifying and differentiating different types of leukemias.[11] These stains are cheap, time saving, easy to perform, and yet effective tools in differentiating different types of leukemias. These include:

- Leukocyte alkaline phosphatase (LAP) to differentiate chronic myeloid leukemia (CML)—chronic phase from neutrophilic leukemoid reaction
- Myeloperoxidase stain—to diagnose acute myeloblastic leukemia
- Sudan black B—to diagnose acute myeloblastic leukemia
- Acid phosphatase (ACP)—to diagnose hairy cell leukemia
- Esterases—to diagnose acute monocytic leukemia (AML-M4 or AML-M5)
- Periodic acid–Schiff block positivity is indicative of acute lymphoblastic leukemia.
- Toluidine blue—for rapid detection and species identification of malarial parasites

REFERENCES

1. Lippi G, Salvagno GL, Montagnana M, Franchini M, Guidi GC. Phlebotomy issues and quality improvement in results of laboratory testing. Clinical Laboratory. 2006;52:217-30.
2. Baskin L, Dias V, Chin A, Abdullah A, Naugler C. Effect of Patient Preparation, Specimen Collection, Anticoagulants, and Preservatives on Laboratory Test Results. Accur Res Clin Lab. 2013:19-34.
3. Plebani M. Quality Indicators to Detect Pre-Analytical Errors in Laboratory Testing. Clin Biochem Rev. 2012;33(3):85-8.
4. Gulati G, Song J, Florea AD, Gong J. Purpose and criteria for blood smear scan, blood smear examination, and blood smear review. Ann Lab Med. 2013;33(1):1-7.
5. Perkins SL, Nakashima MO, Agarwal AM, Olteanu H, Bhargava P, Pozdnyakova O, et al. (2019). Hematology, Clinical Microscopy, and Body Fluids Glossary. [online] Available from https://documents.cap.org/documents/2019-hematology-clinical-microscopy-glossary.pdf [Last accessed April, 2024].
6. Zandecki M, Genevieve F, Gerard J, Gordon A. Spurious counts and spurious results on hematology analysers: a review. Part II: white blood cells, red blood cells, hemoglobin, red cell indices and reticulocytes Int J Lab Hematol. 2007;29(1):21-41.
7. Abramson N. Rouleaux formation. Blood. 2006;107(11):4205.
8. Beckman AK, Ng VL, Jaye DL, Gaddh M, Williams SA, Yohe SL, et al. Clinician-ordered peripheral blood smears have low reimbursement and variable clinical value: A three-institution study, with suggestions for operational efficiency. Diagn Pathol. 2020;15:112.
9. Rosenblatt JE, Reller LB, Weinstein MP. Laboratory diagnosis of infections due to blood and tissue parasites. Clin Infect Dis. 2009;49:1103-8.
10. Krafts KP, Pambuccian SE. Romanowsky staining in cytopathology: history, advantages and limitations. Advan Biotech Histochem. 2011;86(2):82-93.
11. Jamal I. Cytochemical stains in hematology. J Evid Based Med Healthc. 2020;7(25):2349-570.

2. White Blood Cells

Mrinalini Kotru, Kaninnika Sanyal, Prarthana

Q1. What are the causes of neutrophilia?

Ans: Neutrophilia is a condition where the neutrophil count in the blood is higher than the normal range, typically above 7,700 neutrophils/µL. It is the most common form of leukocytosis. The normal absolute neutrophil count (ANC) in adults ranges from 2,500 to 7,000 neutrophils/µL.[1]

Mechanism: The production, proliferation, differentiation, and entry of neutrophils in peripheral blood are tightly regulated by cytokines and controlled by various transcription and growth factors. Neutrophilia can be due to aberrant neutrophils' production by the bone marrow, margination of neutrophils into the bloodstream, and reactive response to various stimuli **(Table 1)**.

TABLE 1: Summarizing the causes of neutrophilia.

Category	Subcategory	Cause	Description
Factitious neutrophilia	Handling artifacts	Prolonged tourniquet application during venipuncture	Artificial increase in neutrophil count due to blood sample handling issues
		EDTA-based or improperly anticoagulated blood samples	Platelet clumping leading to falsely elevated neutrophil count; resolved by using properly anticoagulated samples
		Cryoglobulin particles	Falsely high neutrophil count due to cold-insoluble proteins; resolved by obtaining blood sample at room temperature
Primary neutrophilia	Myeloproliferative neoplasms (MPN)	Chronic myeloid leukemia (CML), essential thrombocythemia (ET), polycythemia vera (PV), and chronic myelomonocytic leukemia (CMML), chronic neutrophilic leukemia (CNL), etc.	Excess and autonomous production of blood cells by the bone marrow

Continued

Continued

Category	Subcategory	Cause	Description
	Genetic/Inherited neutrophilia	Leukocyte adhesion factor deficiency	Rare disorder with marked leukocytosis, recurrent infections, and delayed umbilical cord separation
	Chronic neutrophilic leukemia	*CSF3R* gene mutation	Rare disorder with chronic neutrophilia, splenomegaly, and high neutrophil count
	Transient myeloproliferative disorder (TMD)	Down syndrome-related abnormal myelopoiesis	Transient condition resembling leukemia in infants with Down syndrome, may resolve spontaneously or progress to acute leukemia
	Hereditary neutrophilia	Familial cold urticaria	Autosomal disorder with chronic neutrophilia, splenomegaly, and bleeding complications due to platelet dysfunction
Secondary/reactive neutrophilia	Infection/inflammation	Bacterial/viral infections	Common cause of neutrophilia with left shift, toxic granulations, and Döhle bodies
	Leukemoid reaction	*Clostridium difficile*, tuberculosis, and medications	WBC count >50,000 cells/μL due to infections or medications, needs distinction from acute leukemia
	Chronic inflammatory conditions	Still disease, rheumatoid arthritis, vasculitis, hepatitis, and IBD	Neutrophilia due to cytokine release in chronic inflammation
	Nonhematological neoplasms	Solid tumors	Neutrophilia due to paraneoplastic reactions, bone marrow metastasis, or tumor-related inflammation
	Medications	G-CSF, GM-CSF, glucocorticoids, ATRA, lithium, and catecholamines	Increase neutrophil count by stimulating bone marrow or causing release of neutrophils from marrow into circulation
	Smoking	Cigarette smoking	Associated with elevated leukocyte and neutrophil count (up to 25%)
	Stress	Postoperative, acute myocardial infarction	Neutrophilia due to neutrophil redistribution from marginating to circulating pool, possibly related to epinephrine release
	Exercise	Exercise-induced	Neutrophilia due to increased epinephrine and altered cardiac output, leading to neutrophil redistribution

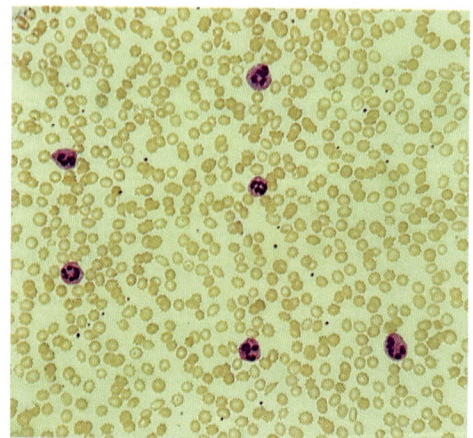

FIG. 1: Peripheral smear showing neutrophilia with segmented neutrophils. (Leishman stain, 1000×).

Q2. How do you classify neutropenia? What are the causes of neutropenia?

Ans: Neutropenia is defined as a reduction in the ANC in peripheral blood, with ANC < 1,500/µL.[2] It is classified based on the severity of ANC depression **(Table 2)**. There could be multiple causes of neutropenia **(Table 3)**.

TABLE 2: Classification of neutropenia.	
Classification	ANC count
Mild neutropenia	$1.0–1.5 \times 10^9$/L
Moderate neutropenia	$0.5–1.0 \times 10^9$/L
Severe neutropenia	$<0.5 \times 10^9$/L

TABLE 3: Causes of neutropenia.		
Category	Specific causes/disorders	Key features
Immune-associated neutropenia	• Isoimmune neonatal neutropenia • Chronic autoimmune neutropenia • Transfusion neutropenia • Chronic idiopathic neutropenia	Autoimmune destruction or alloimmune reaction against neutrophils, often resolving spontaneously in primary cases
Nonimmune hematologic disorders	• Myelodysplastic syndromes • Aplastic anemia • Leukemia • Bone marrow fibrosis or metastasis • Hypersplenism	Disorders causing ineffective hematopoiesis or bone marrow failure, often requiring careful management
Congenital neutropenia	• Kostmann syndrome • Congenital cyclic neutropenia	Genetic disorders causing profound neutropenia with frequent severe infections, often presenting in infancy

Continued

Continued

Category	Specific causes/disorders	Key features
Other congenital anomalies	• Shwachman–Diamond syndrome • Cartilage-hair hypoplasia	Congenital disorders with associated neutropenia and other systemic abnormalities
Functional abnormalities	• Chédiak–Higashi syndrome • Myelokathexis	Neutrophil functional defects, leading to recurrent infections and associated with specific genetic syndromes
Nutritional deficiencies	• Vitamin B12 deficiency • Folate deficiency	Deficiencies in essential nutrients leading to impaired neutrophil production
Drug-induced neutropenia	• Chemotherapy • Antibiotics (e.g., penicillins and cephalosporins)	Neutropenia due to bone marrow suppression or immune-mediated destruction, often reversible upon discontinuation of the offending drug
Infections	• Viral infections (e.g., HIV and hepatitis) • Severe bacterial infections (e.g., sepsis)	Infections leading to neutrophil destruction or sequestration, potentially causing severe neutropenia
Endocrine disorders	• Hypothyroidism • Addison's disease	Hormonal disorders that may affect neutrophil production or lifespan
Nonimmune chronic idiopathic neutropenia	Idiopathic neutropenia	A benign acquired syndrome with no underlying autoimmune or clonal bone marrow disorder, often asymptomatic with an incidental finding of neutropenia
Neutropenia associated with bone marrow disorders	• Aplastic anemia • Fanconi anemia • Myelodysplastic syndromes • Leukemias • Postchemotherapy neutropenia	Severe conditions impairing bone marrow function, leading to reduced neutrophil production and increased infection risk
Congenital disorders of vesicular trafficking	• Chediak–Higashi syndrome • Griscelli syndrome type II • Hermansky–Pudlak syndrome type II	Disorders affecting neutrophil granule function, often associated with albinism, bleeding disorders, and increased infection susceptibility
Postinfectious neutropenia	Postinfectious neutropenia	Neutropenia following severe infections, often transient and resolving as the infection clears
Other specific conditions	• Kostmann syndrome • Myelokathexis • Lazy leukocyte syndrome • Glycogen storage disease type Ib • Pure white cell aplasia • Acquired cyclic neutropenia • Transfusion reactions	Rare syndromes with distinct genetic or metabolic causes of neutropenia, often presenting with recurrent infections and specific bone marrow findings

Q3. What is congenital neutropenia?

Ans: Congenital neutropenias are a group of disorders characterized by abnormally low neutrophil counts, leading to increased susceptibility to infections. The two major forms are severe congenital neutropenia (SCN) and cyclic neutropenia (CN).

Severe Congenital Neutropenia

The SCN is a serious genetic disorder marked by extremely low neutrophil counts (typically under 500 cells/µL), leading to recurrent, severe bacterial infections in neonates and infants.[3]

Clinical Features
- *Onset*: Symptoms usually appear within the first 3 months of life.
- *Infections*: Common pathogens include *Staphylococcus aureus*, *Escherichia coli*, and *Pseudomonas aeruginosa*. Infections often start in early infancy and include omphalitis, perirectal abscesses, otitis media, pneumonia, gingivitis, and urinary tract infections.
- *Severe infections*: Septicemia, peritonitis, and enteritis
- *Bone marrow findings*: Severe neutropenia (ANC < 0.2×10^9/L), with increased monocytes and eosinophils

Pathophysiology

The SCN is associated with increased apoptosis of myeloid precursors, despite normal granulocyte colony stimulating factor (G-CSF) receptor function.

Genetic mutations → defects in neutrophil development → severe neutropenia → increased infection susceptibility → increased risk of myelodysplastic syndrome/acute myeloid leukemia (MDS/AML).

Genetics

The SCN can be inherited in autosomal dominant, autosomal recessive, or X-linked patterns, linked to mutations in several genes affecting neutrophil development and function **(Table 4)**.

TABLE 4: Genetic associations in severe congenital neutropenia.		
Gene	**Syndrome/Condition**	**Key features**
HAX-1	Kostmann's syndrome	Severe neutropenia, increased susceptibility to bacterial infections, and mitochondrial-dependent apoptosis
WASP	Wiskott–Aldrich syndrome	Thrombocytopenia, small platelets, sinopulmonary infections, and eczema
GFI1	–	Regulates genes involved in granulopoiesis (production of granulocytes)
SBDS	Shwachman–Diamond syndrome	Pancreatic insufficiency, skeletal abnormalities, and bone marrow dysfunction
G6PC3	–	Impaired neutrophil function, associated with SCN

Mutation impact: ELANE mutations may lead to defective protein accumulation, causing apoptosis of neutrophil precursors.

Risk of Malignancy
Patients with SCN have an increased risk of developing MDS and AML, with an annual risk of approximately 2–8%.

Cyclic Neutropenia
Cyclic neutropenia is a periodic hematological disorder characterized by recurrent episodes of severe neutropenia (ANC ≤ 0.2 × 10^9/L), which typically occur in cycles of approximately 21 days.[4]

Clinical Features
- *Cycle duration*: Neutropenic episodes typically recur every 21 days but can vary from 12 to 36 days.
- *Neutropenic nadirs*: Each episode of severe neutropenia lasts approximately 3–5 days.
- *Symptoms include*:
  - Recurrent fevers
  - Aphthous ulcers
  - Infections affecting the skin, upper respiratory tract, and ears
- The severity of infections correlates with the depth and duration of the neutropenia during each cycle.

Inheritance and Genetics
- *Inheritance*: CN is primarily inherited in an autosomal dominant pattern, although sporadic cases have been reported. CN can also be acquired in association with other conditions, such as large granular lymphocytosis.
- *Genetics*: Nearly all congenital cases of CN are linked to mutations in the *ELANE* gene, which encodes neutrophil elastase.

Diagnostic Approach
- *Blood counts*: Serial blood counts, taken every 2–3 weeks over a 6-week period, are used to document CN.
- *Genetic testing*: Identification of pathogenic mutations consistent with cyclic white blood cell (WBC) fluctuations.
- *Bone marrow biopsies*: Characteristically show a lack of neutrophils before neutropenic episodes, followed by an increase in neutrophil precursors as recovery begins.

Q4. Describe the various morphological changes in neutrophils and the conditions associated with them.

Ans: The various qualitative or morphologic neutrophil abnormalities that can be identified are shown in **Table 5**.[5]

CHAPTER 2: White Blood Cells

TABLE 5: The morphologic abnormalities seen in neutrophils.

Category	Abnormality	Description
Nuclear abnormalities	Pelger–Huët anomaly	Hyposegmented neutrophil nuclei
	Hypersegmentation	Neutrophils with more than five nuclear segments
	Pyknotic nuclei	Condensed, fragmented nuclei often seen in dying neutrophils
Cytoplasmic abnormalities	Döhle bodies	Blue-gray cytoplasmic inclusions, often seen in infections
	Toxic granules	Dark-staining granules, and indicative of severe infection or stress
	Cytoplasmic vacuoles	Vacuoles in the cytoplasm, often associated with phagocytosis
	Intracellular organisms	Presence of fungi or bacteria within neutrophils
Inherited functional abnormalities	Alder–Reilly anomaly	Large, dark-staining granules due to mucopolysaccharidosis
	Chediak–Higashi disease	Giant granules in neutrophils, associated with albinism and infections.
	May–Hegglin anomaly	Large platelets and Döhle–like bodies in neutrophils
	Chronic granulomatous disease	Defective intracellular killing of pathogens
	Myeloperoxidase deficiency	Lack of enzyme critical for microbial killing
	Adhesion deficiency	Defective leukocyte adhesion and migration

Q5. What is Pelger–Huët anomaly?

Ans: Pelger–Huët anomaly (PHA) is a genetic disorder named after Karl Pelger and G Huët who first described the condition, characterized by abnormal nuclear development in WBCs, particularly neutrophils.[5]

Etiology and Genetics

- *Inheritance*: Autosomal dominant disorder.
- *Gene involved*: Mutations in the *Lamin B receptor (LBR)* gene on chromosome 1q42.1.
- *Function*: The *LBR* gene encodes a protein essential for the nuclear envelope's structural integrity and chromatin organization.
- *Pathology*: Mutations disrupt normal nuclear development, leading to the characteristic nuclear abnormalities of PHA.

Pathology

- *Nuclear appearance*:
  - *Neutrophils*: Bilobed or unilobed nuclei with rod-like, dumbbell-shaped, peanut-shaped, or spectacle-like ("pince-nez") appearances **(Table 6)**.

- *Chromatin*: Coarse chromatin clumping helps differentiate PHA cells from immature forms.
- *Functionality*: Neutrophil function remains normal despite abnormal morphology.
- *Misdiagnosis risk*: The abnormal appearance can be mistaken for immature or dysplastic cells seen in conditions such as myelodysplastic syndromes and acute leukemia.

TABLE 6: Types of Pelger–Huët anomaly (PHA).

Type	Characteristics
Heterozygous PHA	- More common - Neutrophils exhibit bilobed "pince-nez" (eyeglass-shaped) nuclei - Other leukocytes may show mild nuclear abnormalities
Homozygous PHA	- Rare - Neutrophils have round or oval nuclei with no segmentation - Dense chromatin in eosinophils, basophils, and megakaryocytes - Normal myeloid precursor morphology in bone marrow

Clinical Presentation

Symptoms: PHA is usually asymptomatic and often discovered incidentally during routine blood smears.

TABLE 7: Diagnosis of Pelger–Huët anomaly.

Diagnostic method	Key features
Peripheral blood smear	Presence of neutrophils with bilobed or unilobed nuclei and condensed chromatin
Family history	PHA often runs in families, making a thorough family history helpful for diagnosis
Genetic testing	Identification of mutations in the *LBR* gene confirms the diagnosis, especially in atypical cases

Diagnostic Process for Pelger–Huët Anomaly (Table 7)

- *Routine blood smear*: Presence of abnormal neutrophil nuclei (bilobed or unilobed nuclei). These cells are typically mature with condensed chromatin.[6]
- *Family history*: Check for PHA in relatives.
- *Genetic testing*: Confirm *LBR* mutation

TABLE 8: Differential diagnosis of Pelger–Huët anomaly.

Condition	Key Features
Pseudo–Pelger–Huët anomaly	- Morphological changes similar to PHA - Seen in myeloid leukemias, myelodysplasia, or after chemotherapy - Nuclei often resemble the single oval type characteristic of homozygous PHA
Other disorders	Neutrophil nuclear abnormalities can also occur in infections, drug reactions, and severe inflammatory states

Pseudo–Pelger–Huët Anomaly

Pseudo–Pelger–Huët anomaly (PPHA) refers to the presence of WBCs with abnormal nuclear shapes, resembling the PHA **(Table 8)**. This morphological change is observed in various conditions, including myxedema, acute enteritis, agranulocytosis, multiple myeloma (MM), malaria, leukemoid reactions (LRs), drug reactions, and chronic lymphocytic leukemia. However, pseudo–Pelger–Huët cells are most seen in myeloid leukemias, both acute and chronic, and in myeloid metaplasia. These cells typically emerge in the advanced stages of the disease, often following extensive chemotherapy, and predominantly exhibit nuclei similar to those in the homozygous state of PHA.[6]

Q6. What is Alder–Reilly anomaly?

Ans: Alder–Reilly anomaly is an inherited recessive disorder characterized by the presence of large, dark-staining granules in leukocytes. Despite the abnormal morphology, leukocyte function is typically not impaired. The condition is commonly associated with mucopolysaccharidosis (MPS), a group of lysosomal storage disorders.[7]

Associated Conditions

- *Commonly seen in*: Patients with bone and cartilage abnormalities.
- *Linked to MPS*: A group of lysosomal storage disorders due to enzyme deficiencies that impair the breakdown of glycosaminoglycans (GAGs) **(Table 9)**.

Mechanism

GAG accumulation: Due to enzyme deficiencies in MPS, partially degraded GAGs accumulate within lysosomes, leading to the formation of characteristic granules in leukocytes **(Table 10)**.

TABLE 9: Types of mucopolysaccharidosis (MPS) associated with Alder–Reilly anomaly.

MPS type	Syndrome name
MPS I	Hurler syndrome
MPS II	Hunter syndrome
MPS III	Sanfilippo syndrome
MPS IV	Morquio syndrome
MPS VI	Maroteaux–Lamy syndrome
MPS VII	Sly syndrome

TABLE 10: Morphologic features.

Feature	Description
Granules	Large, coarse, and dark-staining granules in leukocytes; stain dark lilac with Wright–Giemsa stains
Distribution	Present in neutrophils, eosinophils, basophils, monocytes, and occasionally lymphocytes
Appearance	Unlike toxic granulation, these granules are persistent and appear in all leukocytes regardless of clinical condition

Clinical Features

Symptoms primarily related to the underlying MPS, including developmental delay, skeletal abnormalities, and organomegaly. The diagnosis is confirmed by genetic studies **(Table 11)**.

TABLE 11: Diagnosis of mucopolysaccharidosis.	
Diagnostic method	**Key features**
Peripheral blood smear	Identification of characteristic granules in leukocytes on a stained blood smear
Bone marrow examination	Not typically required, but can show similar granules
Enzyme assays	Diagnose specific types of MPS by identifying deficient enzyme activity
Genetic testing	Confirms diagnosis by identifying mutations in genes responsible for enzyme deficiencies

Q7. What do you understand by hypersegmentation of neutrophils?

Ans: Neutrophil hypersegmentation can be defined as the presence of neutrophils with six or more lobes or the presence of >3% of neutrophils with at least five lobes.[5] The presence of hypersegmented neutrophil is an important diagnostic feature of megaloblastic anemias. In florid megaloblastic states, neutrophils are often enlarged, and their nuclei may have six or more segments connected by particularly fine chromatin bridges.

Etiology

- *Megaloblastic anemia*: Commonly seen in conditions such as vitamin B12 or folate deficiency due to impaired DNA synthesis, leading to ineffective hematopoiesis and nuclear maturation defects.
- *Myelodysplastic syndromes* can be indicative of bone marrow dysplasia.
- *Hereditary hypersegmentation*: A rare genetic condition with benign clinical implications.
- *Chronic infections and inflammation*: Occasionally, observed due to increased demand for neutrophils.

A right shift with moderately hypersegmented neutrophils may also be seen in uremia and not infrequently in iron deficiency. Hypersegmentation can be seen after cytotoxic and antimetabolite treatment, especially with methotrexate, hydroxycarbamide, and other drugs that induce megaloblastosis.

Hereditary Hypersegmentation of Neutrophils

Hereditary hypersegmentation of neutrophils is an autosomal dominant condition characterized by an increased number of nuclear lobes in neutrophils.[8] This genetic anomaly is important for distinguishing from other conditions associated with neutrophil hypersegmentation, such as folate or vitamin B12 deficiencies.

Key Characteristics

- *Neutrophil features*:
  - Neutrophils exhibit six to ten nuclear lobes, compared to the typical three to four lobes.
  - Despite the increased nuclear segmentation, the overall size of neutrophils remains normal.
- *Genetic inheritance*:
  - The condition is inherited in an autosomal dominant pattern.
  - Heterozygotes display >10% of neutrophils with five or more lobes.
  - Homozygotes may show even higher percentages, exceeding 14%.

- *Bone marrow findings*: Bone marrow shows nuclear indentation in early myeloid cells, including neutrophils, eosinophils, and basophils.
- *Additional observations*: Increased nuclear drumsticks (Barr bodies) have been noted, particularly in female carriers.

Q8. What is May–Hegglin anomaly?

Ans: May–Hegglin anomaly (MHA) is a rare autosomal dominant genetic disorder characterized by the presence of large basophilic cytoplasmic inclusions in leukocytes, particularly neutrophils, along with giant platelets **(Table 12)** and thrombocytopenia.[9] May–Hegglin anomaly is caused by mutation in *MYH9* gene which encodes for nonmuscle myosin heavy chain IIA (NMMHC-IIA). This affects the cytoskeleton of megakaryocytes and leukocytes, leading to abnormal platelet morphology and characteristic inclusions.

TABLE 12: Morphologic features of neutrophils and platelets in May–Hegglin anomaly.

Feature	Description
Döhle–like bodies	Large, pale blue inclusions in neutrophils, eosinophils, and monocytes. These are larger and more prominent than typical Döhle bodies
Giant platelets	Platelets are significantly larger than normal, often larger than a red blood cell
Thrombocytopenia	Reduced platelet count, with variability in severity among individuals

Clinical Features

Patients with *MYH9*-related disorders may experience bleeding tendencies, such as easy bruising, nosebleeds (epistaxis), and heavy menstrual bleeding (menorrhagia), primarily due to thrombocytopenia. However, some individuals may be asymptomatic or have only mild symptoms, with severe bleeding being rare. Additionally, these disorders can include kidney disease (nephropathy) and sensorineural hearing loss, although these complications are less common in pure May–Hegglin anomaly (MHA).

Q9. What is Jordan Anomaly?

Ans: Jordan Anomaly is characterized by the presence of vacuoles within the cytoplasm of granulocytes, monocytes, and sometimes lymphocytes and plasma cells.[10] Neutrophils and monocytes show lipid filled vacuoles which are confirmed through histochemical and fluorescence microscopic analysis. Lipid accumulation is not observed in myeloblasts, erythroblasts, or megakaryocytes.

Q10. What are Döhle bodies?

Ans: Döhle bodies are small, light gray-blue oval inclusions in the cytoplasm of neutrophils and eosinophils, typically found near the cell periphery. They indicate cellular stress or altered granulocyte maturation.[11] They are aggregates of rough endoplasmic reticulum and free ribosomes. There can be various causes of Döhle bodies **(Table 13)**.

TABLE 13: The etiology of Döhle bodies.

Condition	Associated with Döhle bodies
Infections	Severe bacterial infections
Inflammatory states	Conditions like rheumatoid arthritis
Toxic states	Burns, trauma, chemotherapy
Pregnancy	Sometimes noted during normal pregnancy

Q11. What are toxic granules?

Ans: Toxic granules are dark, coarse granules found in neutrophils and their precursors, such as myelocytes and metamyelocytes, during severe infections or inflammatory states. They represent primary (azurophilic) granules that are more prominent and intensely stained and are seen in about 66–75% of patients with sepsis, and can also be seen after burns or trauma. They reflect increased lysosomal enzyme content and indicate accelerated neutrophil maturation under stress.

Diagnostic significance:
- *Indicator of severe inflammation*: Presence of toxic granules helps in diagnosing severe infectious or inflammatory conditions.
- *Correlated findings*: Often seen alongside Döhle bodies and cytoplasmic vacuolization, suggesting a robust inflammatory response.

Note: Toxic-like granules or inclusions can also appear as artifacts due to increased staining or low pH of the stain in a peripheral smear.

Q12. What are the disorders of neutrophil function defects? Discuss in brief common phagocytic disorders.

Ans: Neutrophils work in a systemic manner to perform the function of chemotaxis and phagocytosis using different ligands and molecules.[12] Defects in neutrophil functions can cause various diseases **(Table 14)**.

TABLE 14: Common neutrophil function defects.

Defect	Description	Clinical implications	Associated diseases
Adhesion defects	Impaired ability of neutrophils to adhere to endothelial cells and migrate to infection sites	Recurrent bacterial infections, delayed wound healing	Leukocyte adhesion deficiency (LAD)
Chemotaxis defects	Reduced or absent neutrophil movement toward chemical signals (chemoattractants)	Increased susceptibility to infections due to impaired immune response	Chediak–Higashi syndrome, Job syndrome (Hyper-IgE syndrome)
Phagocytosis defects	Defective engulfment of pathogens by neutrophils	Persistent infections, especially with encapsulated bacteria	Chediak–Higashi syndrome, chronic granulomatous disease (CGD)

Continued

Continued

Defect	Description	Clinical implications	Associated diseases
Degranulation defects	Inability to release antimicrobial granules after engulfing pathogens	Ineffective pathogen killing, leading to recurrent infections	Specific GRANULE DEFICIENCY, Chediak–Higashi syndrome
Oxidative burst defects	Impaired production of reactive oxygen species necessary for pathogen destruction	CGD, increased susceptibility to catalase-positive organisms	CGD
Killing defects	Deficient intracellular killing of pathogens after phagocytosis	Recurrent, severe bacterial and fungal infections	CGD, myeloperoxidase deficiency

Q13. What is leukocyte adhesion deficiency?

Ans: Defect in adhesion of leukocytes to vascular endothelium affecting their subsequent migration to extravascular space gives rise to a group of rare primary immunodeficiency diseases (PIDs) known as leukocyte adhesion defects (LADs) **(Table 15)**. In patients with LAD, the neutrophils fail to migrate to the site of infection leading to a state of tissue neutropenia.[13]

Aspect	LAD type 1	LAD type 2	LAD type 3
TABLE 15: Summary of types of leukocyte adhesion deficiency (LAD).			
Genetic defect	Mutations in *ITGB2* gene	Mutations in *FUCT2* gene	Mutations in *FERMT3* gene
Defective molecule	CD18 (β2 integrins)	Sialyl Lewis X (fucosylated glycan)	All integrins (defective activation)
Pathophysiology	Impaired leukocyte adhesion and migration	Defective leukocyte rolling on endothelium	Defective integrin activation affecting adhesion and migration
Clinical features	Recurrent bacterial infections, poor wound healing, and delayed umbilical cord separation	Recurrent bacterial infections, delayed wound healing, severe mental retardation, short stature, distinct facial features, and Bombay blood phenotype	Severe recurrent infections, Glanzmann thrombasthenia, and delayed umbilical cord separation
Diagnostic methods	<ul><li>Flow cytometry: Reduced CD18/CD11b expression on leukocytes</li><li>Neutrophil characteristics: Deficient motility, impaired phagocytosis, reduced granule secretion, and impaired microbial killing</li><li>Normal immunoglobulin levels</li><li>Normal complement function</li><li>Normal lymphocyte responses</li><li>Genetic testing: ITGB2 mutations confirmation</li></ul>	<ul><li>Phagocytosis: Normal, but with defects in neutrophil motility and aggregation</li><li>Flow cytometry</li><li>Surface expression analysis: Absence of CD15s, normal CD18</li><li>Genetic testing: FUCT2 mutations confirmation</li></ul>	<ul><li>Genetic testing: FERMT3 mutations confirmation</li><li>Platelet aggregation studies: It may reveal Glanzmann thrombasthenia</li></ul>

Q14. What is chronic granulomatous disease?

Ans: Chronic granulomatous disease (CGD) is a primary immunodeficiency disorder characterized by the inability of phagocytes, particularly neutrophils, to effectively kill certain bacteria and fungi. This defect is due to a malfunction in the NADPH oxidase complex, which is essential for the production of reactive oxygen species (ROS) required for the destruction of ingested pathogens.[14] CGD is a genetic disorder with both X-linked and autosomal recessive inheritance patterns.

Etiology and Genetic Basis

- *Genetic mutations*: CGD arises due to mutations in genes encoding components of the NADPH oxidase complex. The key components and their associated genes include:
  - gp91^{phox} *(CYBB gene)*: The most common mutation site, leading to X-linked CGD
  - p22^{phox} *(CYBA gene)*: Associated with autosomal recessive CGD
  - p47^{phox} *(NCF1 gene)*, p67^{phox} *(NCF2 gene), and Rac2 (RAC2 gene)*: Other components involved in autosomal recessive CGD
- *Inheritance patterns*:
  - *X-linked CGD*: Accounts for approximately 65–70% of cases and is caused by mutations in the *CYBB* gene, which encodes gp91^{phox}.
  - *Autosomal recessive CGD*: Makes up the remaining 30–35% of cases, resulting from mutations in other NADPH oxidase components.

Pathophysiology

The NADPH oxidase complex is crucial for the oxidative burst within phagocytes, leading to the generation of ROS, such as superoxide anions and hydrogen peroxide. These ROS are vital for killing ingested pathogens. In CGD, mutations in NADPH oxidase components disrupt this process, leading to impaired microbial killing and chronic granuloma formation.

- *Defective ROS production*: In CGD, the defective NADPH oxidase complex fails to produce ROS, impairing the oxidative burst.
- *Incomplete microbial killing*: The failure to generate ROS results in incomplete degradation of phagocytosed pathogens, particularly catalase-positive organisms.
- *Chronic inflammation and granuloma formation*: Persistent infection and immune activation lead to the formation of granulomas, which are clusters of macrophages attempting to contain the infection.
- *Can lead to autoimmunity*: In CGD, chronic inflammation, continuous immune activation, and altered cytokine profiles can lead to immune dysregulation, may promote development of autoimmune diseases.

Diagnosis

- *Nitroblue tetrazolium (NBT) test*: The NBT test assesses the ability of neutrophils to produce ROS. In CGD, neutrophils fail to reduce NBT to its blue formazan product, indicating a defective oxidative burst.
- *Dihydrorhodamine 123 (DHR) test*: The DHR test, which is currently the preferred diagnostic method, evaluates the oxidative burst in neutrophils by measuring the conversion of DHR to a fluorescent compound in the presence of ROS. A reduced fluorescence signal indicates CGD.

- *Genetic testing*: Genetic testing is used to confirm the specific mutation in NADPH oxidase components, helping to differentiate between X-linked and autosomal recessive forms of CGD.

Q15. What are the tests for neutrophil function defects?

Ans: Primary disorders of neutrophil function result from impairment in neutrophil responses that are critical for host defense.[15] Defects of neutrophil number and function commonly present with recurrent and severe bacterial and fungal infections, often involving the skin and respiratory tract as well as deep tissue sites. There are various tests useful for assessment of neutrophil function **(Table 16)**.

TABLE 16: The various tests useful for assessment of neutrophil function.

Test	Purpose	Method	Interpretation	Associated conditions
Nitroblue tetrazolium (NBT) test	Evaluate oxidative burst activity	Neutrophils incubated with NBT dye. Normal neutrophils reduce dye to blue-black formazan in response to a stimulus (e.g., PMA, bacteria). Patients with CGD show no or minimal color change	• Positive (blue formazan) = normal • Negative (no color change) = oxidative burst defect	Chronic granulomatous disease (CGD)
Dihydrorhodamine 123 (DHR) flow cytometry	Assess oxidative burst capacity	Neutrophils stained with DHR 123, which becomes fluorescent when oxidized by ROS. Fluorescence measured by flow cytometry	• Reduced fluorescence = oxidative burst defect • Can detect carrier state	CGD
Chemotaxis assay	Evaluate neutrophil migration	Neutrophils placed in a chamber with a gradient of chemoattractant (e.g., fMLP and IL-8). The distance or speed of migration is measured, often using a Boyden chamber or underagarose method	Impaired migration = chemotaxis defect	LAD, other chemotactic defects
Phagocytosis assay	Assess ability to engulf pathogens	Neutrophils incubated with opsonized particles (e.g., latex beads, bacteria). The number of engulfed particles is quantified by microscopy or flow cytometry	Reduced phagocytosis = phagocytic function defect	Neutrophil dysfunctions, including specific phagocytic disorders
Oxidative burst test (flow cytometry)	Measure generation of reactive oxygen species (ROS)	Neutrophils stimulated with agents like PMA. ROS production is detected using fluorescent probes (e.g., DCFH-DA). Fluorescence intensity is measured by flow cytometry	Decreased fluorescence = oxidative burst defect	CGD

Continued

Test	Purpose	Method	Interpretation	Associated conditions
Surface marker expression (flow cytometry)	Assess expression of surface markers important for neutrophil function	Flow cytometry used to measure markers like CD11b, CD18 (integrins), CD15 (Sialyl Lewis X), which are involved in adhesion and migration	Abnormal marker expression = adhesion/migration defects	LAD
Degranulation assay	Assess ability to release granules	Neutrophils stimulated (e.g., with fMLP, PMA) to release granules. Granule content (e.g., elastase, lactoferrin, myeloperoxidase) is measured using ELISA or other biochemical assays	Reduced degranulation = granule release defect	Specific granule deficiency (SGD), other degranulation defects
Bactericidal assay	Evaluate ability to kill bacteria	Neutrophils incubated with bacteria. After a set period, the number of surviving bacteria is quantified by plating and counting colony-forming units (CFUs)	Reduced bacterial killing = defect in phagocytosis, oxidative burst, or granule content	CGD, LAD, and other neutrophil dysfunctions

Q16. What is Chediak–Higashi syndrome?

Ans: Chediak–Higashi syndrome (CHS) is a rare, autosomal recessive disorder characterized by immunodeficiency, neurological abnormalities, and other systemic features due to defects in lysosomal trafficking.[16] It is caused by mutations in the *CHS1/LYST* gene on chromosome 1q42-43, which encodes the lysosomal trafficking regulator protein **(Table 17)**. This protein is essential for the proper synthesis, transport, and fusion of cytoplasmic vesicles.

Characteristic triad:
- Albinism
- Recurrent pyogenic infections
- Peripheral neuropathy

TABLE 17: Pathophysiology of Chediak–Higashi syndrome.	
Aspect	**Details**
Genetic cause	Mutations in the *LYST (lysosomal trafficking regulator)* gene
Lysosomal abnormalities	Defective LYST protein leads to abnormal fusion and function of lysosomes, resulting in large, and dysfunctional granules
Accelerated phase	Can terminate as lymphoma-like syndrome, leading to infiltration of nodes, liver, spleen, and marrow; often fatal

Q17. What are the causes of lymphocytosis?

Ans: Lymphocytosis, defined by an increase in absolute lymphocyte count (ALC) to >4,000 lymphocytes/µL in adult patients, is a common hematologic abnormality.[17] Different lymphocyte subsets (T cells, B cells, or NK cells) may be increased depending on the etiology

(**Table 18**). Lymphocytes represent around 20–40% of WBC. The definition of relative lymphocytosis is an increase in WBC of >40% in the presence of a normal absolute white cell count. Normal B:T cell ratio in children is 2:1 while in adults its 1:4.

Category	Condition/Disorder	Description/Key characteristics
TABLE 18: Causes of lymphocytosis.		
Infections	Viral infections	Epstein–Barr virus (EBV) (infectious mononucleosis), cytomegalovirus (CMV), human immunodeficiency virus (HIV) (acute infection), influenza, hepatitis, mumps, measles, rubella, human T-lymphotropic virus type 1 (HTLV-1), adenovirus, etc.
	Bacterial infections	*Bartonella henselae* (cat scratch disease), *Bordetella pertussis* (pertussis), brucellosis, syphilis, and malaria
	Parasitic infections	*Toxoplasma gondii* (toxoplasmosis), babesiosis
	Mycobacterial infections	*Mycobacterium tuberculosis* (tuberculosis)
Chronic inflammatory conditions	Chronic inflammatory diseases	Rheumatoid arthritis and inflammatory bowel disease
	Autoimmune disorders	Systemic lupus erythematosus (SLE) and Sjögren's syndrome
Drug reactions	Drug-induced lymphocytosis	Reactions to allopurinol, carbamazepine, vancomycin, sulfa drugs, and ibrutinib [associated with drug reaction with eosinophilia and systemic symptoms (DRESS) syndrome and redistribution of chronic lymphocytic leukemia (CLL) cells]
Stress	Severe/emergency conditions	Cardiac conditions, status epilepticus, and epinephrine use (transient lymphocytosis preceding neutrophilia)
Asplenia	Postsplenectomy	Lymphocyte count may increase after spleen removal but usually stabilizes over time
Lymphoproliferative disorders	Adult T-cell leukemia/lymphoma (ATLL)	Caused by HTLV-1, characterized by proliferation of T-cells
	Large granular lymphocyte leukemia (LGL)	T-LGL cells are large with azurophilic granules; associated with pancytopenia, splenomegaly, and rheumatoid arthritis
	Acute lymphoblastic lymphoma (ALL)	Characterized by increased lymphoblasts rather than mature lymphocytes
	Monoclonal B lymphocytosis (MBL)	Presence of monoclonal B cells (<5,000 cells/µL) without features of lymphoproliferative disorders, splenomegaly, or cytopenias
	Congenital B-cell lymphocytosis	Due to a germline mutation in CARD11; progresses to chronic lymphocytic leukemia (CLL) by the fourth decade of life
	Persistent polyclonal B-cell lymphocytosis	Rare, associated with polyclonal binucleated lymphocytes, occurs in young smoking women, associated with HLA-DR7 and IgM polyclonal gammopathy, and stable clinical course

PBS findings provide critical insights into the underlying cause of lymphocytosis, as summarized in **Table 19**.

TABLE 19: Types of lymphocytes and associated conditions.

Lymphocyte form	Associated condition
Reactive lymphocytes	Variable in size, abundant cytoplasm, indented nucleus; seen in viral infections such as Epstein–Barr virus (EBV), cytomegalovirus (CMV), and early human immunodeficiency virus (HIV)
Clonal lymphocytes	Small mature lymphocytes, "smudge cells" seen in lymphocytic leukemia (CLL) and monoclonal B-cell lymphocytosis (MBL)
Atypical large lymphocytes	Seen in EBV and other viral infections like CMV or early HIV
Cleaved/angulated/indented nucleus	Present in conditions such as pertussis or malignancies such as follicular lymphoma
"Hairy cells"	Regular cytoplasmic projections characteristic of hairy cell leukemia
Sezary cells	Cribriform nuclei with compact chromatin, seen in Sezary syndrome, a type of cutaneous T-cell lymphoma.
"Villous" lymphocytes	Observed in marginal zone lymphoma (MZL), with distinctive cytoplasmic projections
Large lymphocytes with azurophilic granules	Seen in T-cell large granular lymphocytic leukemia (T-LGL)
Lymphoblasts	Indicative of acute lymphoblastic leukemia (ALL)

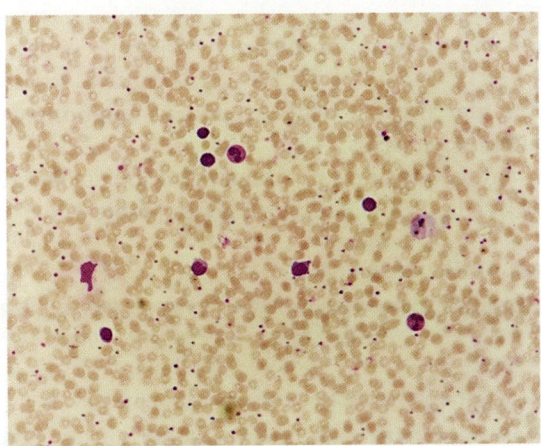

FIG. 2: Reactive lymphocyte with abundant cytoplasm and irregular nucleus (Leishman stain, 1000×).

Q18. What are large granular lymphocytes?

Ans: Large granular lymphocytes (LGL) are larger than typical lymphocytes, measuring about 15–18 μm in diameter.[18] They have a round to oval nucleus, sometimes slightly indented, with condensed chromatin. The cytoplasm is abundant and pale blue, containing coarse azurophilic granules, which are rich in enzymes such as perforin and granzymes, crucial for their cytotoxic function.[18] They play a crucial role in the immune system, particularly in combating viral infections and tumor cells.

Types of Large Granular Lymphocytes

The LGLs are primarily divided into two major types: (1) Natural killer (NK) cells and (2) cytotoxic T lymphocytes (CTLs) **(Table 20)**.

TABLE 20: Types of large granular lymphocytes and their key characteristics.

Type	Function	Markers	Mechanism of action
Natural killer (NK) cells	Involved in innate immunity; target virus-infected; and tumor cells without prior sensitization	CD56 and CD16 (lack CD3)	Induce apoptosis via release of perforin and granzymes
Cytotoxic T lymphocytes (CTLs)	Part of adaptive immunity; recognize antigens on infected/malignant cells presented by MHC class I molecules	CD3 and CD8	Similar mechanism as NK cells; kill target cells through perforin and granzymes

Clinical Significance

- *Reactive conditions*: LGLs can increase in number in various reactive conditions, including:
  - Viral infections, e.g., infectious mononucleosis (IM)
  - Autoimmune diseases, e.g., rheumatoid arthritis
  - *Postvaccination*: Temporary increases following certain vaccinations.
- *Autoimmune disorders*: Rheumatoid arthritis—LGLs can contribute to the pathology through their cytotoxic activity.
- *LGL leukemia*:
  - *Description*: A rare chronic lymphoproliferative disorder with a persistent increase in LGLs.
  - *Symptoms*: Patients may present with cytopenias, splenomegaly, and autoimmune disorders like rheumatoid arthritis.
  - *Diagnosis*: Confirmed through flow cytometry and molecular studies detecting clonal rearrangements of T-cell or NK-cell receptor genes **(Table 21)**.

Diagnosis and Evaluation Process

TABLE 21: Laboratory evaluation techniques for large granular lymphocytes (LGLs).

Technique	Purpose
Peripheral blood smear	Identify the presence of large granular lymphocytes
Flow cytometry	Characterize the immunophenotype of LGLs (e.g., CD3, CD8, and CD56)
Molecular studies	Assess clonality using T-cell receptor gene rearrangement in suspected LGL leukemia

Flow Cytometry Insights

- *Markers*: NK cells often express CD16 and CD57. CD56 is expressed by normal NK cells but downregulated in CLPD-NK. T-LGLs generally express a specific phenotype (e.g., CD3+, TCR αβ+, and CD8+).
- *Prognostic indicators*: Downregulation of certain markers, such as CD56 in NK cells or expression profiles in T-LGLs, can indicate prognosis.

Role of LGLs in Infection and Cancer Surveillance
The LGLs are critical for:
- *Infection surveillance*: Detecting and eliminating virus-infected cells
- *Cancer surveillance*: Early detection and destruction of tumor cells

Q19. **What are Downey cells?**

Ans: Downey cells, also known as reactive lymphocytes or atypical lymphocytes, are a type of lymphocyte that appears in response to viral infections, most notably Epstein–Barr Virus (EBV), which causes IM. These cells exhibit distinctive morphological features that help in their identification and are indicative of an activated immune response.

Clinical Relevance
- *Infectious mononucleosis*:
  - Downey cells are a hallmark of IM caused by EBV.
  - Their presence supports the diagnosis, especially when seen in conjunction with clinical symptoms and serological tests.
- *Other viral infections*: Downey cells can also be seen in other viral infections such as cytomegalovirus (CMV), hepatitis, rubella, and toxoplasmosis.
- *Immune response*:
  - These cells represent the body's immune response to viral antigens.
  - They are typically CD8+ cytotoxic T cells or CD4+ helper T cells activated in response to infection.

Q20. **Enlist the hematological changes associated with Epstein–Barr virus.**

Ans: Key hematologic features in IM are:[19]
- *Atypical lymphocytosis*: Hallmark of IM is the presence of atypical lymphocytes (Downey cells), primarily CD8+ T cells, and less commonly CD16+CD56+ NK cells. These cells exhibit variability in size and shape with abundant cytoplasm and irregular, scalloped edges.
- *Lymphocytosis*: Significant increase in lymphocyte count, often exceeding 50% of total WBCs, with atypical lymphocytes constituting >10%. Peak lymphocytosis typically occurs around the onset of symptoms.
- *White blood cell count*: Typically ranges from 10.0 to 20.0×10^9 cells/L, with some cases exceeding 20.0×10^9/L. The ALC generally surpasses 5.0×10^9 cells/L.

Hematologic Complications
- *Immune hemolytic anemia*: Autoimmune destruction of red blood cells, leading to anemia
- *Immune thrombocytopenia*: Immune-mediated reduction in platelet count, increasing the risk of bleeding
- *Leukopenia*: Less common but can include lymphopenia and granulocytopenia. Severe neutropenia and thrombocytopenia are rare and may indicate hemophagocytic syndromes.
- *Marrow aplasia*: Failure of bone marrow to produce blood cells, leading to pancytopenia
- *Virus-associated hemophagocytic syndrome*: A severe inflammatory condition characterized by the excessive activation of immune cells that engulf other blood cells.
- *Acquired immune deficiencies*: EBV can lead to immune suppression, increasing vulnerability to infections and other complications.

EBV-associated Lymphoproliferative Disorders[20]

- *Chronic active EBV infection*: Persistent atypical lymphocytes and clonal expansion of EBV-infected T or NK cells, leading to chronic symptoms and immune dysfunction.
- *Post-transplant lymphoproliferative disorder (PTLD)*: Proliferation of large immunoblasts in immunocompromised patients (e.g., post-transplant) with a risk of progression to aggressive lymphoma
- *Hodgkin lymphoma*: Characterized by the presence of Reed–Sternberg cells, with approximately 40–50% of cases associated with EBV.
- *Diffuse large B-cell lymphoma (DLBCL)*: It includes EBV-positive variants with clonal expansion of large B lymphocytes, often seen in immunocompromised individuals.
- *Burkitt lymphoma*: Highly associated with EBV, especially in endemic areas, and commonly presents with abdominal tumors
- *Hemophagocytic lymphohistiocytosis (HLH)*: Triggered by EBV, this disorder is characterized by excessive inflammation and tissue damage due to overactive immune cells.

Q21. Discuss morphology of plasma cells.

Ans: There can be multiple morphological variants of plasma cells **(Table 22)**.

TABLE 22: Morphological variants of plasma cells.

Variant	Features
Plasmablasts	Intermediate stage in B cell to plasma cell maturation; larger cells with less condensed chromatin and prominent nucleoli
Plasmacytoid lymphocytes	Intermediate between lymphocytes and plasma cells; seen in conditions like Waldenström macroglobulinemia
Flame cells	Plasma cells with bright red/pink cytoplasm due to increased immunoglobulin content; seen in multiple myeloma
Binucleated/multinucleated cells	Plasma cells with more than one nucleus, often seen in plasma cell neoplasms like multiple myeloma

Immunoglobulin Inclusions in Plasma Cells

Types of inclusions:
- *Dutcher bodies*: Intranuclear inclusions, periodic acid-Schiff (PAS)-positive, representing intranuclear accumulations of immunoglobulins, commonly seen in MM.
- *Russell bodies*: Large, eosinophilic, homogeneous inclusions in the cytoplasm due to immunoglobulin accumulation, often in chronic antigenic stimulation.
- *Mott cells/grape cells*: Plasma cells with multiple, large, round cytoplasmic inclusions due to immunoglobulin accumulation.
    - Mature plasma cells are observed in MM.
    - Mature plasma cells corresponding to the lymphoplasmacytoid subtype exhibit mature chromatin and a high nuclear-to-cytoplasmic (N/C) ratio.
    - Mott cells in MM contain a variable number of round inclusions.
    - Dutcher bodies are inclusions seen in the nucleus.
    - Vacuolated plasma cells are present.
    - Tadpole plasma cells are noted.

- Flaming plasma cells are characterized by bright eosinophilic cytoplasm.
- Plasma cells with irregular nuclear outlines are observed, and the presence of at least 5% of such cells is related to adverse prognosis.
- Crystalline inclusions can be found in plasma cells.
- Abnormal plasma cells that are difficult to ascertain morphologically may lead to a hypothesis of metastatic carcinoma.
- Peripheral blood plasma cells in plasma cell leukemia (PCL) exhibit variable morphology, which corresponds to the aggressive behavior of the disease.
- Plasmablasts show variable morphology.
- Immature plasma cells display one prominent nucleolus with either condensed or fine chromatin.

Immunophenotype of Plasma Cells (Table 23)

TABLE 23: Immunophenotype of reactive versus malignant plasma cells.[21]		
Marker	**Reactive plasma cells**	**Malignant plasma cells**
CD19	Positive	Negative
CD20	Negative (occasionally weakly positive)	Negative
CD27	Positive	Negative or diminished
CD38	Brightly positive	Brightly positive
CD45	Positive (typically weak)	Negative or weakly positive
CD56	Negative	Positive (aberrant expression)
CD117 (c-Kit)	Negative	Positive (aberrant expression)
CD138 (Syndecan-1)	Positive (bright expression)	Positive (bright expression)
Cyclin D1	Negative	Positive (especially in mantle cell lymphoma)
Immunoglobulin light chains (kappa/lambda)	Polyclonal (ratio typically within normal range)	Monoclonal (skewed kappa/lambda ratio)

Key Points

- CD19 and CD27 are typically positive in reactive plasma cells but are often negative or diminished in malignant plasma cells.
- CD56 and CD117 are markers that are aberrantly expressed in malignant plasma cells but not in reactive plasma cells.
- CD45 expression is generally weak in reactive plasma cells and is often negative or weak in malignant plasma cells.
- CD138 is expressed in both reactive and malignant plasma cells, but its presence alone is not sufficient to distinguish between them.
- Immunoglobulin light chain restriction (monoclonality) is a hallmark of malignant plasma cells, while reactive plasma cells typically exhibit a polyclonal distribution of light chains.

These immunophenotypic differences are used to differentiate between reactive and malignant plasma cells in clinical practice, aiding in the accurate diagnosis of plasma cell dyscrasias, including MM.

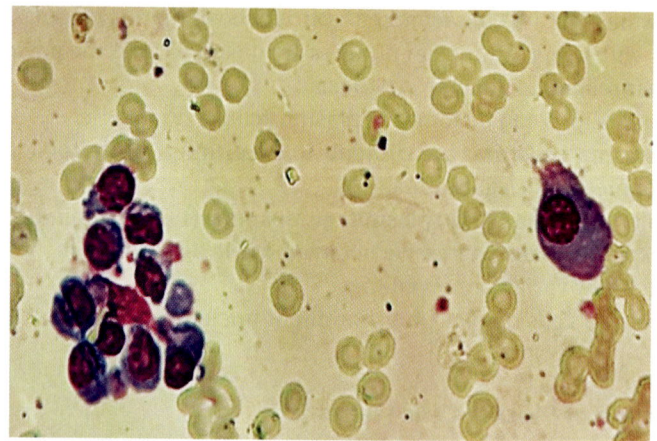

FIG. 3: Plasma cell with eccentric nucleus and perinuclear hof (Bone marrow smear, 1000×).

Q22. What hematological changes are seen in sepsis?

Ans:

- *White blood cell count and differential:*[22]
  - *Leukocytosis/leukopenia*: Both can indicate sepsis.
  - *Neutrophil count*: Neutrophilia or neutropenia suggests infection.
  - *Immature to total neutrophil (I/T) ratio*: An increased I/T ratio is a significant marker for sepsis, especially in neonates.
  - Thrombocytopenia is common in sepsis, particularly in fungal infections.
- *Morphological changes in blood cells as shown in* **Table 24**.

TABLE 24: Morphological changes in various blood cells during sepsis.		
Cell type	**Change**	**Significance**
Neutrophils	Left shift (increased immature forms)	Early release from bone marrow due to infection
	Toxic granulation	Reflects active inflammation
	Döhle bodies	Seen in severe infections
	Cytoplasmic vacuolization	Suggests phagocytic activity and severe infection
Monocytes	Increased numbers	Reflects immune response to infection
Lymphocytes	Reactive lymphocytes	Indicates activation, often seen in viral infections
Erythrocytes	Anemia, spherocytes, and schistocytes	Signs of hemolysis or bone marrow suppression
Platelets	Thrombocytopenia, large/giant platelets	Indicates platelet consumption/destruction, often in sepsis

- *Emerging biomarkers in sepsis*: Certain biomarkers are being developed to predict or evaluate sepsis **(Table 25)**.

TABLE 25: Biomarkers in sepsis.

Biomarker	Significance
CD64	Increased expression on neutrophils, indicating sepsis within 4–6 hours
Serum amyloid A (SAA)	Early acute phase reactant indicating inflammation
Cytokines (IL-6, TNF-α, IL-8)	High sensitivity for diagnosing EOS when combined with CRP
Cell surface markers (CD11b, CD64)	Aids in sepsis diagnosis through flow cytometry

Scoring System for Neonatal Sepsis

Monroe devised a criteria which used three parameters of total PMN count, immature PMN count, and I:T ratio for scoring neonatal sepsis, whereas in the hematologic scoring system, more indices can be used.[23]

Q23. Enumerate work-up for leukemoid reactions.

Ans: Leukemoid reactions are characterized by an excessive increase in WBC count, often exceeding 50,000 cells/μL. They can mimic clonal disorders such as chronic myelogenous leukemia (CML) or chronic neutrophilic leukemia (CNL), making accurate diagnosis essential. The diagnostic approach includes a thorough history, physical examination, imaging, and specific laboratory tests to differentiate LRs from these conditions.

Key Diagnostic Steps

- *History and physical examination*:
  - Fever, drug, or toxin exposures: Investigate any history of fever, drug use, or exposure to toxins.
  - Organomegaly: Assess for enlargement of organs, which may indicate underlying pathology.
- Lab parameters **(Table 26)**

TABLE 26: The various laboratory parameters useful in evaluation of leukemoid reaction.

Parameter	Details	Significance
Complete blood count (CBC) with differential	• *Leukocytosis*: WBC > 50,000/μL • *Neutrophilia with left shift*: Increased immature neutrophils (bands, metamyelocytes, and myelocytes)	Indicates a strong reactive process; helps differentiate from leukemia
Peripheral blood smear	• *Toxic granulation*: Coarse, dark granules in neutrophils • *Döhle bodies*: Light blue-gray cytoplasmic inclusions • *Cytoplasmic vacuolization*: Presence of vacuoles in neutrophils • *Absence of blasts*: Blasts typically <5%	Suggests an inflammatory or infectious cause; absence of significant blasts helps rule out leukemia
Leukocyte alkaline phosphatase (LAP) score	Elevated LAP score	High LAP score supports a reactive process; low in CML

Continued

Parameter	Details	Significance
C-reactive protein (CRP) and erythrocyte sedimentation rate (ESR)	Elevated CRP and ESR	Elevated in infections or inflammation; supportive of a reactive process
Molecular testing (BCR-ABL1 fusion gene)	BCR-ABL1 negative	Absence of the Philadelphia chromosome differentiates from CML
Bone marrow examination (if indicated)	*Hypercellularity*: Increased myeloid precursors with normal maturation. Absence of dysplasia or blast increase	May be necessary if there is suspicion of malignancy; helps rule out leukemia
Imaging studies (if required)	Chest X-ray, CT scan, abdominal ultrasound	Used to detect underlying infections, inflammation, or malignancy
Cytochemical staining	• *Myeloperoxidase (MPO)*: Positive in myeloid cells, typically strong in CML • *Sudan black B (SBB)*: Positive in myeloid cells, strong in CML	MPO and SBB are typically strongly positive in CML but may show weak or variable positivity in reactive conditions
Flow cytometry	*Immunophenotyping*: Analysis of surface markers to identify clonal populations (e.g., CD13, CD33 for myeloid lineage in CML)	Helps differentiate clonal hematologic disorders from reactive processes
Other relevant tests	• *Serum vitamin B12 and uric acid levels*: Often elevated in CML • *LDH (lactate dehydrogenase)*: Elevated in both CML and leukemoid reactions, higher in malignancies	Elevated vitamin B12 and uric acid levels can suggest a myeloproliferative disorder like CML rather than a reactive leukemoid reaction

Key Points

- *CBC and peripheral smear*: Focus on identifying reactive neutrophilia and excluding significant blasts.
- *LAP score and cytochemistry (MPO and SBB)*: Elevated LAP and weak/variable MPO and SBB positivity suggest LR, while low LAP and strong positivity suggest CML.
- *Flow cytometry*: Useful for identifying clonal hematologic disorders, helping to rule out CML.
- *Additional lab tests*: Elevated B12, uric acid, and LDH can indicate CML over a LR.

Q24. What is mild, moderate, and severe eosinophilia? What are the causes of eosinophilia?

Ans: In healthy state, eosinophils comprise 1–6% of the total WBCs. The normal acceptable range of absolute eosinophil count (AEC) is 0.02–0.5 × 10^9/L. Eosinophilia refers to an AEC > 0.5 × 10^9/L **(Table 27)**.[24] There can be multiple causes of eosinophilia **(Table 28)**.

TABLE 27: The following table states the various degrees of eosinophilia according to the absolute eosinophil count in peripheral blood.

Degree of eosinophilia	Absolute eosinophil count
Mild	$0.5–1.0 \times 10^9/L$
Moderate	$1.0–5.0 \times 10^9/L$
Severe	Greater than $5.0 \times 10^9/L$

TABLE 28: The causes of eosinophilia.

Category	Condition/Disorder	Description/Key characteristics
Infections	Parasitic infections	Moderate-to-high eosinophilia
	Mycobacterial infection	Eosinophilia secondary to drug therapy
	Invasive fungal infections	• Due to allergic response • Especially in coccidioidomycosis patients
	Yeast	CSF eosinophilia in Cryptococcus infection
	Viral infections	Herpes, HIV infection, and COVID-19
Allergic diseases	Allergic rhinitis	Mild eosinophilia
	Atopic dermatitis	• Mild-to-moderate eosinophilia • Common in children
	Urticarial/angioedema	• Mild eosinophilia • Normal blood count of eosinophils but increased infiltration of eosinophils in skin
	Fungal allergy	• Mild-to-moderate eosinophilia • Due to IgE sensitization
	Asthma chronic rhinosinusitis	Mild-to-moderate eosinophilia
Drug reactions	Antibiotics, NSAIDs, antipsychotic drugs	• Asymptomatic eosinophilia to life-threatening complications • Drug rash, eosinophilia-myalgia syndrome • Counts return to normal on stopping the drug
Neoplasms	Acute eosinophil leukemia	Rare cause but when associated with eosinophilia, it is usually high
	Chronic eosinophil leukemia	Rare cause but when associated with eosinophilia, it is usually high
	• Pre B cell ALL • Myeloid leukemia	Moderate to high eosinophilia in CML
	Lymphomas	• Most common is Hodgkin disease • Intense tissue eosinophilia • Moderate blood eosinophilia
	Histiocytosis X	Intense tissue eosinophilia
	Solid tumors, especially adenocarcinoma	

Continued

Continued

Category	Condition/Disorder	Description/Key characteristics
Musculoskeletal	Rheumatoid arthritis	Rare cause but when associated with eosinophilia, can be mild to even severe
	Eosinophilic fasciitis	Rare cause but when associated with eosinophilia, can be mild to even severe
Gastrointestinal	Eosinophilic gastroenteritis	Mild-to-moderate eosinophilia
	Eosinophilic esophagitis	Marked tissue eosinophilia with mild or absent blood eosinophilia
	Celiac disease	Tissue eosinophilia
	Inflammatory bowel disease	Tissue eosinophilia in both Crohn's disease and ulcerative colitis
	Allergic gastroenteritis	• Mild to high eosinophilia • Common in children
Autoimmune disorders	Sarcoidosis IgG4 disease	Clinical sequelae of eosinophilia may or may not be present

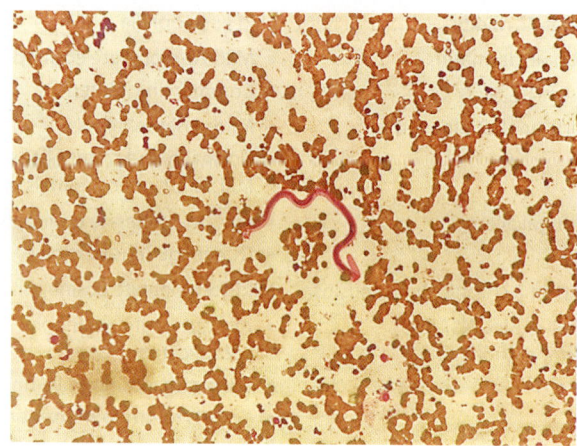

FIG. 4: Microfilaria of Wuchereria bancrofti identified in a peripheral smear (Giemsa stain, 1000×).

Q25. What is hypereosinophilic syndrome? How do you approach a case with eosinophilia?

Ans: Hypereosinophilia (HES) refers to an AEC > 1.5×10^9/L on two examinations at least 1 month apart. Hypereosinophilic syndrome includes a group of heterogenous disorders that are characterized by persistent and marked elevation of eosinophil levels and mediators, leading to infiltration into the tissues and consequent end-organ damage.[25] There are many clinical subtypes of HES **(Table 29)**.

TABLE 29: Clinical subtypes of HES.

Subtype	Definition	Genetics	Manifestations	Laboratory findings
Myeloid hypereosinophilia/hypereosinophilic syndrome (HE/HES)	Suspected or proven eosinophilic myeloid neoplasm, including those associated with rearrangements of PDGFRA and other recurrent molecular abnormalities	• *FIP1L1-PDGFRA fusion gene* • JAK2 point mutation and translocation formed by t(8;9) • FGFR1 rearrangements such as (8p11-12) • PDGFRB rearrangements such as t(5;12) • Chronic eosinophilic leukemia (CEL) • HES with myeloid features without known mutation	• Anemia • Thrombocytopenia • Hepatosplenomegaly	• Dysplastic eosinophils • Elevated serum tryptase and B12 levels • Bone marrow features suggestive of a myeloid neoplasm
Lymphocytic HE/HES	Presence of a clonal or phenotypically aberrant T cell population that produces type 2 cytokines (IL-5) that drive the eosinophilia and raised IgE levels	Most common CD3–CD4+ but other populations such as CD3+CD4 CD8– and CD4+CD7– can also be seen	Dermatologic manifestations including angioedema, nodules, eczematous dermatitis, and erythroderma	Aberrant T Cells detected in skin biopsies from affected areas
Overlap HES	Single organ restricted eosinophilic disorders and clinically defined eosinophilic syndromes that overlap in presentation with idiopathic HES	–	• Eosinophilic gastrointestinal disorders • Eosinophilic granulomatosis with polyangiitis	• Laboratory markers of inflammation • Raised erythrocyte sedimentation rate (ESR) • Raised C-reactive protein (CRP) • Levels are affected by disease severity and treatment status • Tissue HES is present • HES blood criteria are unmet

Continued

Continued

Subtype	Definition	Genetics	Manifestations	Laboratory findings
Associated HE/HES	In the context of a defined disorder, such as a helminth infection, neoplasm, immunodeficiency, or hypersensitivity reaction			
Familial HE/HES	Occurrence in >1 family member while excluding associated HE/HES			
Idiopathic HE/HES	Unknown cause and exclusion of other subtypes			

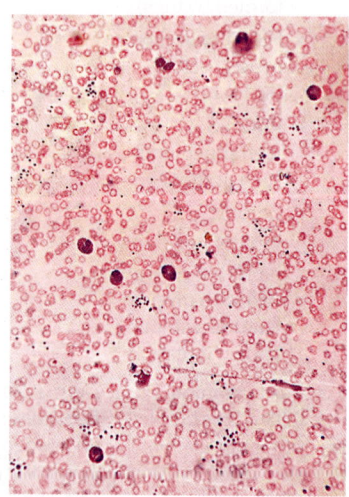

FIG. 5: Peripheral smear showing marked eosinophilia with increased eosinophils, some showing bilobed nuclei and coarse granules (Leishman stain, 1000×).

Q26. What is basophilia and what are the causes of basophilia?

Ans: Basophilia refers to peripheral blood basophil count generally >0.1×10^9 /L, and basophils comprising >2% of the total leukocyte count.[26] There can be multiple causes of basophilia **(Table 30)**.

TABLE 30: Causes of basophilia.		
Category	**Condition/Disorder**	**Description/Key characteristics**
Allergy/Inflammation	Ulcerative colitis	• Most common cause of nonclonal basophilia • Show increased expression of basophil activation markers (CD63 and CD203c)
	Drug or food hypersensitivity	• Associated with increased IgE levels • Increased expression of FcεRI on basophils • In Th2-mediated allergic responses, basophilia promoted by IL-3 and thymic stromal lymphopoietin
	Erythroderma/Urticaria	
Endocrinopathy	Diabetes mellitus	• High basophil count in diabetic patients (type 1 and type 2) as compared to non-diabetics • Even higher counts in patients with diabetic ketoacidosis
	Exogenous estrogen administration	
	Hypothyroidism	

Continued

Continued

Category	Condition/Disorder	Description/Key characteristics
Infections	Chicken pox	Due to trigger of inflammatory response
	Influenza	
	Small pox	
	Tuberculosis	
Anemia	Iron deficiency anemia	
Radiation exposure	Ionizing radiation	
Leukemia	Chronic myeloid leukemia	• Basophilia is most common blood count abnormality in both chronic and blast phase • Derived from the malignant clone • Can contain Philadelphia chromosome • Basophil count is prognostic marker • Used to measure treatment response • Contain higher levels of tryptase in their granules • Express α-tryptase mRNA
	AML with t(9,22), t(6,9), t(3,6), and 12p abnormalities	
	Acute basophilic leukemia	• Lacks defining cytogenetics • Immature basophils comprise 20–80% of bone marrow cellular elements • Irregular/segmented nuclei with relatively clumped chromatin, coarse basophilic granules • Sparse mature basophils • Show metachromatic staining with toluidine blue • Negative for MPO, SBB, Naphthol AS-D CAE, and NSE • Positive for CD11b, CD13, CD33, CD34, CD38, CD123, CD203c, and CD9 • Weak positive for CD117 • Negative for HLA-DR
Myeloproliferative neoplasms	Primary myelofibrosis	Slight increase in blood basophils
	Polycythemia vera	
	Essential thrombocythemia	

Q27. What is monocytosis?

Ans: World Health Organization defines persistent monocytosis as an absolute monocyte count $> 1 \times 10^9$/L with monocytes comprising >10% of the total leukocytes. This rise must be sustained and should persist for >3 months.

Q28. What is monocytopenia? What are its causes?

Ans: Monocytopenia is a condition characterized by a decrease in the number of monocytes circulating in the blood with levels below 0.2×10^9/L. The causes of monocytopenia are enumerated in **Table 31**.

TABLE 31: Causes of monocytopenia.

Causes	Remarks
Infections	Human immunodeficiency virus (HIV), Epstein–Barr virus (EBV), adenovirus infection, and military tuberculosis
Medication	Corticosteroids and immunoglobulin therapy
Neoplastic disorders	Hairy cell leukemia, acute lymphoblastic leukemia (ALL), and Hodgkin lymphoma
Chemotherapy induced	Myelosuppression, other cytopenias also occur
Hematopoietic cell mutation	GATA2 mutations
Postsurgical procedure	After gastric or intestinal resection

REFERENCES

1. Tahir N, Zahra F. Neutrophilia. In: StatPearls [Internet]. Treasure Island (FL): StatPearls Publishing; 2024.
2. Gibson C, Berliner N. How we evaluate and treat neutropenia in adults. Blood. 2014;124(8):1251-8.
3. Skokowa J, Dale DC, Touw IP, Zeidler C, Welte K. Severe congenital neutropenias. Nat Rev Dis Primers. 2017;3:17032.
4. Dale DC, Bolyard AA, Aprikyan A. Cyclic neutropenia. Semin Hematol. 2002;39(2):89-94.
5. Palmer L, Briggs C, McFadden S, Zini G, Burthem J, Rozenberg G, et al. Nomenclature and grading of peripheral blood cell morphology. Int Jnl Lab Hem. 2015;37:287-303.
6. Colella R, Hollensead SC. Understanding and recognizing the Pelger–Huët anomaly. Am J Clin Pathol. 2012;137(3):358-66.
7. Leal AF, Nieto WG, Candelo E, Pachajoa H, Alméciga-Díaz CJ. Hematological findings in lysosomal storage disorders: A perspective from the medical laboratory. EJIFCC. 2022;33(1):28-42.
8. Manley HR, Keightley MC, Lieschke GJ. The neutrophil nucleus: an important influence on neutrophil migration and function. Front Immunol. 2018;9:2867.
9. Saito H, Kunishima S. Historical hematology: May-Hegglin anomaly. Am J Hematol. 2008;83(4):304-6.
10. Safavi M, Vasei M, Motamed F. Jordans' anomaly as a red flag for neutral lipid storage diseases. Fetal Pediatr Pathol. 2022;41(3):526-8.
11. Neal A, Simon-Lopez R, Barella S. Use of neutrophil cell population data for the detection of neutrophil hypergranulation and other neutrophil inclusions as Döhle bodies, cytoplasm vacuolation. Blood. 2014;124(21):4966.
12. Bouma G, Ancliff PJ, Thrasher AJ, Burns SO. Recent advances in the understanding of genetic defects of neutrophil number and function. Br J Haematol. 2010;151:312-6.
13. van de Vijver E, Maddalena A, Sanal Ö. Hematologically important mutations: leukocyte adhesion deficiency. Blood Cells Mol Dis. 2012;48(1):53-61.
14. Roos D. Chronic granulomatous disease. Br Med Bull. 2016;118(1):50-63.
15. Dinauer MC. Neutrophil Defects and Diagnosis Disorders of Neutrophil Function: An Overview. Methods Mol Biol. 2020;2087:11-29.
16. Nagai K, Ochi F, Terui K, Maeda M, Ohga S, Kanegane H, et al. Clinical characteristics and outcomes of Chédiak-Higashi syndrome: A nationwide survey of Japan. Pediatr Blood Cancer. 2013;60(10):1582-6.
17. Devi A, Thielemans L, Ladikou EE, Nandra TK, Chevassut T. Lymphocytosis and chronic lymphocytic leukaemia: investigation and management. Clin Med. 2022;22(3):225-9.
18. Oshimi K. Clinical Features, Pathogenesis, and Treatment of Large Granular Lymphocyte Leukemias. Intern Med. 2017;56(14):1759-69.
19. Okano M. Haematological associations of Epstein-Barr virus infection. Baillieres Best Pract Res Clin Haematol. 2000;13(2):199-214.
20. Fugl A, Andersen CL. Epstein-Barr virus and its association with disease - a review of relevance to general practice. BMC Fam Pract. 2019;20:62.

21. Flores-Montero J, de Tute R, Paiva B, Perez JJ, Böttcher S, Wind H, et al. Immunophenotype of normal vs. myeloma plasma cells: Toward antibody panel specifications for MRD detection in multiple myeloma. Cytometry B Clin Cytom. 2016;90(1):61-72.
22. Goyette RE, Key NS, Ely EW. Hematologic changes in sepsis and their therapeutic implications. Semin Respir Crit Care Med. 2004;25(6):645-59.
23. Saboohi E, Saeed F, Khan RN, Khan MA. Immature to total neutrophil ratio as an early indicator of early neonatal sepsis. Pak J Med Sci. 2019;35(1):241-6.
24. Butt NM, Lambert J, Ali S, Beer PA, Cross NC, Duncombe A, et al; British Committee for Standards in Haematology. Guideline for the investigation and management of eosinophilia. Br J Haematol. 2017;176(4):553-72.
25. Klion AD. How I treat hypereosinophilic syndromes. Blood. 2015;126(9):1069-77.
26. Feriel J, Depasse F, Geneviève F. How I investigate basophilia in daily practice. Int J Lab Hematol. 2020;42(3):237-45.

3. Red Blood Cells

Bhushan Asthana, Rama Hariharan, Blessy Mathew

Q1. What are target cells?

Ans: Target cells, or codocytes, have an excess of cell membrane relative to cell volume. These cells are red blood cells (RBCs) with solid area in the center of central pallor.[1] They are found in thalassemia, hemoglobin E (HbE) syndromes, hemoglobin C (HbC) disorders, and nonhemolytic states such as obstructive jaundice and postsplenectomy. Macrocytic target cells can be seen in liver disease, and microcytic target cells may be seen in thalassemia. Target cells can also occur as an artifact of slide preparation. Artifactual target cells are generally irregularly distributed on the slide.

Q2. What is the common cause of spiculated appearance of RBCs in peripheral smear?

Ans: The two basic types of spiculated red cells are echinocytes and acanthocytes (from the Greek word 'acantha', which means thorn). Acanthocytes indicate disturbed erythrocyte lipid composition and occur in association with abetalipoproteinemia. Acanthocytic forms, in fact, are determined by a structural pathologic membrane defect, whereas echinocytic forms can be caused and reversed by pH, osmolarity, biochemical, and even electrical variations. The spiculated appearance of RBCs can also result from an ethylenediaminetetraacetic acid (EDTA) artifact resulting due to prolonged storage of >6 hours between sample collection and smear preparation. Therefore, for accuracy, it is important to ensure that the peripheral blood smear is freshly prepared for examination. Spiculated RBCs from EDTA artifact have more uniformly distributed spicules and affect almost all of the RBCs in the film.

Q3. What are Heinz bodies?

Ans: Heinz bodies are inclusions in RBCs that are composed of denatured hemoglobin attached to the erythrocyte cell membrane, are indicative of oxidative injury to the erythrocyte.[2] They are visualized by supravital stains such as methylene blue, bromocresol, or crystal violet. Heinz bodies can be seen in glucose-6-phosphate dehydrogenase (G6PD) deficiency, alpha thalassemia, and chronic liver disease. Their presence may also be an indication of asplenia or hyposplenism. The presence of Heinz bodies can ultimately result in hemolytic anemia.

Q4. What is a fast-moving hemoglobin?

Ans: Fast moving Hb (FMH) is a rare hemoglobin variant that moves faster than HbA on alkaline agarose gel electrophoresis. FMH is caused by a mutation that replaces a negatively charged amino acid in the alpha, beta, or gamma chains. Hb H, Hb Barts, Hb J-Meerut, Hb J-Baltimore, and Hb N-Baltimore are few examples of FMH.

Q5. Why reticulocytes are termed as polychromatophilic cells?

Ans: Reticulocytes occupy the intermediate position between nucleated RBCs and mature red cells and tend to stain bluer than mature RBCs on Romanowsky stain.[3] Depending on their respective RNA content, they exhibit different shades of bluish staining in peripheral blood smear and are thus termed as polychromatophilic cells. They undergo removal of RNA on passing through spleen on first day of being in the circulation and are an important indicator of RBC production. This residual RNA generally is lost progressively during the 24 hours after the cell enters the circulation. All polychromatophils are reticulocytes, however, not all reticulocytes are polychromatophils. Immature reticulocyte fraction (IRF) is the ratio of immature reticulocytes to total number of reticulocytes and is an early indicator of bone marrow regeneration and erythropoiesis and suggests bone marrow responsiveness to various conditions and therapies.

Q6. What is the significance of reticulocyte count?

Ans: The normal life span of RBCs is 120 days and the duration of a reticulocyte in the peripheral blood is 1 day. It follows that reticulocytes at a random time, in a normal subject at a steady state, will be 1/120, or 0.8% of all red cells. The reticulocyte percentage in the peripheral blood is an indication of the rapidity of red cell turnover and reflects the amount of erythropoiesis on a given day. Reduced reticulocyte percentages are seen in bone marrow suppression. Increased reticulocyte percentages are seen in hemolytic disorders, whether intrinsic (e.g., hemoglobinopathy or enzymopathy) or extrinsic (e.g., traumatic, heart valve, and acquired immune hemolytic anemia).[3] Reticulocytes can cause an increase in mean cell volume (MCV) if the percentage is markedly elevated.

Q7. What is eosin-5-maleimide binding test?

Ans: Flow cytometry test based on eosin-5-maleimide (EMA) binds to band 3 cytoskeletal protein of RBC membrane. This is a sensitive and specific test for diagnosis of hereditary spherocytosis (HS). Band 3 is reduced in HS and congenital dyserythropoietic anemia (CDA) type II. Hence, EMA fluorescence is reduced. Other causes of reduced EMA binding are hereditary cryohydrocytosis and South east Asian ovalocytosis. EMA fluorescence is normal or increased in autoimmune hemolytic anemia (AIHA) since there is no band 3 deficiency.[4]

Q8. What is the marker of erythroid precursors identified by immunohistochemistry?

Ans: CD71 is the marker for erythroid precursors and stains all stages of erythroblasts. It is also known as transferrin receptor (TfR).[5] It is present on all actively proliferating cells essential for iron transport into proliferating cells. TfRs are transmembrane glycoprotein present on surface of all body cells, but 80% of the receptors are on erythroid precursors. The concentration of TfR diminishes as normoblasts mature to reticulocytes. The highest concentration is present on intermediate normoblasts. Spectrin and glycophorin are also used for the identification of erythroid precursors in paraffin embedded sections.

Q9. Do valvular prostheses cause thrombotic microangiopathy?

Ans: In patients with valvular prosthesis, when RBCs flow across a pressure gradient created by the prosthesis, the red cells get fragmented leading to intravascular hemolysis. Hemolytic uremic syndrome (typical and atypical), thrombotic thrombocytopenic purpura (caused by

ADAMTS13 deficiency), and HELLP syndrome in pregnancy are known to cause thrombotic microangiopathy (TMA).[6] These conditions lead to platelet aggregation in the microcirculation of capillaries, leading to thrombocytopenia and schistocytes on peripheral blood film.

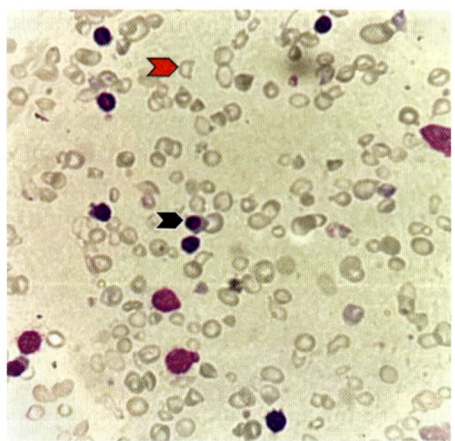

FIG. 1: Peripheral smear (100×) reveal hemolytic blood picture with microcytic hypochromic red blood cells, fragmented cells (red arrowhead), nucleated RBC (black arrowhead).

Courtesy: Dr Abhishek Purohit.

Q10. A 32-year-old woman with a history of irritable bowel syndrome is found to have iron deficiency anemia and a serum folate of 1 µg/L (2–11 µg/L). Her serum vitamin B12 is normal. What is the probable cause?

Ans: The clinical history suggests celiac disease. A major milestone in the history of celiac disease was the identification of tissue transglutaminase as the autoantigen, thereby confirming the autoimmune nature of this disorder.[7] The recommended first-line test [National Institute for Health and Care Excellence (NICE) guidelines] is IgA antitissue transglutaminase antibodies. If this is negative, IgA should be assayed and, in deficient patients (2% of those with celiac disease), tests for IgG antitissue transglutaminase and antiendomysial antibodies should be done. About 5% of patients with celiac disease do not have antibodies to tissue transglutaminase. Diagnosis then depends on antibodies to endomysium or to deamidated gliadin peptide. It is important that patients continue on a gluten-containing diet until serological evaluation and duodenal biopsy are done.

Q11. A 6-month-old baby boy born to South East Asian parents presents with failure to thrive. He had been weaned on to cow's milk at an early age. He is found to have pallor and hepatosplenomegaly. His RBC profile shows Hb 7.8 g/L (99–141 g/L), MCV 65 fL (71–84 fL), and MCH 18 pg (24–34 pg). His blood film shows anisocytosis, poikilocytosis, hypochromia, microcytosis, and some nucleated RBCs. Serum ferritin is 250 µg/L (14–200 µg/L).

Ans: The findings are those of beta-thalassemia major. Beta-thalassemia major typically shows markedly elevated HbF (30–95%) with normal to mildly elevated HbA2. The pathogenesis of beta-thalassemia is two-fold. First, there is decreased hemoglobin synthesis causing anemia and an increase in HbF and HbA2 as there are decreased beta chains for HbA formation.[8] Second, and of most pathologic significance in beta-thalassemia major and intermedia, the relative excess alpha chains form insoluble alpha chain inclusions that cause marked intramedullary hemolysis. Alpha-thalassemia would either present in utero or at birth with hydrops fetalis (deletion of all four alpha genes) or later in life as hemoglobin H disease (deletion of three of four alpha genes), which has a less severe phenotype. CDA is associated with normocytic or macrocytic red cells and congenital sideroblastic anemia with a dimorphic blood film. Severe iron deficiency anemia would have ferritin levels of <14 µg/L. A common confounding factor in hemoglobin electrophoresis is a concomitant iron deficiency that masks an underlying beta-thalassemia minor. The resultant electrophoresis pattern appears normal. This is because iron deficiency anemia normalizes the HbA2 percentage that is the key finding in beta-thalassemia minor.[8]

Q12. A 31-year-old woman known to have elevated transaminases for several years but not been followed up. She is found to have hemoglobin of 74 g/L and a reticulocyte count of 270×10^9/L (50–100×10^9/L). She has developed recent onset tremors. A blood film shows irregularly contracted cells, polychromasia, and nucleated RBCs. A Heinz body preparation is positive. What is the probable diagnosis?

Ans: The patient seems to have Wilson disease. In Wilson disease, there is a faulty copper excretory mechanism, leading copper to accumulate in the liver and spill into the blood where it begins to accumulate in other organs and tissues-like subthalamus, cortex of the brain, and cornea.[9] Wilson disease is inherited as autosomal recessive condition caused by a mutation in the Wilson disease protein (*ATP7B*) gene. Symptoms usually are related to the brain and liver. Liver-related symptoms include vomiting, ascites, pedal edema, yellowish skin, and itchiness. Brain-related symptoms include tremors, muscle stiffness, trouble speaking, personality changes, and auditory or visual hallucinations. The majority of patients present with liver dysfunction within the first decade of life.[9] The neuropsychiatric features are seen in the third or fourth decade of life. The acute hemolysis is due to release of copper from dying liver cells. The presence of irregularly contracted cells and the positive Heinz body preparation indicate oxidant damage to red cells, Heinz bodies represent oxidized hemoglobin. Ceruloplasmin level will be <20 mg/dL (normal 20–40 mg/dL). Urinary copper levels will be raised > 100 µg/dL. These two laboratory findings with Kayser–Fleischer rings in cornea are usually enough for diagnosis of Wilson disease.

Q13. Why sickle cell disease with hereditary persistence of fetal hemoglobin (S/HPFH) is less severe than Hb Sβ0 or Hb Sβ+?

Ans: The severity of sickle cell disease is ameliorated by increasing the level of fetal Hb (HbF) in RBCs because HbF acts as an antisickling hemoglobin. A coexisting state of hereditary persistence of fetal hemoglobin (HPFH) and therapy with hydroxyurea, in a patient with SCD, both lead to reduced severity of the disease.

Q14. What is mitochondrial poisoning seen in chronic alcoholics?

Ans: Chronic alcoholics are associated with sideroblastic anemias. Due to toxic effects of alcohol on the mitochondria, it causes mitochondrial poisoning in the bone marrow ultimately leading to impaired heme synthesis and accumulation of iron in the mitochondria—contributing to the formation of ringed sideroblasts, identified on Perls stain performed on bone marrow aspirates. The sideroblastic anemias are a heterogeneous group of inherited and acquired disorders characterized by anemia and the presence of ring sideroblasts in the bone marrow. Ring sideroblasts are abnormal erythroblasts with iron-loaded mitochondria that are visualized by Prussian blue staining as a perinuclear ring of green-blue granules.[10] The mechanisms that lead to the ring sideroblast formation are heterogeneous, but in all of them, there is an abnormal deposition of iron in the mitochondria of erythroblasts.

REFERENCES

1. Bain BJ, Bates I, Laffan MA. Blood Cell Morphology in Health and Disease. Dacie and Lewis Practical Haematology, 12th edition. Philadelphia: Elsevier; 2017. pp. 61-92.
2. Jacob H, Winterhalter K. Unstable hemoglobins: The role of heme loss in Heinz body formation. Proc Natl Acad Sci U S A. 1970;65(3):697-701.
3. Peebles DA, Hochberg A, Clarke TA. Analysis of manual reticulocyte counting. Am J Clin Pathol. 1981;76: 713-17.
4. Park SH, Park CJ, Lee BR, Cho YU, Jang S, Kim N, et al. Comparison Study of the Eosin-5'-Maleimide Binding Test, Flow cytometric osmotic fragility test, and cryohemolysis test in the diagnosis of hereditary spherocytosis. Am J Clin Pathol. 2014:142;474-84.
5. Marsee DK, Pinkus GS, Yu H. CD71 (Transferrin Receptor): An effective marker for erythroid precursors in bone marrow biopsy specimens. Am J Clin Pathol. 2010;134:429-35.
6. Arnold DM, Patriquin CJ, Nazy I. Thrombotic microangiopathies: a general approach to diagnosis and management. CMAJ. 2017;189(4):E153-9.
7. Caio G, Volta U, Sapone A, Leffler DA, De Giorgio R, Catassi C, et al. Celiac disease: a comprehensive current review. BMC Med. 2019;17;142.
8. Needs T, Gonzalez-Mosquera LF, Lynch DT. Beta Thalassemia. In: StatPearls [Internet]. Treasure Island (FL): StatPearls Publishing; 2024.
9. Immergluck J, Anilkumar AC. Wilson Disease. In: StatPearls [Internet]. Treasure Island (FL): StatPearls Publishing; 2024.
10. Rodriguez-Sevilla JJ, Calvo X, Arenillas L. Causes and Pathophysiology of Acquired Sideroblastic Anemia. Genes (Basel). 2022;13(9):1562.

4. Basics of Complete Blood Count

Jitender Mohan Khunger

Q1. How should a peripheral blood smear be reported?

Ans: A peripheral blood smear is reported in view of the following:[1]
- *Red blood cells*: Morphology, immature forms, inclusion bodies, and arrangement of cells.
- *White blood cells*: Differential count, morphology, abnormal or immature forms.
- *Platelets:* Adequacy, abnormal forms
- *Hemoparasites*: Malaria, filaria

Q2. What is packed cell volume (PCV) (hematocrit)?

Ans: PCV is the volume occupied by the red cells when a sample of anticoagulated blood is centrifuged. It indicates relative proportion of red cells to plasma. PCV is also called hematocrit.

Q3. What is mean corpuscular volume (MCV)?

Ans: MCV is a measure of average size of the red cells. It is measured directly by automated instruments from the measurement of mean volume of each red blood cell.

$$MCV = \frac{PCV \text{ in \%}}{\text{Red cell count in millions/mm}^3} \times 10$$

Q4. What is red cell distribution width (RDW)? What is its significance?

Ans: RDW is a measure of degree of variation in red cell size (anisocytosis) in a blood sample. It is measured by automated analyzers.[2]
Normal RDW is 9.0–14.5

Significance: It is helpful in differential diagnosis of some types of anemia. Among microcytic anemia RDW is low in beta thalassemia trait, high in Iron deficiency anemia, and normal in anemia of chronic disease.

Q5. What disease can be diagnosed by measuring red cell distribution width?

Ans: RDW blood test is useful in the following conditions:[2]
- A high RDW help provide a clue for a diagnosis of early nutritional deficiency such as iron, folate, or vitamin B12 deficiency, as it becomes elevated earlier than other red blood cell parameters.

- It aids in distinguishing between uncomplicated iron deficiency anemia (elevated RDW, normal to low MCV) and uncomplicated heterozygous thalassemia (normal RDW, low MCV): However, definitive tests are required.
- It can also help distinguish between megaloblastic anemia such as folate or vitamin B12 deficiency anemia (elevated RDW) and other causes of macrocytosis (often normal RDW).
- RDW can be used as guidance for flagging samples that may need manual peripheral blood smear examination, since elevated RDW may indicate red cell fragmentation, agglutination, or dimorphic red blood cell populations.

Q6. What is reticulocyte index?

Ans: Reticulocyte index or reticulocyte production index (RPI) is a parameter that provides an assessment for adequate bone marrow response to anemia.[3]

Reticulocyte production index (RPI) and corrected reticulocyte count are essentially the same. The corrected reticulocyte count is basically correcting the reticulocyte count for patient's degree of anemia (Patient's PCV).

Corrected reticulocyte count (percentage) = Reticulocyte count (percentage) of patient × PCV of patient/normal PCV.

This correction formula produces the corrected reticulocyte count.

Q7. What are the causes of high and low reticulocyte index?

Ans:
High reticulocyte index is seen in the following:
- Hemolytic anemia
- Recent blood loss
- Hemoglobinopathies, e.g., sickle cell anemia
- Following specific therapy of nutritional anemia (e.g., iron in iron deficiency anemia, vitamin B12/folate in vitamin B12, and folate deficiency anemia)

Low reticulocyte index is seen in:
- Aplastic anemia, pure red cell aplasia
- Ineffective erythropoiesis (e.g., megaloblastic anemia)
- Bone marrow infiltration (leukemia, lymphoma, myelofibrosis, and metastasis)
- Renal failure, anemia of chronic disease

Q8. What is erythrocyte sedimentation rate (ESR)? How is it measured? What is its significance?

Ans: ESR measures the rate of setting of erythrocytes in anticoagulated whole blood.[4] Anticoagulated blood is allowed to stand in a glass tube for 1 hour and the length of column of plasma above the red cells is measured in millimeters; this corresponds to ESR. Different methods for estimation of ESR are:
- Westergren method
- Wintrobe method
- Zeta sediment ratio
- Micro-ESR

Signification of erythrocyte sedimentation rate: ESR is elevated in a wide range of organic diseases. Raised ESR (>100 mm at 1 hour) is seen in infection, paraproteinemias, and malignancies.

Q9. What is immature platelet fraction?

Ans: The immature platelet fraction (IPF) is a parameter that measures young and more reactive platelets in peripheral blood. Platelets newly released from the bone marrow are larger and more reactive than mature platelets and contain larger amounts of ribonucleic acid (RNA).
- *Clinical implications:*
    - Differential diagnosis of thrombocytopenia
    - Clinical evaluation of myelodysplastic syndromes
    - Recovery after marrow/stem cell transplantation/chemotherapy
    - Predicting sepsis in critically-ill patients

Q10. How is antinuclear antibody identified?

Ans: Antinuclear antibody (ANA) test is a part of an evaluation for part of an evaluation for possible autoimmune disease.

The ANA test identifies autoantibodies that target substances contained inside cells.[5] Connective tissue diseases (CTD) are a group of autoimmune disorders which are characterized by presence of ANAs in the blood of patients. ANAs are a specific class of autoantibodies that have the capability of binding and destroying certain structures within the nucleus of the cells.

In general, there are two ways of test to identify ANA. Results depend upon which type of test is done to identify ANA.

1. *Indirect immunofluorescence (IF):* This type of ANA test uses IF. A titer measures a pattern where the ANA is detected in the cells. In this test, antinuclear (or anticytoplasmic) antibodies bind to the cells that have been fixed and permeablized on a slide. The addition of a secondary antibody (with an attached fluorescent dye) is directed against human antibodies and may reveal staining of the nucleus or cytoplasm as detected using a fluorescent microscope. Although IF-ANA test is widely used and considered to be gold standard still the results may sometimes be misinterpreted. As it detects several different antibodies cross-reactions can occur.
2. *Solid-phase assays:* The other type of ANA tests uses solid-phase assays. In these tests, a panel of autoantigens is attached to a solid surface. Next, the patient's sample and a secondary antibody directed against human antibodies (with an attached fluorescent dye or an enzyme that catalyzes a colorimetric reaction) are added. The result may be reported as being within a "positive," "intermediate," or "negative" range for each specific autoantibody.

There are two types of enzyme immunoassay (EIA) or enzyme-linked immunosorbent assay (ELISA) methods currently used for ANA testing. One is called generic assay which detects ANA of broad specificity similar to IF-ANA and other is antigen specific assay that detects ANA and reacts with a single autoantigen, i.e., double-stranded deoxyribonucleic acid (dsDNA), Sjögren's syndrome anti-Ro (SS-A/Ro), SS-B/La, scleroderma (Scl-70), systemic lupus erythematosus (Sm), Sm/RNP, etc.

REFERENCES

1. Jaso J, Nguye A, Nguyen AN. A synoptic reporting system for peripheral blood smear interpretation. Am J Clin Pathol. 2011;135(3):358-64.
2. Das Gupta A, Hegde C, Mistri R. Red cell distribution width as a measure of severity of iron deficiency in iron deficiency anaemia. Indian J Med Res. 1994;100:177-83.
3. D´Onofrio G, Zini G, Rowan RM. Reticulocyte counting: methods and clinical applications. Advanced laboratory methods in haematology. 2002:78-126.
4. Kratz A, Plebani M, Peng M, Lee YK, McCafferty R, Machin SJ; International Council for Standardization in Haematology (ICSH). ICSH recommendations for modified and alternate methods measuring the erythrocyte sedimentation rate. Int J Lab Hematol. 2017;39(5):448-57.
5. Kumar Y, Bhatia A, Minz RW. Antinuclear antibodies and their detection methods in diagnosis of connective tissue diseases: a journey revisited. Diagn Pathol. 2;4:1.

5. Rare Causes of Anemia

Sanjeev Kumar Sharma, Anamika Bakliwal

Q1. What is aplastic anemia?

Ans: Aplastic anemia (AA) is marked by pancytopenia with markedly hypocellular marrow and normal marrow cell cytogenetics.[1] Peak incidences occur between ages 15 and 25 years, and 65 and 69 years. Emerging use of molecular cytogenomics is helpful in delineating immune mediated AA from inherited bone marrow failures (IBMF). The standard first-line treatment for newly diagnosed acquired severe/very severe AA patients is horse antithymocyte globulin and ciclosporin-based immunosuppressive therapy (IST) with eltrombopag or allogeneic hematopoietic stem cell transplant (HSCT) from a matched sibling donor.

Q2. What are the bone marrow findings in aplastic anemia?

Ans: A good-quality trephine biopsy specimen of at least 2 cm is essential to assess the overall cellularity and morphology of residual hematopoietic cells and to exclude an abnormal infiltrate. Care should be taken to avoid tangential biopsies, as subcortical marrow is normally hypocellular.[1] The cellularity could also be misleadingly low in patients who had pelvic radiotherapy.

In most cases, the biopsy specimen is hypocellular throughout; sometimes hypocellularity is patchy with both hypocellular and residual cellular areas. In such cases, an overall average cellularity of <30% should be ascertained after excluding lymphocytes and plasma cells. Small lymphoid aggregates may occur, particularly in the acute phase of the disease or when AA is associated with systemic autoimmune diseases such as rheumatoid arthritis or systemic lupus erythematosus. Increased reticulin staining, dysplastic megakaryocytes (best assessed by immunohistochemistry) and blasts are not seen in AA; their presence either indicates a hypoplastic myelodysplastic syndrome (MDS) or evolution to MDS or leukemia.[2] Dyserythropoiesis is very common in AA and does not distinguish MDS from AA.[1]

Q3. What is hypocellular myelodysplastic syndrome?

Ans: Most cases of MDS have a normocellular or hypercellular bone marrow (BM); however, 10–20% of cases have decreased cellularity. Integrating cytohistological and genetic features led to criteria (the hg-score) to define hypocellular (h)-MDS. Acquired somatic mutations, such as *DNMT3A*, *ASXL1*, *PIGA*, and *BCOR/BCORL1*, can be present at low variant allele frequency in approximately 20–30% of idiopathic AA.[3] Quantitative CD34 enumeration can help in discriminating h-MDS from AA.[4]

Q4. What is the association between aplastic anemia and paroxysmal nocturnal hemoglobinuria?

Ans: Paroxysmal nocturnal hemoglobinuria (PNH) is a complement-driven hemolytic anemia resulting from the clonal expansion of stem cells harboring a somatic PIGA mutation.[5] Approximately, 50–60% of patients with AA have a PNH clone. So, actually there is deletion of stem cells in AA but in PNH there is selective proliferation of these PIGA mutated stem cells. PNH testing should be performed by flow cytometry. PNH is not associated with inherited forms of AA such as dyskeratosis congenita, Fanconi anemia, or Shwachman-diamond syndrome.[6]

Q5. What is stress cytogenetics?

Ans: Fanconi anemia (FA) is a disease characterized by genomic instability, increased sensitivity to deoxyribonucleic acid (DNA) cross-linking agents, and the presence of clonal chromosomal abnormalities. The gold standard diagnostic assay for FA patients is cytogenetic analysis, revealing chromosomal breaks induced by DNA cross-linking agents such as mitomycin C (MMC) or diepoxybutane (DEB).[7] Metaphases are observed under microscope for detecting the presence of gap, break, and radial structure (biradial, triradial, and higher order radial structures) suggestive for FA.

The chromosome breakage test using peripheral blood T-lymphocytes is the accepted screening assay for FA. Primary skin fibroblasts have also been used as a readily available screening alternative, particularly if the T-cell analyses are ambiguous or do not give a clear result that the patient has FA, especially when there is a question of mosaicism.

Q6. What is the role of next-generation sequencing in diagnosing inherited bone marrow failure syndromes?

Ans: Next-generation sequencing (NGS) encompasses a broad range of techniques that enable the simultaneous sequencing of a massive amount of nucleic acid molecules.[8] These complementary approaches include targeted gene sequencing, whole-exome sequencing (WES), and whole-genome sequencing (WGS).

Recent advances in genetic research have identified a large number of causative genes of IBMFS and reinforced the need for a comprehensive genetic diagnostic system in both clinical practice and research. Molecular findings have become a part of the gold standard in IBMFS diagnostics. These data can not only provide diagnoses in patients without classic IBMFS presentations but also define deficient pathways crucial for therapeutic decision-making.

In addition, WES/WGS applications will certainly identify novel IBMFS causative genes, which should continue to increase the genetic diagnostic rate of NGS.[9]

Q7. What are congenital dyserythropoietic anemias?

Ans: The congenital dyserythropoietic anemias (CDAs) are a group of rare hereditary disorders characterized by congenital anemia, ineffective erythropoiesis with distinct morphologic features in BM, late erythroblasts, and the development of secondary hemochromatosis. CDAs are classified into the three major types (type I, II, III), plus the transcription factor-related CDAs, and the CDA variants, on the basis of the distinctive morphological, clinical, and genetic features.[10] NGS has revolutionized the field of diagnosis and research into CDAs, with reduced time to diagnosis, and ameliorated differential diagnosis in terms of identification of new causative/modifier genes and polygenic conditions. CDA type II is the most common form among the CDAs. The genes mutated in the major CDA subgroups include *CDAN1* in type I and *SEC23B* in type II and *KIF23* gene in type III.[11] CDA type II is also known by its acronym HEMPAS for hereditary erythroblastic multinuclearity associated with a positive acidified serum test.

Q8. What is sideroblastic anemia?

Ans: Sideroblastic anemia (SA) consists of a group of inherited and acquired anemias of ineffective erythropoiesis characterized by the accumulation of ring sideroblasts in the BM due to disrupted heme biosynthesis. Congenital sideroblastic anemia (CSA) is rare and has three modes of inheritance: X-linked (XLSA), autosomal recessive (ARCSA), and maternal.[12] Acquired SA is more common and can be a result of MDS or other, generally reversible causes. Congenital XLSA is characterized by the accumulation of ring sideroblasts in the BM owing to a hereditary defect in the heme biosynthesis caused by missense mutations in the gene encoding 5′-aminolevulinate synthase 2 (*ALAS2*). This alteration leads to ineffective erythropoiesis and anemia-related symptoms.

Q9. How chronic alcoholism leads to anemia?

Ans: Chronic alcohol ingestion is often associated with anemia, which may be a result of multiple causes:
- Nutritional deficiencies
- Chronic gastrointestinal bleeding
- Hepatic dysfunction and alcoholic liver disease
- Hemolytic anemia
- Hypersplenism from portal hypertension
- Direct toxic effects of ethanol on erythropoiesis (and thrombopoiesis) and on folate metabolism.

Q10. How is hereditary spherocytosis diagnosed?

Ans: Spherocytes on the blood film are the hallmark of the disease. "Pincered" red cells may be seen in individuals with AE1 (band 3) deficiency, whereas, spherocytic acanthocytes are associated with β-spectrin mutations. Hereditary spherocytosis (HS) red cells are osmotically fragile, and this has been exploited in various laboratory tests, including the acid glycerol lysis test (AGLT) and the cryohemolysis test. The standard osmotic fragility test measures the premature lysis of HS red cells in hypotonic salt solutions. Incubation of cells for 24 hours prior to measuring osmotic fragility improves sensitivity of the test. Eosin 5′-maleimide (E5M) is a fluorescent dye that binds to erythrocyte transmembrane proteins, and HS patients exhibit decreased fluorescence. Red cell membrane proteins analysis by quantitative sodium dodecyl sulfate polyacrylamide gel electrophoresis (SDS-PAGE) can be used to identify the underlying defective protein.

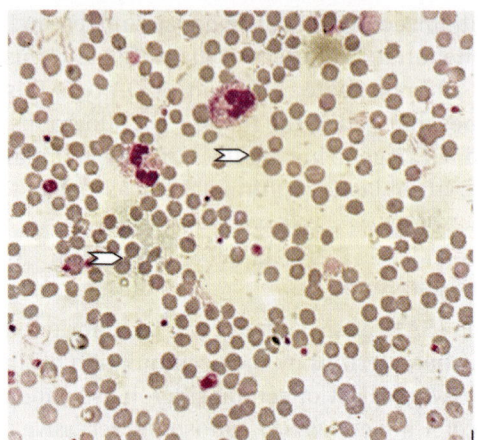

FIG. 1: Peripheral smear (100×) reveals numerous spherocytes (arrowhead).
Courtesy: Dr Abhishek Purohit.

REFERENCES

1. Kulasekararaj A, Cavenagh J, Dokal I, Foukaneli T, Gandhi S, Garg M, et al. Guidelines for the diagnosis and management of adult aplastic anaemia: A British Society for Haematology Guideline. Br J Haematol. 2024;204(3):784-804.
2. Bono E, McLornan D, Travaglino E, Gandhi S, Galli A, Khan AA, et al. Clinical, histopathological and molecular characterization of hypoplastic myelodysplastic syndrome. Leukemia. 2019;33(10):2495-505.
3. Kulasekararaj AG, Jiang J, Smith AE, Mohamedali AM, Mian S, Gandhi S, et al. Somatic mutations identify a subgroup of aplastic anemia patients who progress to myelodysplastic syndrome. Blood. 2014;124(17):2698-704.
4. Matsui WH, Brodsky RA, Smith BD, Borowitz MJ, Jones RJ. Quantitative analysis of bone marrow CD34 cells in aplastic anemia and hypoplastic myelodysplastic syndromes. Leukemia. 2006;20(3):458-62.
5. Luzzatto L. PNH phenotypes and their genesis. Br J Haematol. 2020;189(5):802-5.
6. DeZern AE, Symons HJ, Resar LS, Borowitz MJ, Armanios MY, Brodsky RA. Detection of paroxysmal nocturnal hemoglobinuria clones to exclude inherited bone marrow failure syndromes. Eur J Haematol. 2014;92(6):467-70.
7. Ketan J, Patel A, Joenjeb H. Fanconi anemia and DNA replication repair. Genes Dev. 2007;6(7):885-90.
8. Bamshad MJ, Ng SB, Bigham AW, Tabor HK, Emond MJ, Nickerson DA, et al. Exome sequencing as a tool for Mendelian disease gene discovery. Nat Rev Genet. 2011;12(11):745-55.
9. Hideki M, Yusuke Okuno Y, Shiraishi Y, Doisaki S, Narita A, Sakaguchi H, et al. Clinical utility of next-generation sequencing for inherited bone marrow failure syndromes. Genet Med. 2017;19(7):796-802.
10. Iolascon A, Andolfo I, Russo R. Congenital dyserythropoietic anemias. Blood. 2020;136(11):1274-83.
11. Iolascon A, Heimpel H, Wahlin A, Tamary H. Congenital dyserythropoietic anemias: molecular insights and diagnostic approach. Blood. 2013;122(13):2162-6.
12. Abu-Zeinah G, DeSancho MT. Understanding Sideroblastic Anemia: An Overview of Genetics, Epidemiology, Pathophysiology and Current Therapeutic Options. J Blood Med. 2020;11:305-18.

6. Thalassemias

Gurmeet Singh

Q1. What are the common mutations seen in β-thalassemias?

Ans: *β-thalassemias* are caused by mutations in the *HBB* gene that reduce or abolish the production of the β-globin chains of hemoglobin.[1,2] These mutations can be classified into two types:
1. *β0 mutations*: These result in no production of β-globin. Common β0 mutations include:
    i. Nonsense mutations [e.g., CD17 (A>T), CD 39 (C>T)]
    ii. Frameshift mutations [e.g., CD44 (–C), CD 8/9 (+G)]
    iii. Splice site mutations [e.g., intervening sequence (IVS)-I-1 (G>A)]
2. *β+ mutations*: These allow for some production of β-globin, but at reduced levels. Common β+ mutations include:
    i. Promoter region mutations [e.g., –28 (A>G), –29 (A>G)]
    ii. Splice site mutations [e.g., IVS-I-5 (G>C), IVS-II-654 (C>T)]
    iii. Polyadenylation signal mutations [e.g., poly A (A>G)]

These mutations lead to an imbalance in the α/β-globin chain ratio, resulting in ineffective erythropoiesis and hemolysis.

Q2. How is the lab diagnosis of β-thalassemias made?

Ans: The diagnosis of β-thalassemia typically involves the following laboratory investigations:[3,4]
- *Complete blood count (CBC)*: Shows microcytic hypochromic anemia with a low mean corpuscular volume (MCV) and mean corpuscular hemoglobin (MCH).
- *Peripheral blood smear*: Reveals microcytes, target cells, and sometimes nucleated red blood cells.
- *Hemoglobin electrophoresis*: This is the key diagnostic test that identifies abnormal hemoglobin patterns. In β-thalassemia, there is a reduced or absent HbA (α2β2) with increased levels of HbA2 (α2δ2) and/or HbF (α2γ2).
- *High-performance liquid chromatography (HPLC)*: This can accurately quantify HbA2, HbF, and detect variant hemoglobins, playing a crucial role in diagnosis.
- *Genetic testing*: Identifies specific mutations in the *HBB* gene. This is particularly useful for prenatal diagnosis and in cases where the diagnosis is uncertain.

Peak name	Calibrated area (%)	Area (%)	Retention time (min)	Peak area
P1	---	0.0	0.85	754
Unknown	---	0.1	0.99	2029
F	0.8	---	1.11	16725
Unknown	---	1.2	1.21	26964
P2	---	4.4	1.33	98529
P3	---	5.1	1.74	113948
Ao	---	83.0	2.41	1864118
A2	5.1*	---	3.70	121790

Total area: 2,244,857

F concentration = 0.8%
A2 concentration = 5.1*%

*Values outside of expected ranges
Analysis comments:

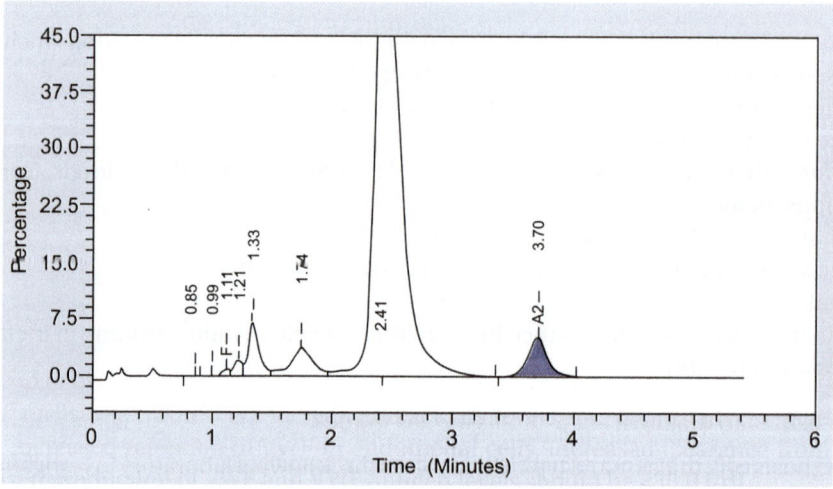

FIG. 1: Hemoglobin HPLC of a patient with beta-thalassemia trait.

Courtesy: Dr Anil Handoo.

Q3. What is the role of high-performance liquid chromatography in diagnosing thalassemias?

Ans: High-performance liquid chromatography plays a critical role in diagnosing thalassemias by:[3,4]
- *Quantifying hemoglobin fractions*: HPLC provides precise quantification of hemoglobin fractions, including HbA, HbA2, and HbF, which is essential in diagnosing thalassemias.
- *Differentiating between thalassemia and iron deficiency anemia*: Elevated HbA2 (>3.5%) is a key indicator of β-thalassemia trait, while normal or low HbA2 suggests iron deficiency anemia.
- *Identifying hemoglobin variants*: HPLC can detect and differentiate between various hemoglobin variants such as hemoglobin S (HbS), hemoglobin C (HbC), hemoglobin D (HbD), and hemoglobin E (HbE), aiding in the diagnosis of compound hemoglobinopathies.

Q4. How hemoglobin electrophoresis is different from high performance liquid chromatography?

Ans: *Hemoglobin electrophoresis* and *HPLC* are both used to analyze hemoglobin variants, but they differ in several ways:[5]
- *Principle*:
  - *Hemoglobin electrophoresis*: Separates hemoglobin molecules based on their charge by applying an electric field.
  - *HPLC*: Separates hemoglobin based on their interaction with the stationary phase of the chromatographic column under high pressure.

Peak name	Calibrated area (%)	Area (%)	Retention time (min)	Peak area
Unknown	---	0.1	0.99	1531
F	0.4	---	1.08	9224
Unknown	---	1.0	1.19	22388
P2	---	4.0	1.31	86783
P3	---	4.1	1.69	88751
Ao	---	87.4	2.36	1893742
A2	3.0	---	3.62	64209

Total area: 2,166,628

F concentration = 0.4%
A2 concentration = 3.0%

Analysis comments:

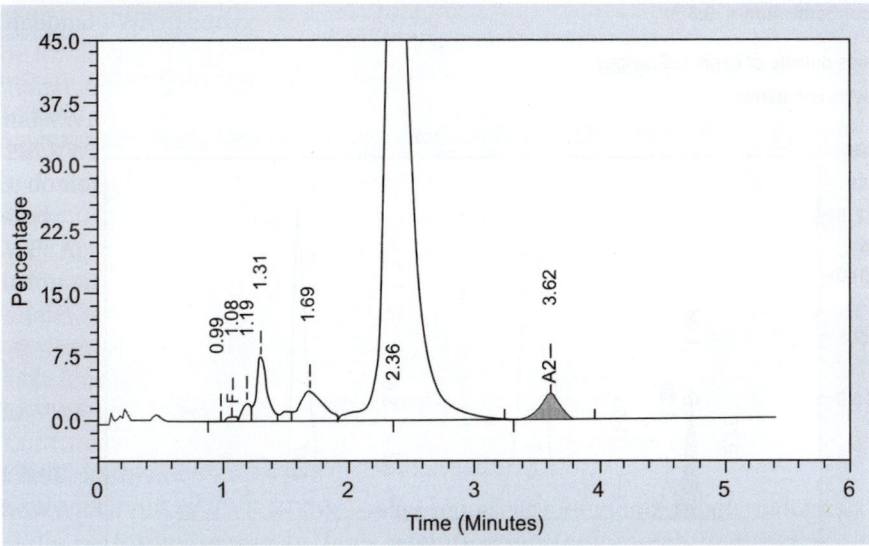

FIG. 2: Normal hemoglobin high-performance liquid chromatography (HPLC).
Courtesy: Dr Anil Handoo.

- *Resolution*:
  - *Hemoglobin electrophoresis*: Has lower resolution and may not accurately differentiate between some hemoglobin variants.
  - *HPLC*: Offers higher resolution and precision in quantifying different hemoglobin fractions and detecting variants.
- *Time and automation*:
  - *Hemoglobin electrophoresis*: Generally manual, time-consuming, and interpretation can be subjective.
  - *HPLC*: Automated, faster, and provides quantifiable results, making it more suitable for high-throughput screening.

Q5. Which tests are used for confirmation of hemoglobin S?

Ans: The confirmation of HbS, the variant associated with sickle cell disease, involves:[6]
- *Hemoglobin electrophoresis*: Identifies the presence of HbS by its characteristic migration pattern.

Peak name	Calibrated area (%)	Area (%)	Retention time (min)	Peak area
P1	---	0.0	0.75	805
F	10.2*	---	1.08	151176
P2	---	2.9	1.28	55139
P3	---	3.4	1.69	65977
Ao	---	50.9	2.40	980624
A2	3.5*	---	3.61	70006
S-window	---	31.2	4.37	601415

Total area: 1,925,141

F concentration = 10.2*%
A2 concentration = 3.5*%

*Values outside of expected ranges

Analysis comments:

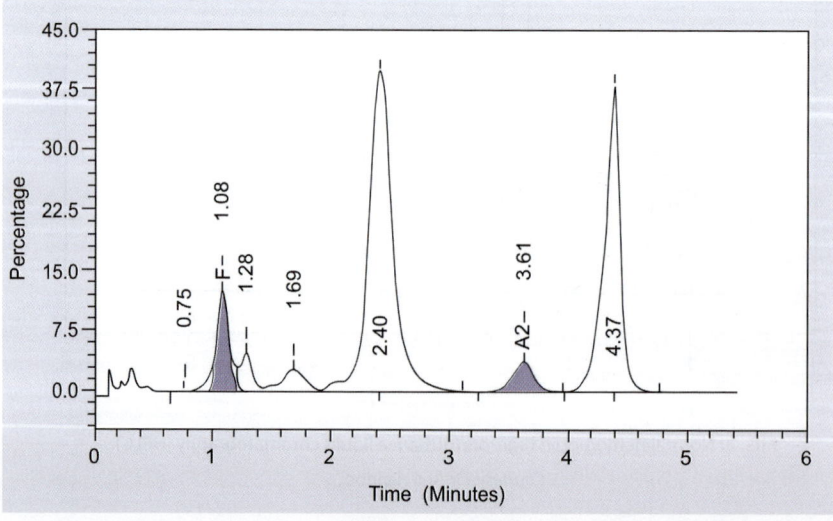

FIG. 3: Hemoglobin HPLC of a patient with sickle cell trait.

Courtesy: Dr Anil Handoo.

- *High-performance liquid chromatography*: Precisely quantifies HbS and distinguishes it from other hemoglobin variants.
- *Sickle solubility test*: A rapid screening test where HbS forms a turbid solution in the presence of a reducing agent, confirming the presence of HbS.
- *Deoxyribonucleic acid (DNA) analysis*: Confirms the diagnosis by detecting the specific point mutation (GAG → GTG) in the *HBB* gene responsible for HbS.

Peak name	Calibrated area (%)	Area (%)	Retention time (min)	Peak area
Unknown	- - -	0.1	0.96	1878
F	1.8*	- - -	1.09	30558
P2	- - -	0.2	1.25	2936
Unknown	- - -	0.1	1.36	1416
P3	- - -	7.5	1.83	130847
Ao	- - -	5.1	2.23	88580
Unknown	- - -	0.6	2.68	9740
A2	80.4*	- - -	3.70	1477441

Total area: 1,743,396

F concentration = 1.8*%
A2 concentration = 80.4*%

*Values outside of expected ranges
Analysis comments:

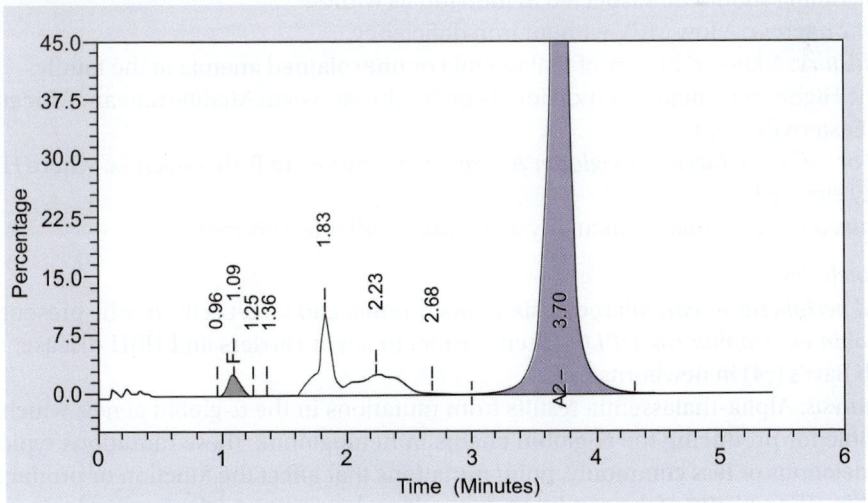

FIG. 4: Hemoglobin HPLC of a patient with homozygous HbE.
Courtesy: Dr Anil Handoo.

Q6. What is hemoglobin E disease?

Ans: Hemoglobin E disease is caused by a mutation in the *HBB* gene (GAG→AAG at codon 26), leading to the production of an abnormal hemoglobin variant, HbE. This variant is common in Southeast Asia and leads to mild hemolytic anemia. Individuals can present in three forms:[7]
1. *HbE trait (heterozygous)*: Usually asymptomatic with microcytosis and mild anemia.
2. *HbE disease (homozygous)*: Causes mild hemolytic anemia and microcytosis.
3. *HbE-β-thalassemia*: A more severe condition resulting from the coinheritance of HbE and β-thalassemia, leading to moderate-to-severe anemia with clinical variability.

Q7. What are the modifiers of HbE-β-thalassemia?

Ans: HbE-β-thalassemia is a compound heterozygous condition with a wide spectrum of clinical severity. Modifiers include:[8]
- *α-thalassemia*: Coinheritance can ameliorate the severity by reducing the α-globin chain excess.
- *XmnI polymorphism*: An XmnI site in the Gγ-globin gene promoter is associated with increased HbF levels, which can mitigate disease severity.
- *Haplotypes and coinheritance of other hemoglobinopathies*: Certain genetic backgrounds and the coinheritance of other hemoglobin variants can influence disease severity.
- *Environmental and nutritional factors*: Iron status, infections, and other external factors can impact clinical presentation.

Q8. When will you suspect α-thalassemia? How is α-thalassemia diagnosed?

Ans: *Suspicion of α-thalassemia*:
Alpha-thalassemia should be suspected in individuals with:[9,10]
- *Microcytic anemia*: A low MCV without iron deficiency.
- *Family history*: A known history of thalassemia or unexplained anemia in the family.
- *Ethnicity*: Higher prevalence in individuals of Southeast Asian, Mediterranean, African, or Middle Eastern descent.
- *Normal or mildly reduced hemoglobin A2 levels*: In contrast to β-thalassemia, where HbA2 is usually elevated.
- *Unexplained mild anemia*: Particularly when iron studies are normal.

Diagnosis includes:
- *CBC and peripheral smear*: Microcytosis, hypochromia, and target cells may be present.
- *Hemoglobin electrophoresis/HPLC*: Often normal in silent carriers and HbH disease; may show Hb Bart's (γ4) in newborns.
- *DNA analysis*: Alpha-thalassemia results from mutations in the α-globin genes, which are responsible for producing the α-globin chains in hemoglobin. These mutations typically involve deletions or less commonly, point mutations that affect the function or production of α-globin. The severity of the condition depends on how many of the four *α-globin* genes (two on each chromosome 16) are affected.
  - *Common mutations*:
    - Gene deletions:
      - *-α3.7 and -α4.2 deletions*: These are the most common types of single-gene deletions, often leading to α-thalassemia trait when one gene is deleted.

- *Southeast Asian (--SEA), Mediterranean (--MED), Filipino (--FIL), Thai (--THAI)*, and *--SA*: These are common two-gene deletions found in different ethnic groups (e.g., --SEA, --MED, and --THAI). Homozygosity or compound heterozygosity for these deletions can cause more severe forms of α-thalassemia, including HbH disease.
  - *Point mutations*:
    - *αCS (Constant Spring)*: A point mutation that produces an elongated and unstable α-globin protein, which can result in a nondeletional form of HbH disease.
    - *αQS (Quong Sze)*: Another point mutation leading to an unstable α-globin chain, often resulting in mild-to-moderate anemia.
  - *Other less common mutations*:
    - *α-thalassemia mental retardation syndrome (αTα)*: Caused by a mutation that involves both deletion and nondeletional mechanisms, leading to severe syndromic forms of the disease.
    - *αPolyA*: Mutations in the polyadenylation signal of the α-globin gene can also lead to decreased α-globin production and contribute to the disease phenotype.

These mutations vary in frequency across different populations, with specific deletions being more prevalent in certain ethnic groups. Genetic testing can identify these mutations to confirm a diagnosis of α-thalassemia.
- *Newborn screening*: Detection of Hb Bart's in newborns can indicate α-thalassemia.

Q9. What are the causes of elevated hemoglobin A2?

Ans: Elevated HbA2 levels (>3.5%) are typically seen in:
- *β-thalassemia trait*: The most common cause.
- *Megaloblastic anemia*: Due to vitamin B12 or folate deficiency.
- *Hyperthyroidism*: Can also result in increased HbA2.
- *Antiretroviral therapy*: Particularly in patients receiving zidovudine.
- *Hereditary persistence of fetal hemoglobin (HPFH)*: Can coexist with slightly elevated HbA2.

Q10. What are the newborn screening methods for hemoglobinopathies?

Ans: Newborn screening for hemoglobinopathies involves:[11]
- *Isoelectric focusing*: Separates hemoglobin based on charge differences, suitable for newborn screening.
- *HPLC*: Widely used for screening due to its high resolution and ability to quantify hemoglobin fractions.
- *Capillary electrophoresis*: Offers precise separation and is increasingly used in newborn screening programs.
- *DNA testing*: Used for confirmatory testing in positive screens, especially when multiple hemoglobinopathies are suspected.

Q11. What is Hb Barts?

Ans: Hb Barts (γ4) is a form of hemoglobin composed of four gamma (γ) chains. It is typically present:[12]
- *In newborns*: Especially in those with α-thalassemia, indicating the absence of sufficient α-globin chains.
- *In hydrops fetalis syndrome*: A severe form of α-thalassemia (usually due to deletion of all four α-globin genes) where Hb Barts is the predominant hemoglobin, leading to fatal anemia.

Q12. **What are the various automatic devices for hemoglobinopathy diagnostics?**

Ans: The various automatic devices for hemoglobinopathy diagnostics are:[13]
- *High-performance liquid chromatography systems*:
  - *Functionality*: HPLC systems are widely used for screening and diagnosing hemoglobinopathies, including thalassemias. They separate hemoglobin variants based on their interaction with a stationary phase under high pressure, providing precise quantification of hemoglobin fractions such as HbA2, HbF, and other abnormal hemoglobins.
  - *Applications*: Commonly used in clinical laboratories for routine diagnosis and monitoring of patients with hemoglobinopathies.
- *Capillary electrophoresis (CE) systems*:
  - *Functionality*: Capillary electrophoresis systems separate hemoglobins based on their charge as they move through a capillary tube filled with an electrolyte solution. These systems offer high-resolution separation, allowing for the accurate identification of various hemoglobin variants.
  - *Applications*: These systems are employed in both high-throughput laboratories and smaller clinics due to their efficiency and reliability.
- *Isoelectric focusing (IEF) systems*:
  - *Functionality*: Isoelectric focusing systems separate hemoglobin variants based on their isoelectric points (the pH at which they carry no net charge). This technique is particularly effective in identifying hemoglobinopathies in newborns and in specific diagnostic scenarios where high resolution is required.
  - *Applications*: Primarily used in newborn screening programs to detect disorders such as sickle cell disease and other hemoglobinopathies.
- *Automated hemoglobin electrophoresis systems*:
  - *Functionality*: These systems separate hemoglobin variants based on their charge by applying an electric field to a gel or other medium. Automated electrophoresis systems are designed for routine analysis, offering clear and reliable separation of hemoglobin variants.
  - *Applications*: Commonly used in clinical settings for the diagnosis of hemoglobinopathies, especially where HPLC or CE is not available.
- *Mass spectrometry*:
  - *Functionality*: Mass spectrometry provides precise identification of hemoglobin variants by measuring the mass-to-charge ratio of ionized particles. This technique offers high specificity and sensitivity, making it useful in complex diagnostic cases.
  - *Applications*: Primarily used in research settings or specialized laboratories due to their advanced capabilities and detailed analysis.
- *Point-of-care devices*:
  - *Functionality*: Point-of-care devices are designed for rapid, on-site testing of hemoglobin variants. They typically use immunoassay techniques or other simple methods to detect common variants such as HbA, HbS, and HbC.
  - *Applications*: Ideal for use in resource-limited settings, emergency situations, or remote locations where quick results are necessary.

These automated systems cater to different clinical needs, from high-throughput laboratory testing to rapid point-of-care diagnostics, ensuring comprehensive and efficient screening, and diagnosis of hemoglobinopathies.

Peak name	Calibrated area (%)	Area (%)	Retention time (min)	Peak area
Unknown	- - -	0.0	0.59	1029
Unknown	- - -	0.1	1.02	2024
F	0.3	- - -	1.08	5960
Unknown	- - -	1.9	1.19	45906
P2	- - -	7.7	1.31	188754
P3	- - -	6.5	1.73	159189
Ao	- - -	81.8	2.36	1998653
A2	1.7*	- - -	3.63	43138

Total area: 2,444,653

F concentration = 0.3%
A2 concentration = 1.7*%

*Values outside of expected ranges
Analysis comments:

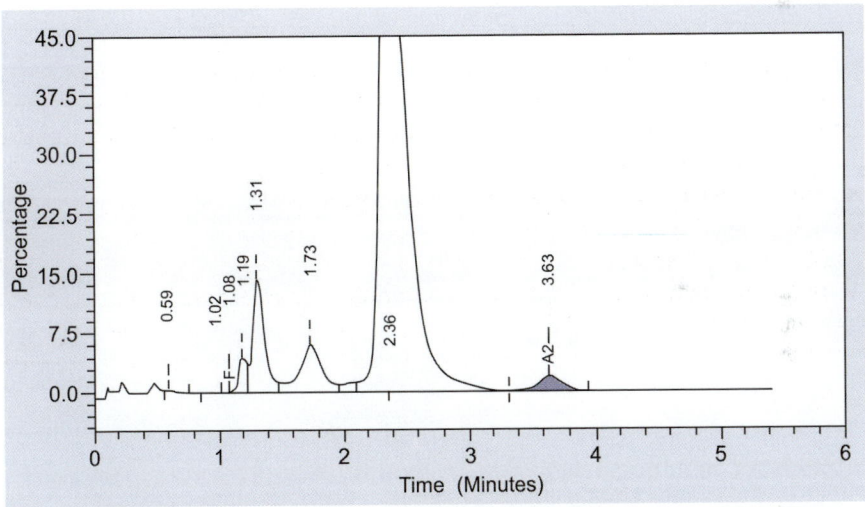

FIG. 5: HPLC of a diabetic patient showing elevated P3 suggestive of increased HbA1c.
Courtesy: Dr Anil Handoo.

REFERENCES

1. Jaing TH, Chang TY, Chen SH, Lin CW, Wen YC, Chiu CC. Molecular genetics of β-thalassemia: A narrative review. Medicine (Baltimore). 2021;100(45):e27522.
2. Thein SL. The molecular basis of β-thalassemia. Cold Spring Harb Perspect Med. 2013;3(5):a011700.
3. Brancaleoni V, Di Pierro E, Motta I, Cappellini MD. Laboratory diagnosis of thalassemia. Int Jnl Lab Hem. 2016:38;32-40.
4. Munkongdee T, Chen P, Winichagoon P, Fucharoen S, Paiboonsukwong K. Update in Laboratory Diagnosis of Thalassemia. Front Mol Biosci. 2020;7:74.
5. Ou CN, Rognerud CL. Diagnosis of hemoglobinopathies: electrophoresis vs. HPLC. Clinica Chimica Acta. 2001;313(1-2):187-94.
6. Arishi WA, Alhadrami HA, Zourob M. Techniques for the Detection of Sickle Cell Disease: A Review. Micromachines (Basel). 2021;12(5):519.

7. Fucharoen S, Weatherall DJ. The hemoglobin E thalassemias. Cold Spring Harb Perspect Med. 2012;2(8):a011734.
8. Premawardhena A, Fisher CA, Olivieri NF, de Silva S, Arambepola M, Perera W, et al. Haemoglobin E beta thalassaemia in Sri Lanka. Lancet. 2005;366(9495):1467-70.
9. Motiani A, Zubair M, Sonagra AD. Laboratory Evaluation of Alpha Thalassemia. Treasure Island (FL): StatPearls Publishing; 2024.
10. Vijian D, Wan Ab Rahman WS, Ponnuraj KT, Zulkafli Z, Mohd Noor NH. Molecular Detection of Alpha Thalassemia: A Review of Prevalent Techniques. Medeni Med J. 2021;36(3):257-69.
11. Ghosh K, Colah R, Manglani M, Chaudhary VP, Verma I, Madan N, et al. Guidelines for screening, diagnosis and management of hemoglobinopathies. Indian J Hum Genet. 2014;20(2):101-19.
12. Chui DHK. α-Thalassemia: Hb H Disease and Hb Barts Hydrops Fetalis. Ann NY Acad Sci. 2005;1054:25-32.
13. Harteveld CL, Achour A, Arkesteijn SJG, Ter Huurne J, Verschuren M, Bhagwandien-Bisoen S, et al. The hemoglobinopathies, molecular disease mechanisms and diagnostics. Int J Lab Hematol. 2022;44 (Suppl 1):28-36.

7. Hemostasis

Ankur Ahuja, Gurpreet Kaur, Metaanksha Ahuja

Q1. A sample of 32-year-old male was received as a part of the routine procedure for the dental extraction. The sample initially was taken by the training nurse in ethylenediaminetetraacetic acid (EDTA). However, the sample was returned by the coagulation lab because of the wrong vacutainer. The sister did not realize the importance and poured the same sample into the light blue-topped sodium citrate vacutainer. The sample showed prothrombin time (PT) of 70 seconds against the control of 13 seconds (reference range: 11–14 seconds) and activated partial thromboplastin time (APTT) of 84 seconds against the control of 32 seconds (reference range: 31–35 seconds). The patient never had any bleeding episodes. He got extracted his tooth 2 weeks later when his PT/APTT were within normal limits.

(a) What is the possible cause of prolonged PT/APTT?
(b) What other precautions should be taken while collecting samples for coagulation testing?

Ans:
(a) EDTA and sodium citrate are known for chelating calcium, so the coagulation process is inhibited as soon as the samples are collected. But, while the sodium citrate has the light chelating effect which becomes reversible soon after the recalcification of the plasma, EDTA causes a strong inhibitory effect which will cause inhibition even after recalcification. Here, the sample was taken first in EDTA which already chelated the calcium in an irreversible manner whose irreversible effect persisted even after the recalcification during the testing.

The blood samples should not be transferred from one collection vacutainer to another.[1-3] This holds even for the mixing of two sodium citrate samples, as this may cause a doubling up of citrate levels and dilution of the plasma samples.

The contamination can also occur if proper draw order is not being done. The correct order of drawing of blood is depicted in **Fig. 1**.

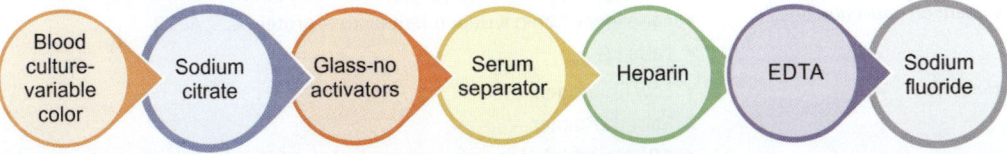

FIG. 1: Order of drawn of sample.
(EDTA: ethylenediaminetetraacetic acid)

(b) The other preanalytical technical factors which can interfere with the tests and their interferences over the tests are depicted in **Table 1**. There can also preanalytical patient's factors **(Table 2)** or incomplete sample processing **(Table 3)** which can interfere with coagulation parameters.

TABLE 1: Preanalytical technical factors and their interferences in coagulation parameters.

Preanalytical factors	Interferences in parameters
Timing of the sample	• Fibrinolytic activity trough is at 06 AM. • If patient is on factor replacement, then • FVIII is estimated after 15 minutes, and • FIX is estimated after 30 minutes.
Traumatic venipuncture Improper mixing of the sample with the anticoagulants in the vacutainer	Because of the consumption of the coagulation factors it leads to prolonged PT, APTT
Contamination of sample by EDTA Assessment of K$^+$ (very high) and Ca^{2+} (very low) indicates its presence	• Raised PT, APTT • False low factor levels • False time-dependent factors inhibition • False lupus anticoagulant (LA)
Partially clotted sample Testing after using heparin neutralizer	• False raised APTT> PT, TT • False shortening of APTT • False low FII, V, VIII factors • False high FVII levels • False time-dependent factors inhibition • False LA
Underfilled citrate tube (Filling the vacutainer to the mark)	• False raised PT, APTT, TT • False low fibrinogen, D-dimers and factors
Heparin contamination (Flushing of lines is important before withdrawing the samples)	• False raised TT>APTT>PT • False low factors (FVIII, IX, XI, XII) • False low antithrombin • False LA • False imprint of factors inhibition
Delayed transport	• Reduced FV, FVIII (Labile factors) • Activation of FVII

(APTT: activated partial thromboplastin time; EDTA: ethylenediaminetetraacetic acid; PT: prothrombin time; TT: thrombin time)

TABLE 2: Preanalytical patient's factors and their interferences in coagulation parameters.

Preanalytical factors	Interferences in parameters
Vitamin K deficient (liver disease, patient on anticoagulants)	• Prolongs PT, APTT (PT>APTT) • False low vitamin K dependent factors, protein C, S, APCR • False LA
Hemolysis	• Low fibrinogen, PT • Raised D-dimer • APTT low/high depending upon the loss of fibrinogen or its activation

Continued

Continued

Preanalytical factors	Interferences in parameters
High hematocrit (>55%)	*Due to reduced plasma:* Citrate ratio, PT, APTT tests are prolonged[*]
High fatty diets	• High FVIIa and fibrinogen leading to shorten PT, TT • Interference with the platelet factors • Low FII, FIX, FX, FVII, FVIIa, FXIIa
Physical activity, stress, illness	High vWF, FVIII, and fibrinogen (acute phase reactants)
Prolonged fasting	Low F II, VII, and X
Circadian rhythm	Fibrinogen and plasminogen activator inhibitor-I highest in the morning
Anticoagulant therapy	Effects LA, APCR, antithrombin, protein C, and protein S
Acute thrombotic episodes	• Increased FVIII • Reduced protein C, S

[*]Relationship of haematocrit values and citrate concentration in a 5 mL sample (Adapted from Dacie & Lewis Practical Haematology 12th Edn).
(APCR: activated protein C resistance; APTT: activated partial thromboplastin time; LA: lupus anticoagulant; PT: prothrombin time; TT: thrombin time)

TABLE 3: Inappropriate sample processing factors and their interferences in coagulation parameters.

Factors	Interferences in parameters
Whole blood refrigerated before centrifugation	• FVII and platelet (Plt) activation (any refrigerated samples to be avoided) • Decreased FVIII and vWF
Delayed testing/poor storage/several freeze-thaw events, storage in frost-free freezer	• Reduced FV, FVIII (Labile factors) • Activation of FVII
Poor centrifugation Platelet poor plasma (PPP) preparation—centrifugation at 2,000 g for 15 minutes at 4°C[*] (approximately 4,000 rev/min)	• Plt contamination • Hemolysis • False low APTT • False reduced heparin levels • False negative LA • False increased factor levels
Filtered plasma (used for lupus anticoagulants)	Raised APTT (due to loss of FVIII and vWF)

[*]4°C for all assays except prothrombin test, lupus anticoagulant (LAC), factor VII assays, activated PC resistance (APCR) which requires room temperature as the platelets gets activated at 4°C which releases phospholipids, factor V, and will hamper these tests.
LAC tests also require double centrifugation to ensure the platelet count to be <10,000/mm^3.

Q2. A 54-year-old lady with a known case of seizures on phenytoin was admitted for recurrent cerebral vein thrombosis (CVT) episodes. Her last episode was just a week back when she was admitted to an intensive care unit (ICU). A sample was taken from the central line in the peripheral veins. While taking the samples, the nurse noticed a small clot. She heparinized the central line to get a normal flow sample. A sample was sent for the workup for the thrombosis. The laboratory diagnosed her as a case of lupus anticoagulant positive because of raised APTT and

positive lupus tests. Subsequently, the lady was retested after 12 weeks as per the diagnostic protocol for antiphospholipid syndrome (APS) and was found negative.
(a) What were the factors involved in the misdiagnosis in her case?
(b) What are the other factors which can lead to interference in lupus anticoagulant tests?

Ans:
(a) In this case, certain factors led to the false positive lupus anticoagulant test which are as given in the following text:[4,5]
- The patient was on phenytoin which is known to cause false positive lupus anticoagulant.
- Heparin contamination has been there in this case which is known for inhibition of clotting factors like FXa (indirectly through binding with antithrombin, which further inactivates FXa); direct inhibition of thrombin by binding to it and indirectly by binding to antithrombin which further inhibits thrombin; prevents prothrombin activation by disrupting prothrombin activator complexes.
- Lupus test was done in an acute thrombotic event which may also lead to false positivity. In acute thrombotic events, FVIII levels are increased along with C reactive protein (CRP) which interferes with lupus anticoagulant tests.

(b) Factors leading to interference of lupus anticoagulant tests are:
- *Sampling issues*:
  - Platelets contamination—corrective action is by keeping platelets to <10,000/mm³ by double centrifugation 1500 × g (approximately 3000 RPM) for 15 minutes. A correct centrifugation speed is essential else the phospholipid-containing vesicles released from platelets can bind to lupus anticoagulants (LAs).
  - Repeated freezing-thawing cycle may lead to disruption of the platelets membrane which will bind to LAs. Corrective action is a single cycle of freezing-thawing, with freezing plasma sample within 4 hours of the collection and when required for the testing, then thawing the sample rapidly for 5 minutes in the water bath of temperature 37°C and analyzing within 4 hours.
  - Improper storage—the corrective action is storing the plasma sample for 14 days if kept at −20°C and for 6 months if kept at −70°C. PT test have to be conducted within 24 hours at room temperature or 4°C else FVII will get activated and lead to shortening of PT.
- *Interfering factors*:
  - Factors leading to increased FVIII levels—acute thrombotic episodes, pregnancy, cancers
    – Corrective action avoidance during acute episodes or use with caution.
  - C-reactant protein leading to false positive LA assays because of affinity with phospholipids.
  - Infections—Coronavirus disease of 2019 (COVID-19), infectious mononucleosis
  - Drugs—antibiotics, antiepileptics, antiarrhythmics, and anticoagulants

Q3. Can the serum sample measure coagulation parameters PT, APTT, TT?

Ans: No, as there is a removal of coagulation factors in the serum sample, it can cause prolongation of these parameters.

Q4. Can the blood sample be stored in cold storage?

Ans: Yes, cold storage is acceptable for various coagulation tests except for the PT. The sample needs to be centrifuged and then the plasma is aliquoted.[6]

Q5. What precaution should be taken for the samples for unfractionated heparin therapy?

Ans: Samples should be centrifuged within 1 hour else platelet factor 4 released from the platelets will neutralize heparin and interfere with the tests.

Q6. How is prothrombin time measured?

Ans: Prothrombin time is measured by using a prothrombin reagent which is comprised of calcium chloride which overcomes the citrate anticoagulant to initiate the coagulation process, recombinant tissue factor, and phospholipids. This when added to the patient's plasma activates the clotting process.[7] The time it takes for the patient's plasma to clot is called PT and is measured in seconds. The clot is detected mechanically or optically depending upon the automated coagulometer available.

Q7. What is the clinical use of prothrombin time?

Ans: Prothrombin time measures extrinsic and common pathway activity which involves FVIIa activity.[7] Thus, whatever inherited or acquired factors which cause deficiency of FVII will lead to prolonged PT. These causes are enumerated in **Table 4**.

TABLE 4: Causes of prolonged prothrombin time (PT).

Cause	Reason for prolonged PT
Liver dysfunction	Reduction of the production of most coagulation factors
Vitamin K deficiency	Reduction of vitamin K-dependent coagulation factors such as factors II, VII, IX, and X
Vitamin K-antagonist therapy	The same reasons mentioned above
Disseminated intravascular coagulation	Wide systemic activation of the coagulation process leads to depletion of the coagulation factors
Antiphospholipid antibody syndrome (APS)	APS causes the conversion of prothrombin to thrombin in vivo, which subsequently leads to a decrease in prothrombin thus leading to an increased PT
Inherited deficiency of FII, V, VII, X	Extrinsic and common factors deficiency lead to prolonged PT

Q8. What is the use of PT mixing studies?

Ans: Mixing studies of PT are required to differentiate between inhibitors or deficiency of clotting factors when PT is prolonged.

Q9. What is APTT?

Ans: APTT is an abbreviation for activated partial thromboplastin time. Activated means an activator such as celite, silica, ellagic acid, or kaolin is added which activates contact-dependent factor XII and thus the intrinsic coagulation pathway. The partial is added to emphasize the fact that there is an absence of the tissue factor in the thromboplastin. Overall, APTT measures the functionality of all coagulation factors except FVII (where PT is prolonged) and FXIII [where PT, APTT, and thrombin time (TT) all are normal, and clot solubility and FXIII assays are the screening and confirmatory tests respectively for FXIII assessment].[7]

Q10. **How is APTT measured?**

Ans: APTT test uses decalcified blood (because of sodium citrate) to avert clotting in the tube itself. Thereafter, plasma is separated by centrifugation. Further, calcium and activators are added to the plasma which begins the intrinsic coagulation pathway. Cephalin is the alternative for platelet phospholipids. APTT is the time in seconds required to form a clot.[7]

Q11. **What are the clinical uses of the APTT?**

Ans: The clinical uses of the APTT test are summarized in **Table 5**.

TABLE 5: Clinical uses of activated partial thromboplastin time (APTT).	
Indication	**Remarks**
Preoperative testing	Not recommended in low-risk or elective surgery, noncardiac surgery unless clinically indicated
Unfractionated heparin monitoring	Therapeutic APTT range for heparin is 60–100 seconds (normal APTT is between 25 and 35 seconds)
Screening for bleeding disorders	Deficiency of clotting factors or presence of inhibitors to intrinsic and common factors, von Willebrand factor, disseminated intravascular coagulation
Screening of thrombotic disorders	Antiphospholipid syndrome

Q12. **What precautions should be taken while measuring APTT?**

Ans: While measuring APTT, it is very important to take certain precautions that may have an impact on its results. These are summarized in **Table 6**.

TABLE 6: Conditions affecting activated partial thromboplastin time (APTT).	
Patient factors	• Diseases—liver disorders, bleeding disorders • Drugs—anticoagulants, replacement therapy
Specimen collection factors	• Poor venipuncture—hemolysis, activation of coagulation process before transferring to vacutainer • Inaccurate sample in vacutainer • Wrong vacutainer • Wrong order of sample collection in vacutainer • Incomplete mixing of sample in vacutainer
Specimen transport factors	• Old sample • Improper temperature • Inappropriate handling
Specimen processing and storage	• Inadequate centrifugation speed, time • Inappropriate temperature storage • Presence of platelets >1,000/µL • Presence of neutralizing agents • Use of filters

Q13. What is APTT mixing study?

Ans: APTT mixing study is done when there is prolonged APTT either due to deficiency of coagulation factors or there are inhibitors to coagulation factors.[8] The coagulation factors that are involved are both intrinsic factors of coagulation cascade which will prolong isolated APTT or common factors of the coagulation cascade which prolong both PT and APTT.

After prolonged APTT, it is desired to discriminate between the deficiency and inhibitors by correcting the APTT in the former and unable to correct APTT in the latter.

In the final step, using specific factor deficient plasma the factor (s) involved is (are) diagnosed.

Q14. How is APTT mixing study performed?

Ans: The method of mixing study includes mixing the patient plasma with normal pooled plasma **(Table 7)**.

TABLE 7: The process of mixing study is depicted in the table at 0 and 2 hours.	
Mixing patient plasma with normal pool plasma (1:1) and incubate	Control plasma is prepared from 20 donors having normal coagulation screen
Clotting time accessed immediately	FVIII inhibitors corrects immediately rest all factor inhibitors are not corrected
Clotting time accessed after 2 hours	FVII inhibitors are time dependent and takes 2 hours for inhibitory effect

Q15. Why is it very essential to ensure strict quality control while performing coagulation workup?

Ans: Coagulation process evolves numerous enzymes and unstable factors which can influence the results of the coagulation tests, and impact the diagnosis and management, hence there is a dire requirement to have the quality control. The aim of quality control while performing coagulation work is to:
- Augment the diagnostic accuracy.
- Improve patient care and safety.

Q16. What are the conditions which lead to prolongation of both PT and APTT?

Ans: The conditions and the specific workup is explained in the given **Table 8**.

TABLE 8: Workup for prolonged prothrombin time (PT) and activated partial thromboplastin time (APTT).	
Multiple factor deficiency	• Rule out vitamin K deficiency by giving a trial of vitamin K • Access liver function tests
Anticoagulants (warfarin, direct acting, heparins)	• History of drugs • Anti-Xa assay, anti-IIa assay
Factor V, X, or II or combined FV and FVIII deficiency	Specific factor assays
Fibrinogen deficiency/disorder	• Thrombin time, D-dimer • Fibrinogen assays
Disseminated intravascular coagulation	• History • Platelet count, D-dimer, fibrinogen

Q17. **What are the assays available for the fibrinogen estimation?**

Ans: Fibrinogen can be assessed qualitatively and quantitatively.

While fibrinogen antigen is quantified by immunological assay [enzyme-linked immunosorbent assays (ELISA), radial immunodiffusion, and electrophoresis] and is used to differentiate congenital dysfibrinogenemia from congenital afibrinogenemia.[9]

Q18. **Which functional assay is recommended for fibrinogen?**

Ans: Clauss assay is commonly done for fibrinogen assessment.[9] Though PT based fibrinogen assay is easy and inexpensive, but it is not recommended because of the following reasons:
- Highly dependent upon the reagents and the analyzers and thus its results may vary between labs, over time-to-time, between batch-to-batch.
- Overestimation of fibrinogen levels especially when patient is on anticoagulants or thrombolytics and in dysfibrinogenemia.

Q19. **What are the clinical uses of fibrinogen assays?**

Ans: Fibrinogen assays are used for the work up of following **(Fig. 2)**:

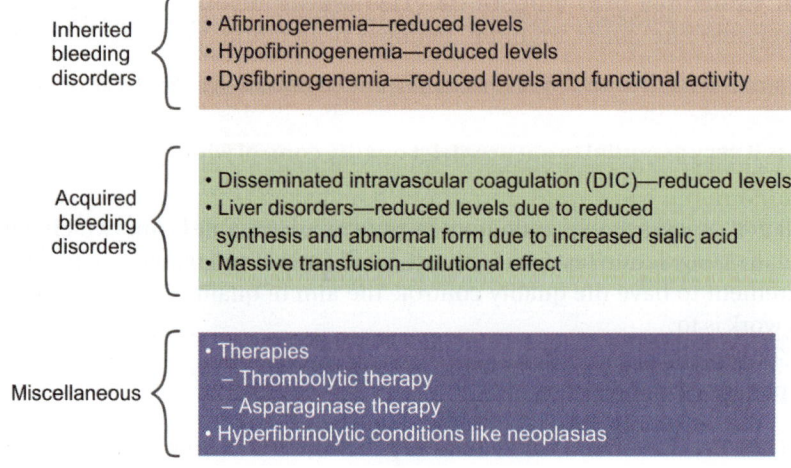

FIG. 2: Uses of fibrinogen assay.

Q20. **A patient was referred to you for the fibrinogen estimation. What physiological and pathological factors would you like to know prior to the test?**

Ans: Various factors can increase fibrinogen levels which are:
- *Physiological*:
    - Age—with age it increases
    - Gender—females have increased levels
    - Postmenopausal status
    - Ladies on oral contraceptives
    - Pregnancy
- *Pathological*:
    - Any infection/inflammatory condition as fibrinogen, is an acute phase reactant.

Q21. A 4-year-old child on workup was found to have abnormal Clauss assay. How will you differentiate between afibrinogenemia, hypofibrinogenemia, and dysfibrinogenemia?

Ans: While afibrinogenemia will show absolute absent fibrinogen, dysfibrinogenemia will have functional: Immunological ratio of <0.7 and hypofibrinogenemia will have >0.7.

Q22. What are one-stage and two-stage clotting assays?

Ans: Factors are measured by assays which are one stage clotting assay (OSCA) or two stage clotting assay (TSCA)/chromogenic assays (CA).[10,11] APTT-based clotting assays measures intrinsic factors and common coagulation cascade factors. **Table 9** compares these assays.

TABLE 9: Comparison of one stage clotting assay (OSCA) and two stage clotting assays (TSCA).

	OSCA	TSCA/chromogenic assay (CA)
Steps	One step	Two steps
Principle (s)	Degree correction of clotting time when patient's plasma is added to another plasma which is deficient in that factor which is needed to be measured	• In the first step coagulation initiated by FXIa with FVIII as the rate limiting step for FXa formation • In the second step, FXa is measured which correlates with FVIII activity after addition of first stage sample to the normal plasma • FXa is measured by reference curve in TSCA and by chromogenic substrate in CA • CA are preferred over TSCA
Preferred	Yes	No
Requirements	• APTT reagents • Standard reference plasma[1] (SRP) • Factor deficient plasma[2] • Patient plasma	• Activated serum[3] • Factor V[4] • Adsorbed patient plasma[5] • Normal plasma[6] • $CaCl_2$ and phospholipid
Advantages	• Labs are familiar to it • Protocols of equipment are set • Automation is easier • Inexpensive • Can detect factor VIII levels <1% of normal • FDA approved for FVIII and FIX	• Three dilutions of sample and factor deficient plasma not required • Less interference by nonspecific inhibitors • Accurate for recombinant replacement therapy[7] • FDA approved for FVIII • Bleeding phenotypes correlate better than one stage • 16% of mild hemophilia cases can be missed by the one stage assay wherein CAs are useful

[1] The clotting time of SRP and the patient plasma are compared to derive the factor concentration of patient plasma.
[2] Factor deficient plasma is targeting factor <0.01 IU/mL with normal levels of other factors.
[3] This provides FIX (in case of factor VIII assays), FX, and FXIa which starts coagulation process. It is available commercially prepared or can be prepared in lab itself by incubating whole blood in glass tube followed by centrifugation and lastly following the serum.
[4] Commercially available. Required as a cofactor to initiate the coagulation reaction.
[5] Adsorbed plasma is done by adsorbing with $Al(OH)_2$ which removes vitamin K dependent factors (FII, VII, IX, and X) thus preventing progression of the first stage beyond the prothrombinase complex.
[6] Normal plasma provides fibrinogen and prothrombin so that the coagulation proceeds to form the clot.
[7] With recombinant up to 40% discrepancy can occur which can be overcome by using recombinant FVIII reference instead of standard plasma.

CHAPTER 7: Hemostasis

Q23. What are chromogenic assays?

Ans: Chromogenic assays are one of the types of two stage assay where the amount of FXa (directly proportional to FVIII levels) is measured by action on a chromogenic substrate which releases color.[10,11] The intensity of color is directly related to FXa levels, thus FVIII levels. The absorbance of the sample at a specific wavelength which is usually 405 nm is measured and compared to a reference curve. Commonly one stage assay shows higher values of FVIII:C than the CA, however, reverse can happen sometimes.

Q24. Can the genetic mutation cause false negativity in the estimation of FVIII in chromogenic assay and hence become the limitation?

Ans: Yes, when this can happen when certain mutations like in GLA domain of the vitamin K dependent proteins lead to dysfunctional protein. Because of the dysfunctional protein activation, enzymatic activity does not occur and hence no color formation, leading to false normal results. In those cases, clotting based assay are useful.

Q25. What makes chromogenic assays advantageous for the various inhibitors?

Ans: Chromogenic assay procedure encounters a high dilution of plasma which causes the dilution of inhibitors like lupus anticoagulants, various anticoagulant drugs which makes them insensitive, except direct oral anticoagulants which remains sensitive.

Q26. As per European Pharmacopoeia and the International Society on Thrombosis and Haemostasis (ISTH) subcommittee, which method is a reference method for FVIII and FIX assessment?

Ans: Chromogenic assay is a reference method as per European Pharmacopoeia and ISTH subcommittee because the one stage method is susceptible to interference by analytical factors such as lipids, heparin, and other anticoagulants, and high chances of preactivation of FVIII. Besides, CA is based upon two factor assays and is very precise.

Q27. A 12-year-old known case of hemophilia A on factor replacement was referred to ascertain the requirement of testing for factor inhibitors. What are the indications for getting him screened for FVIII inhibitors?

Ans: The indications of testing of clotting factor inhibitor assays are mentioned in **Table 10**.[12,13]

TABLE 10: Indications of clotting factor inhibitor assays testing.	
Patient clinical scenario	**Clotting factor concentrate (CFC) related**
Newly diagnosed every 6–12 months then annually	After initial factor exposure
Target joint bleeds unresponsive/partially responsive to CFC	Intensively treated (>5 days)
Recurrent bleeds unresponsive/partially responsive to CFC	Within 4 weeks of the last infusion
Before surgery	Suboptimal postoperative response

Q28. A 2-year-old child was diagnosed as a case of hemophilia A. His mother was a noncarrier and there was no significant family history. What could be the inheritance of hemophilia A?

Ans: Probably the child is a sporadic case of hemophilia A which could be due to the following factors:[14,15]

- Haldane hypothesis—which predicted that to maintain a consistent frequency of a genetic disorder in the population it requires one-third cases to have spontaneous mutation. The factors which predispose for the spontaneous mutation are:
  - Presence of large size (186 kb) *FVIII* gene
  - Presence of hot spots region (e.g., CpG dinucleotides)
  - Unpaired X chromosome in males
- Mosaicism—Germline/somatic

Q29. A 13-year-old female was brought with history of episodes of joint bleeding. On workup, she was found to have FVIII—4%, VWF:FVIIIB/VWF:Ag ratio of 1.6 (Normally >1) suggesting mild-moderate hemophilia A. What could be the reasons of hemophilia A in females?

Ans: Females with bleeding phenotype (rare to have severe bleeding):[16,17]
- Loss of part of the normal X chromosome, as happens in Turner syndrome.
- Skewed X inactivation
- Coinheritance of hemophilia mutations from an affected father and a carrier mother.
- Chromosomal translocations or pathogenic variants in the *XIST* gene.

Q30. A 25-year-old female with possible carrier status of hemophilia A wishes to know her status before conceiving. What all assays can be used to access her carrier status?

Ans: The following assays can be done to know her carrier status:[18-20]
- *Bioassay and immunoassay—VIIIC to vWF ratio*:
  - Inferior to genetic assays except in cases of hemophilia B wherein coagulation-based assays are slightly superior but still DNA based assays are preferred.
    - Normal—0.74–2.20
    - Obligatory carriers—0.18–0.90
  - Detection rate
    - Obligatory carriers—72–94%
    - Possible carriers—48–51%
  - False positives
    - Stress
    - Pregnancy
    - Blood type
    - Oral contraceptives
    - Contamination of plasma samples with thrombin
  - False negative
    - Proteolytic enzymes
- *DNA based assay*:
  - Polymerase chain reaction (PCR)
    - Amplification of specific regions of a gene
    - Determine variations only (point mutations, intron 22, or intron 1 inversions)
  - Multiplex ligation-dependent probe amplification (MLPA)
    - Quantify the copy number (dosage) of a genomic sequence
    - Useful for identifying gene deletions
    - Identify *F8* and *F9* gene deletions

- Next-generation sequencing (NGS)
  - Whole genome sequencing (WGS) or whole exome sequencing (WES)
  - Identify point mutations, complex changes (deletions, inversions)
  - WGS analyze both coding and noncoding sequence (promoter regions, introns)
  - WES only analyzes coding regions and thus would not detect intron inversions
- Sanger sequencing
  - Considered to be the gold standard for determining sequence.
  - Variants identified by NGS are confirmed by Sanger sequencing.

Q31. An 8-year-old boy presented with soft tissue bleeding. He was found to have prolonged APTT which got corrected on mixing study and except for FVIII which was 8%, his all-other factors were normal. His von Willebrand factor (vWF) antigen was also normal.
(a) What is the differential diagnosis?
(b) What are the parameters required to differentiate them?

Ans:
(a) Differential diagnosis are hemophilia A and von Willebrand disease (VWD) type 2N.
(b) While both hemophilia A and VWD type 2N have prolonged APTT, reduced FVIII with normal vWF antigen (except when type 2N defect is inherited with a vWF null allele), the parameters which will differentiate hemophilia A and VWD are summarized in **Table 11**.

TABLE 11: Difference between hemophilia A and von Willebrand disease (VWD).

Parameters	Hemophilia A	VWD type 2N
Gender	Males predominantly	Both genders
Family history	Generally present	Negative
	X-linked recessive	Autosomal dominant
VWF:FVIII B	Normal	Homozygotes/compound heterozygotes—decreased Heterozygotes—normal/low
VWF: FVIIIB/VWF:Ag ratio (Normally >1)	Normal	Heterozygotes—around 0.5 Homozygotes—<0.3 in the most severe forms
Mutational analysis	F8 gene	VWF D'D3 domain

Q32. What assays are used in the diagnosis of VWD?

Ans: The assays have been tabulated in **Table 12 and Flowchart 1**.

TABLE 12: Various von Willebrand disease (VWD) assays.

Assay	Principle
von Willebrand factor ristocetin cofactor activity (VWF:RCo)	• A functional assay of plasma VWF • Based upon the degree of platelet agglutination induced after the addition of ristocetin
VWF:GPIbR	Based upon ristocetin-induced binding of VWF to a recombinant wild-type (WT) GPIb fragment

Continued

Continued

Assay	Principle
VWF:GPIbM	Based upon spontaneous binding of vWF to a gain-of-function variant GPIb fragment
VWF:GPIBA	Measures the ability of vWF to bind to GPIbα
von Willebrand collagen binding activity (VWF:CB)	Quantifies the ability of vWF to bind to collagen
VWF:RCo	vWF:RCo assays measure the interaction between the A1 domain of vWF and GpIbα receptor to on the surface of the platelet
Von Willebrand activity (VWF:Act)	Uses a monoclonal antibody that targets the part of the vWF molecule that binds to the GpIb receptor
VWF:FVIIIB	An assay that measures the ability of vWF to bind FVIII
von Willebrand Factor antigen (VWF:Ag)	An immunological assay that quantifies the amount rather than the function of vWF in plasma
von Willebrand factor propeptide (VWFpp)	The propeptide of vWF

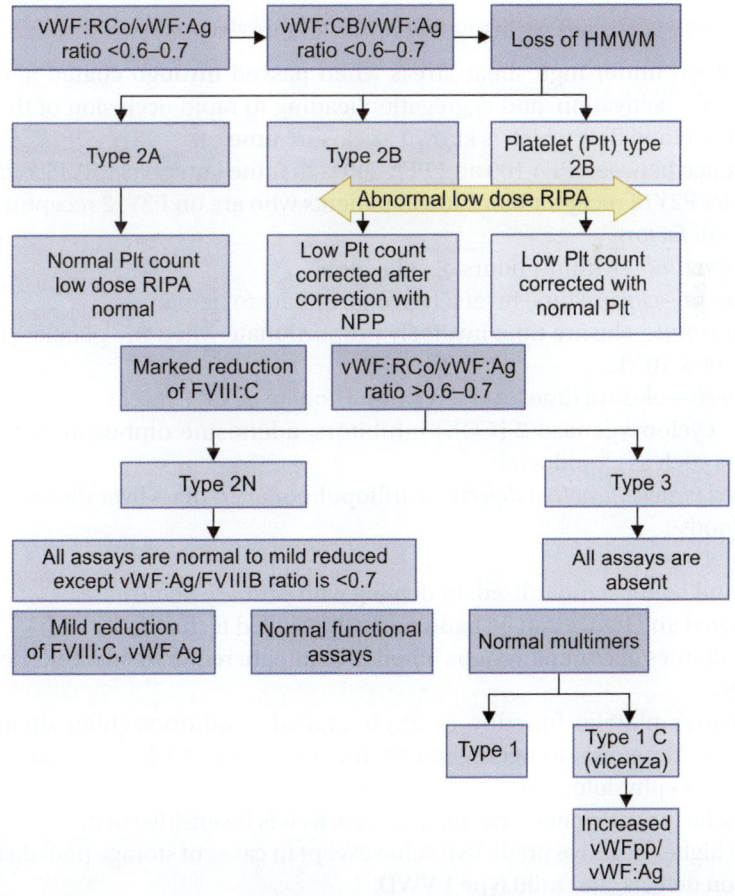

FLOWCHART 1: Algorithm for the diagnosis of vWD.
(HMWM: high-molecular-weight multimers; NPP: normal pooled plasma; RIPA: ristocetin-induced platelet agglutination; VWF:RCo: von Willebrand factor ristocetin cofactor activity; VWF:Ag: von Willebrand factor antigen; VWF:CB: von Willebrand collagen binding activity; VWFpp: von Willebrand factor propeptide)

Q33. A 13-year-old child was brought with a suspected history of platelet function disorder and was advised for PFA-100/200. How will you assess it?

Ans: Platelet function assay (PFA) has many clinical implications:
- *Introduction*:
    - The PFA—100/200 is a device for analyzing platelet function.
    - It detects problems with primary hemostasis.
    - It has replaced the bleeding time.
    - It measures platelet function at high shear rates and hence more physiological **(Fig. 3)**.
- Principle

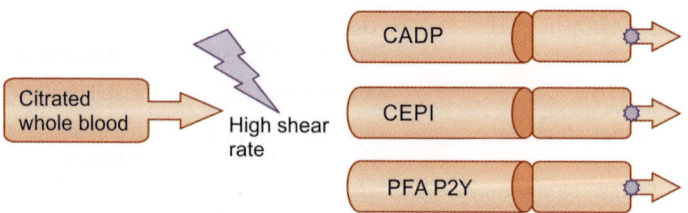

FIG. 3: Platelet function assay (PFA) assessment.
(CADP: collagen and ADP; CEPI: collagen and epinephrine)

Citrated blood under high shear stress when passed through coated agonists induces platelet adhesion, activation, and aggregation leading to rapid occlusion of the aperture and cessation of the blood flow which is known as closure time.

The difference between PFA 100 and PFA 200 is that the latter has PFA P2Y cartridge which detects platelet P2Y12 receptor blockade in patients who are on P2Y12 receptor antagonist.
- *Preanalytical factors*.
    - *Collection time*—within 4 hours of collection.
    - *Hematocrit*—closure time inversely proportionate to hematocrit.
    - *Platelet count*—closure time inversely proportionate when the platelet (Plt) counts fall below $100 \times 10^9/L$.
    - *VWF levels*—closure time inversely proportionate to VWF levels.
    - *Drugs*—cyclooxygenase-2 (COX) inhibitors, adenosine diphosphate (ADP) receptor blockers such as clopidogrel
    - *Acquired platelet function defects*—cardiopulmonary bypass liver disease, uremia.
    - Some foods
- *Advantages*:
    - Rapid and better standardized. In dealing with primary hemostasis.
    - Automated and hence can be handled by nonskilled technician.
    - Small volumes of citrated venous blood (800 μL) are required and hence can be used for children.
    - It measures platelet function at physiological conditions (high shear rates) while luminous transmission aggregometry measures platelet function at low shear rates which is less physiological.
    - Clotting factor deficiencies cannot interfere as it is insensitive to it.
    - It has a higher negative predictive value except in cases of storage pool disorder, primary secretion defects, and mild type 1 VWD.
- *Reference range*:
    - 78–199 seconds for the CEPI cartridge
    - 55–137 seconds for the CADP cartridge

Q34. How is ristocetin-induced platelet agglutination procedure done?

Ans: Principle—ristocetin, an antibiotic which has been removed from the market induces the binding of von Willebrand factor to the GpIb complex.

Sample collection—5-10 mL blood in sodium citrate to make patient-rich plasma. Methodology—ristocetin at varying (low/high) is added to the patient rich plasma and the aggregation is measured by the light transmission aggregometry (LTA) **(Tables 13 and 14)**.

TABLE 13: Interpretation of dose effects of Ristocetin in various subtypes of VWD.

Concentration of ristocetin which is able to induce 30% aggregation	Low dose (<0.5 mg/mL) ristocetin	High dose (1.5, 5 mg/mL)
von Willebrand disease (VWD) subtypes	• Hyper aggregation in • Platelet-type VWD • Type 2B VWD	Reduced aggregation in Type 1, 2A, 2M, 3 VWD

TABLE 14: Differentiation of VWD subtypes after mixing studies.

von Willebrand disease (VWD)	Mixing of patient's plasma with control platelets	Mixing of control plasma + patient's platelets
Platelet-type VWD	Hyper aggregation persists	Normal aggregation
Type 2B VWD	Normal aggregation	Hyper aggregation persists

Q35. How is type 2 VWD classified?

Ans: Type 2 VWD is a form of VWD characterized by a bleeding disorder associated with a qualitative deficiency and functional anomalies of vWF. Depending on the type of functional abnormalities, this form is classified as type 2A, 2B, 2M, or 2N **(Table 15)**.[21]

TABLE 15: Type 2 von Willebrand disease (VWD).

Type	Pattern of inheritance	Pathology	Lab diagnosis

Type 2A	AD	• *Mutations*—A2 domain rarely D1/D2, C-terminal CK
		• *Pathophysiology*
		  ○ Defective intracellular transport leads to reduced secretion of HMW multimers
		  ○ High predisposition for proteolysis
			• vWF:RCo/vWF:Ag<0.6
			• vWF:CBA/vWF:Ag<0.6
			• Multimer electrophoresis— loss of large multimers
			• RIPA—decreased
			• FVIII activity—normal or reduced

Type 2B	AD	*Mutation*—A1 domain mutation *Pathophysiology*—Increased affinity of abnormal VWF for platelet Gp1b receptor leading to thrombocytopenia especially induced during stress situations such as pregnancy and desmopressin	• vWF:RCo/vWF:Ag<0.6 • RIPA—increased at low dose • Multimer electrophoresis— loss of large multimers • CBC/PBS—thrombocytopenia in 40–50% with abnormal morphology platelets • FVIII activity—normal or reduced

Continued

Continued

Type	Pattern of inheritance	Pathology	Lab diagnosis
Type 2M	AD	*Mutations*—A1 domain; rarely A3 domain	• vWF:RCo/vWF:Ag<0.6 • vWF:CBA/vWF:Ag>0.6 • Multimer study—normal multimers but with smeary pattern
Type 2N	AR	*Mutation*—NH2 terminus	vWF:RCo/vWF:Ag>0.6 vWF:CBA/vWF:Ag>0.6 FVIII:C/vWF:Ag<0.5 Multimer study—all multimers present

(CBC: complete blood count; HMWM: high-molecular-weight multimers; PBS: peripheral blood smear; RIPA: ristocetin-induced platelet agglutination; vWF:RCo: von Willebrand factor ristocetin cofactor activity; vWF:Ag: von Willebrand Factor antigen; vWF:CBA: von Willebrand collagen binding activity)

Q36. How is type 3 VWD diagnosed?

Ans: Type 3 VWD patients present markedly reduced levels of vWF and factor VIII.[22]
- *Clinical presentation*:
  ○ Severe bleeding
    – Mucocutaneous bleed depicting absent vWF related platelet binding function (primary hemostatic disorder).
    – Joint/soft tissue bleed depicting absent vWF in the circulation and thus marked reduced FVIII function (secondary hemostatic disorder).
  ○ Pattern of inheritance—autosomal recessive
- *Lab investigations*:
  ○ vWF antigen—methodology
    – Enzyme linked immunosorbent assay
    – Automated method by using latex beads which are coated with antibodies to vWF
      ♦ Comparable with ELISA mostly
      ♦ False negativity because of rheumatoid factors

REFERENCES

1. Levy JH, Szlam F, Wolberg AS, Winkler A. Clinical use of the activated partial thromboplastin time and prothrombin time for screening: a review of the literature and current guidelines for testing. Clin Lab Med. 2014;34(3):453-77.
2. Lippi G, Favaloro EJ. Preanalytical Issues in Hemostasis and Thrombosis Testing. Methods Mol Biol. 2017;1646:29-42.
3. Smock KJ, Moser KA. What have we learned from coagulation laboratory participation in external quality programs? Int J Lab Hematol. 2019;41 Suppl 1:49-55.
4. Molinari AC, Martini T, Banov L, Ierardi A, Leotta M, Strangio A, et al. Lupus anticoagulant detection under the magnifying glass. J Clin Med. 2023;12(20):6654.
5. Devreese KM, de Groot PG, de Laat B, Erkan D, Favaloro EJ, Mackie I, et al. Guidance from the Scientific and Standardization Committee for Lupus Anticoagulant/Antiphospholipid Antibodies of the International Society on Thrombosis and Haemostasis: Update of the Guidelines for Lupus Anticoagulant Detection and Interpretation. J Thromb Haemost. 2020;18:2828-39.

6. Adcock Funk DM, Lippi G, Favaloro EJ. Quality standards for sample processing, transportation, and storage in hemostasis testing. Semin Thromb Hemost. 2012;38(6):576-85.
7. Kamal AH, Tefferi A, Pruthi RK. How to interpret and pursue an abnormal prothrombin time, activated partial thromboplastin time, and bleeding time in adults. Mayo Clin Proc. 2007;82(7):864-73.
8. Adcock DM, Moore GW, Kershaw GW, Montalvao SAL, Gosselin RC. International Council for Standardization in Haematology (ICSH) recommendations for the performance and interpretation of activated partial thromboplastin time and prothrombin time mixing tests. Int J Lab Hematol. 2024;46(5):777-88.
9. Mackie IJ, Kitchen S, Machin SJ, Lowe GD; Haemostasis and Thrombosis Task Force of the British Committee for Standards in Haematology. Guidelines on fibrinogen assays. Br J Haematol. 2003;121(3):396-404.
10. Marlar RA, Strandberg K, Shima M, Adcock DM. Clinical utility and impact of the use of the chromogenic vs one-stage factor activity assays in haemophilia A and B. Eur J Haematol. 2020;104(1):3-14.
11. Potgieter JJ, Damgaard M, Hillarp A. One-stage vs. chromogenic assays in haemophilia A. Eur J Haematol. 2015;94(Suppl 77):38-44.
12. Witmer C, Young G. Factor VIII inhibitors in hemophilia A: rationale and latest evidence. Ther Adv Hematol. 2013;4(1):59-72.
13. Baker P, Platton S, Gibson C, Gray E, Jennings I, Murphy P, et al. British Society for Haematology, Haemostasis and Thrombosis Task Force. Guidelines on the laboratory aspects of assays used in haemostasis and thrombosis. Br J Haematol. 2020;191(3):347-62.
14. Lawn RM. The molecular genetics of hemophilia: blood clotting factors VIII and IX. Cell. 1985;42(2):405-6.
15. Miller CH, Benson J, Ellingsen D, Driggers J, Payne A, Kelly FM, et al. F8 and F9 mutations in US haemophilia patients: correlation with history of inhibitor and race/ethnicity. Haemophilia. 2012;18(3):375-82.
16. Merskey C. The occurrence of haemophilia in the human female. Q J Med. 1951;20(79):299-312.
17. Pavlova A, Brondke H, Müsebeck J, Pollmann H, Srivastava A, Oldenburg J. Molecular mechanisms underlying hemophilia A phenotype in seven females. J Thromb Haemost. 2009;7(6):976-82.
18. Ratnoff OD, Jones PK. The laboratory diagnosis of the carrier state for classic hemophilia. Ann Intern Med. 1977;86(5):521-8.
19. Konkle BA, Johnsen JM, Wheeler M, Watson C, Skinner M, Pierce GF; My Life Our Future programme. Genotypes, phenotypes and whole genome sequence: Approaches from the My Life Our Future haemophilia project. Haemophilia. 2018;24(Suppl 6):87-94.
20. Dutta D, Gunasekera D, Ragni MV, Pratt KP. Accurate, simple, and inexpensive assays to diagnose *F8* gene inversion mutations in hemophilia A patients and carriers. Blood Adv. 2016;1(3):231-9.
21. Tosetto A, Castaman G. How I treat type 2 variant forms of von Willebrand disease. Blood. 2015;125(6):907-14.
22. Tosetto A, Badiee Z, Baghaipour MR, Baronciani L, Battle J, Berntorp E, et al. Bleeding symptoms in patients diagnosed as type 3 von Willebrand disease: Results from 3WINTERS-IPS, an international and collaborative cross-sectional study. J Thromb Haemost. 2020;18(9):2145-54.

8. Heparin-induced Thrombocytopenia

Jatin Munjal

A 56-year-old male was admitted with chest pain. He was diagnosed to have acute coronary syndrome and was started on heparin. Five days later, he developed thrombocytopenia.

Q1. What is the most likely cause of thrombocytopenia in this patient?

Ans: Heparin-induced thrombocytopenia (HIT) is one of the important and frequent drug-induced causes of thrombocytopenia.

The HIT may develop in two distinct forms: (i) type I and (ii) type II. HIT type I (also known as heparin-associated thrombocytopenia) is a nonimmunologic response to heparin treatment, mediated by a direct interaction between heparin and circulating platelets causing platelet clumping or sequestration. HIT type I affects up to 10% of patients, usually occurs within the first 48–72 hours after initiation of heparin treatment, and is characterized by a mild and transient thrombocytopenia (rarely <100,000/mm^3), often returning to normal within 4 days once the heparin is withdrawn.[1] No laboratory tests are required to diagnose HIT type I, and it is not associated with an increased risk of thrombosis, whereas HIT type II is immune-mediated and associated with a risk of thrombosis. It has recently been proposed that the term "HIT type I" be changed to "nonimmune heparin-associated thrombocytopenia" and that the term "HIT type II" be changed to "HIT" to avoid confusion between the two syndromes.[2]

Q2. What is the pathogenesis of heparin-induced thrombocytopenia?

Ans: HIT is caused by the formation of antibodies that activate platelets following heparin administration.[3]

When heparin binds with PF4, it undergoes a conformational change and becomes immunogenic, leading to the generation of heparin-PF4 antibodies, most frequently immunoglobulin G (IgG).[4] The heparin-PF4-IgG multimolecular immune complex then activates platelets via their Fcγ-IIa receptors, causing the release of prothrombotic platelet-derived microparticles, platelet consumption, and thrombocytopenia.[4] The rate of seroconversion varies with extent of preceding platelet activation, duration of heparin exposure, and drug composition (e.g., chain length). The highest rates of seroconversion occur in patients undergoing cardiac surgery, on extracorporeal membrane oxygenation (ECMO), or after insertion of ventricular assist devices, likely due to the combined effects of underlying vascular disease, persistent platelet activation leading to increased PF4 levels, and exposure to high doses of unfractionated heparin (UFH) (~1–4 U/mL).[5] These microparticles in turn promote excessive thrombin generation, frequently resulting in thrombosis.

Q3. Why thrombosis develops in patients with heparin-induced thrombocytopenia?

Ans: As discussed above, binding of heparin or similar polyanions in solution stabilizes the conformation of the PF4 tetramer and nucleates incorporation of additional molecules of heparin and PF4 into a larger antigenic complex.[6] This permits incorporation of multiple IgG anti-PF4 antibodies in each complex forming soluble "ultralarge immune complexes" (ULICs) that reach dimensions exceeding a micron in size.[7]

Soluble ULICs initiate prothrombotic responses, but it is likely that the key event that sustains the risk of thrombosis is the development of large oligomeric immune complexes on the surface of platelets, monocytes, and neutrophils leading to activation of Fcγ-IIA receptors (FcγRIIA).[5]

Activation of monocytes leads to expression of cell surface tissue factor and generation of thrombin. Thrombin generated by activated monocytes augments platelet FcγR-IIA signaling through protease activated receptor 1 to generate highly procoagulant "coated" platelets.[8]

The HIT ULICs stimulate neutrophil adhesion to endothelial cells downstream of thrombi, promote their retrograde migration into venous thrombi, and generate neutrophil extracellular traps (NETs) stabilized by HIT ULICs that develop resistance to degradation by DNase.[9] Injured endothelium releases large multimers of von Willebrand factor (vWF) that binds PF4 and HIT ULICs and propagates thrombosis.[10]

Q4. How is heparin-induced thrombocytopenia diagnosed?

Ans: The criteria for diagnosis of HIT include:[11]
- Normal platelet count before the commencement of heparin
- Thrombocytopenia defined as a drop in platelet count by 30% to <100 × 10^9/L or a drop of >50% from the patient's baseline platelet count
- Onset of thrombocytopenia typically 5–10 days after initiation of heparin treatment, which can occur earlier with previous heparin exposure (within 100 days).
- Acute thrombotic event
- The exclusion of other causes of thrombocytopenia
- The resolution of thrombocytopenia after cessation of heparin
- HIT antibody seroconversion

Current approaches to diagnosis involve use of clinical algorithms, such as the 4Ts to assess pretest probability and confirmation by laboratory testing. The 4Ts incorporates essential features of disease described previously (timing of heparin therapy, complications of thrombocytopenia and thrombosis, and exclusion of other causes) and categorizes disease likelihood based on the cumulative score (low risk: 0–3; intermediate risk: 4–5; high risk: 6–8).[12] As a stand-alone test, a low 4Ts score has excellent sensitivity and a negative predictive value that exceeds 98% outside of the ICU or postcardiopulmonary surgical settings. However, an intermediate or high 4T's score has a much more limited positive predictive value (14% and 64%, respectively) due to low specificity (33–64%).[5]

Q5. What are the laboratory assays for the diagnoses of heparin-induced thrombocytopenia and what is their clinical relevance?

Ans: Various immunoassays have been developed based on detecting binding of HIT antibodies to PF4/heparin (or PF4/polyanion). The following assays are available.

PF4-dependent Immunoassays

The dominant PF4-dependent immunoassay is the enzyme immunoassay (EIA), also called enzyme-linked immunosorbent assay (ELISA). The major advantage of PF4-dependent EIAs is their high sensitivity: At least 97% of patients with HIT will test positive in a solid-phase EIA.[13] A major disadvantage is low diagnostic specificity, especially when only a weak positive result is obtained. Thus, it is recommended to consider strength of reactivity when interpreting an EIA result.[14]

Then there is chemiluminescence assay (CLIA) which detects binding of anti-PF4/heparin antibodies to magnetic particles coated with PF4/polyvinyl sulfonate (PVS). In a study of 509 patient sera ($n = 33$ SRA-positive). The CLIA's sensitivity was 97.0% (32/33) and specificity was also high 98.5% (469/476). Testing is performed "on-demand" with results available in approximately 30 minutes after preparation of serum (or citrated plasma).[15]

Latex immunoturbidimetric assay (LIA) classified as a "functionalized immunoassay" as it detects HIT antibodies based upon their ability to inhibit the aggregation of latex nanoparticles coated with a HIT-like monoclonal antibody (KKO) following addition of PF4/PVS complexes. In theory, this assay will detect anti-PF4/heparin antibodies of IgG, IgA, and/or IgM classes (as any of these could inhibit nanoparticle aggregation), yet the diagnostic specificity of the LIA exceeds that of IgG-specific EIAs. As with the CLIA, testing is usually performed "on-demand" with results available <20 minutes after preparation of patient plasma (serum is not used for the LIA).[14]

With such a rapid test result (assuming local availability of the CLIA or LIA), the physician can order the blood test while performing the usual diagnostic workup for HIT (review heparin exposures, assess timing of platelet count changes, examine the blood film, order duplex ultrasound for deep-vein thrombosis, etc.), and have the HIT test result back in time to impact diagnostic reasoning.

Platelet Activation Assays

Serotonin release assay (SRA), heparin-induced platelet activation assay (HIPA), platelet aggregometry, etc. They are all indirect assays; that is, they test patient serum/plasma against normal donor platelets. However, these are technically demanding (platelet washing) and require selected (pedigree) platelet donors whose platelets react well to HIT antibodies.[16] An advantage of platelet activation assays is their unique role for diagnosis of "autoimmune HIT" (aHIT).

Rapid Screening Tests

Based on qualitative demonstration of anti-PF4–heparin complex antibodies are also available on a range of equipment/devices usually within 1 hour. They have high degree of sensitivity; however, the trade-off is a lack of specificity for those antibodies that cause platelet activation and/or the detection of non-PF4-heparin antibodies. Furthermore, there is no quantification of the antibody concentration present, stratification of which has been used in the assessment of the chances of developing clinical HIT. Amongst these are lateral flow immunoassay (LFIA) which should be performed only on fresh samples and particle immunofiltration assay (PIFA) but PIFA lacks sizeable peer-reviewed data supporting its utility for HIT diagnosis.[15]

Q6. Should the patient with heparin-induced thrombocytopenia be rechallenged with heparin in future?

Ans: Patients who developed HIT should ideally avoid rechallenge with heparin, especially now that several effective alternative anticoagulants are available. For this purpose, they should be given an alert card and informed that they should not receive heparins in the future unless advised by a specialist. If such individuals require thromboprophylaxis, fondaparinux or a direct oral anticoagulant (DOAC) may be considered to prevent the resurgence of the HIT antibodies.

However, UFH is the preferred anticoagulant for patients undergoing cardiac surgery and hemofiltration. In clinical practice, there are data to support the safe use of UFH in patients with previous HIT > 3 months earlier. The basis for this is that (1) there is no relationship between the day of onset and previous heparin exposure; (2) in patients who develop rapid-onset HIT, the previous exposure to heparin is more recent; generally, in the last 100 days; and (3) HIT antibodies are transient and generally disappear with a median of 50–85 days, depending on the assay.[15]

If an individual with a previous diagnosis of HIT requires an intervention where heparin is the most appropriate anticoagulant, first determine whether the antibodies are still present. If the antibodies have cleared, rechallenge with heparin in the perioperative setting has been tried successfully by some experts.

Q7. Which anticoagulants can be used in such patients?

Ans: Current guidelines recommend immediate discontinuation of heparin therapy and institution of nonheparin alternative therapies when HIT is suspected by an intermediate or high 4Ts score; in patients at high risk for bleeding, confirmation by ELISA may be warranted.[17] Parenteral therapies include the DTIs (argatroban and bivalirudin), factor Xa inhibitors such as danaparoid and the synthetic pentasaccharide fondaparinux. The choice of therapeutic agent is guided by drug half-life, patient comorbidities (hepatic or renal disease), and availability.

The DOACs are being increasingly used as first-line therapy for patients who can tolerate anticoagulation.[17] But sufficient clinical data are unavailable to meaningfully assess their safety and efficacy and; most of the published experience is with rivaroxaban.[18]

Warfarin remains a safe alternative oral anticoagulant choice once patients have been bridged with parenteral anticoagulants until platelet counts recover.[17] Warfarin therapy without bridging is associated with complications of warfarin skin necrosis and venous limb gangrene due to reduced synthesis of protein C and impaired generation of activated protein C (aPC), i.e., PF4 binds to chondroitin sulfate residues on thrombomodulin and enhances aPC activation, an effect reversed by HIT antibodies.[13]

REFERENCES

1. Franchini M. Heparin induced thrombocytopenia: an update. J Thrombosis. 2005;3:14.
2. Rice L. Heparin-induced thrombocytopenia: myths and misconceptions. Arch Intern Med. 2004;164:1961-4.
3. Reilly RF. The pathophysiology of immune-mediated heparin-induced thrombocytopenia. Semin Dial. 2003;4:1654-60.
4. Kelton JG, Smith JW, Warkentin T, Hayward CP, Denomme GA, Horsewood P. Immunoglobulin G from patients with heparin-induced thrombocytopenia binds to a complex of heparin and platelet factor 4. Blood. 1994;83:3232-9.

5. Arepally GM, Cines GB. Pathogenesis of Heparin induced thrombocytopenia. Transl Res. 2020;225:131-40.
6. Cai Z, Yarovoi SV, Zhu Z, Rauova L, Hayes V, Lebedeva T, et al. Atomic description of the immune complex involved in heparin-induced thrombocytopenia. Nat Commun. 2015;6:8277.
7. Rauova L, Poncz M, McKenzie SE, Reilly MP, Arepally G, Weisel JW, et al. Ultralarge complexes of PF4 and heparin are central to the pathogenesis of heparin-induced thrombocytopenia. Blood. 2005;105:131-8.
8. Tutwiler V, Madeeva D, Ahn HS, Andrianova I, Andrianova I, Hayes V, et al. Platelet transactivation by monocytes promotes thrombosis in heparin-induced thrombocytopenia. Blood. 2016;127:464-72.
9. Gollomp K, Kim M, Johnston I, Hayes V, Welsh J, Arepally GM, et al. Neutrophil accumulation and NET release contribute to thrombosis in HIT. JCI Insight. 2018;20;3(18):e99445.
10. Johnston I, Sarkar A, Hayes V, Koma GT, Arepally GM, Chen J, et al. Recognition of PF4-VWF complexes by heparin-induced thrombocytopenia antibodies contributes to thrombus propagation. Blood. 2020;135(15):1270-80.
11. Ahmed I, Majeed A, Powell R. Heparin induced thrombocytopenia: diagnosis and management update. Postgrad Med J. 2007;83(983):575-82.
12. Arepally GM. Heparin induced thrombocytopenia. Blood. 2017;129(21): 2864-72.
13. Warkentin TE. Laboratory diagnosis of heparin-induced thrombocytopenia. Int J Lab Hematol. 2019;41: 15-25.
14. Husseinzadeh HD, Gimotty PA, Pishko AM, Buckley M, Warkentin TE, Cuker A. Diagnostic accuracy of IgG-specific versus polyspecific enzyme-linked immunoassays in heparin-induced thrombocytopenia: a systematic review and meta-analysis. J Thromb Haemost. 2017;15(6):1203-12.
15. Sun L, Gimotty PA, Lakshmanan S, Cuker A. Diagnostic accuracy of rapid immunoassays for heparin-induced thrombocytopenia. A systematic review and meta-analysis. Thromb Haemost. 2016;115:1044-55.
16. Cuker A, Arepally GM, Chong BH, Cines DB, Greinacher A, Gruel Y, et al. American Society of Hematology 2018 guidelines for management of venous thromboembolism: heparin-induced thrombocytopenia. Blood Adv. 2018;2:3360-92.
17. Warkentin TE, Pai M, Linkins LA. Direct oral anticoagulants for treatment of HIT: update of Hamilton experience and literature review. Blood. 2017;130:1104-13.
18. Linkins LA, Warkentin TE, Pai M, Shivakumar S, Manji RA, Wells PS, et al. Rivaroxaban for treatment of suspected or confirmed heparin induced thrombocytopenia study. J Thromb Haemost. 2016;14(6):1206-10.

9. Von Willebrand Disease

Preeti Tripathi

CASE

A 30-year-old female presented with menorrhagia since she has achieved menarche. She also complained of epistaxis off and on. Her platelet counts and peripheral blood smear findings were within normal limits.

Screening coagulogram shows normal prothrombin time (PT) but prolonged activated partial thromboplastin time (aPTT) (PT—14 seconds, control 13 seconds, aPTT—45 seconds, control 26–32 seconds). Her mother also had history of menorrhagia. There is no history suggestive of joint bleeding/swelling.

Q1. What is the most likely diagnosis?

Ans: If we analyze the history provided, the most likely diagnosis is von Willebrand disease (VWD). This patient appears to be suffering from an inherited bleeding disorders as indicated by presence of significant family history (mother also having menorrhagia) and repeated episodes of bleedings (off and on epistaxis and continued menorrhagia). The two broad differentials in a case with isolated prolonged aPTT test in such a scenario include hemophilia and VWD.

Hemophilia being an X-linked disorder is more commonly seen in males while VWD is seen in both males and females with equal frequency and is transmitted as autosomal dominant disorder in most cases. In females, VWD is more readily detected due to the presence of bleeding associated with menstrual cycles and childbirth.

The type of bleeding also differs in the two conditions—hemophilia impacts the coagulation cascade and presents with delayed onset large bleeds (e.g., hemarthrosis and large muscle bleeds) whereas, VWD primarily impairs hemostasis through defective platelet adhesion and aggregation and hence presents commonly with mucosal bleeds (epistaxis, menstrual bleeds, and postpartum bleeds). Rare subtype of VWD may have hemarthrosis too.

This patient is a female with a positive family history, history of mucosal bleeds and prolonged aPTT, hence most likely diagnosis is most likely VWD. The subtype may be VWD type 1; however, it needs confirmation with a battery of tests including factor VIII levels and VWD-directed tests.

Q2. When will you suspect von Willebrand disease (VWD)?

Ans: Von Willebrand disease is caused by deficient or defective plasma von Willebrand factor (VWF), a large multimeric glycoprotein that plays an important role in primary hemostasis by mediating platelet hemostatic function and stabilizing blood coagulation factor VIII (FVIII). VWD prevalence estimates range from 1 in 100 to 1 in 10,000 and is inherited equally between men and women; however, women are more likely to come to medical attention because of gynecologic and obstetric bleeding.

The symptoms of VWD can be highly variable ranging from mild-to-severe bleeding based on the subtype, level of VWF activity, age, and sex. It should be suspected in individuals presenting with excessive mucocutaneous bleeding including the following:
- Bruising without recognized trauma
- Prolonged, recurrent nosebleeds
- Bleeding from the gums after brushing or flossing teeth or prolonged bleeding following dental cleaning or dental extractions
- Menorrhagia, particularly if occurring since menarche
- Prolonged bleeding following surgery, trauma, or childbirth
- Gastrointestinal bleeding

The utility of standard clinical assessment tools [bleeding assessment tools (BATs)] to score occurrence of symptoms and their severity as part of VWD diagnosis is increasingly recognized.[1,2] These tools can help in following:
- Determine if there is more bleeding than in the general population.
- Justify the diagnosis of a bleeding disorder.
- Quantify the extent of symptoms; indicate situations requiring clinical intervention.
- Bleeding severity assessment correlates with the long-term probability of bleeding.

A major challenge for affected patients is achieving an accurate and timely diagnosis. Patients with mild bleeding symptoms may experience delays of 15 years or more from the onset of symptoms as disease is quite heterogeneous with a wide spectrum of presentation.

Q3. **Which type of von Willebrand disease is it most likely?**

Ans: This patient seems to have type 1 VWD which is the most common variant of VWD and makes up about 70–80% of the cases.[1,2] It is characterized by a mild-to-moderate decrease in VWF as measured by the VWF antigen and activity levels. The quantitative deficiency may be due to increased retention of VWF in endothelial cells, increased clearance from plasma, or decreased production of VWF and VWF antigen levels should be <30 IU/dL.

The VWF antigen: VWF activity ratio is >0.7.[3] In addition, there is a corresponding decrease in circulating FVIII levels which may lead to prolonged aPTT (present in this case).

Low VWF levels: Patients presenting with moderate levels of VWF antigen (30–50 IU/dL) are common and may pose a significant challenge for a laboratory diagnosis of type 1 VWD. Even though the VWF levels are low and these patients often present with bleeding symptoms, they do not meet the criteria for a diagnosis of VWD type 1 (<30 IU/dL). This group of patients should be considered to have "low VWF" rather than a diagnosis of type 1 VWD.

Q4. **What should be the first and second line of investigations in a patient with suspected VWD?**

Ans: The diagnosis of VWD is established in a patient with excessive mucocutaneous bleeding and characteristic results of assays of hemostasis factors specific for VWD. In addition, a positive family history is supportive of the diagnosis; however, in a small group of cases, family history may not be positive because of incomplete penetrance and variable expressivity.

No single laboratory assay can definitively diagnose VWD and hence a battery of tests are usually performed to reach the diagnosis.[3,4] Clinical laboratory tests can be divided into screening tests and confirmatory tests.

First-line Tests for VWD

Complete blood count (CBC) may be normal, but could also show a microcytic anemia (if the individual is iron deficient) or a low platelet count (thrombocytopenia), specifically in type 2B VWD.

Activated partial thromboplastin time is often normal, but may be prolonged when the factor VIII (FVIII:C) level is reduced to below 30–40 IU/dL, as can be seen in severe type 1 VWD, type 2N VWD, or type 3 VWD. The normal range for FVIII:C clotting activity is approximately 50–150 IU/dL. PT and aPTT are normal in VWD.

Although some laboratories may also include a skin bleeding time and platelet function analysis (PFA closure time) in their evaluation of an individual with suspected VWD, these tests lack sensitivity in persons with mild bleeding disorders.

Factor VIII:C level—functional FVIII assay (i.e., activity of FVIII in the coagulation cascade) (normal range ~50–150 IU/dL) helps in diagnosis of VWD type 1/2N and 3 wherein low VWF levels leads to secondary deficiency of factor VIII. Moreover, low levels of FVIII combined with low levels of VWF increases bleeding risk (representing defects in both primary and secondary hemostasis).

The VWF:Ag levels—quantity of VWF protein (antigen) in the plasma, measured antigenically using enzyme-linked immunosorbent assay (ELISA) or by latex immunoassay (LIA) will establish the quantitative deficiency of VWF (subtype VWD 1 and 3) and should be performed even if the screening tests are normal in an individual in whom VWD is suspected. Normal ranges are determined by the individual laboratory.[4,5] There are many preanalytical/analytical factors which may affect this level. Also, the quantitative levels are not true indicator of functional VWF in body.

The lower the VWF level, the greater the bleeding risk. However, VWF:Ag identifies both functional and nonfunctional VWF forms. Thus, VWF:Ag cannot be used in isolation since normal VWF:Ag levels do not always exclude VWD (levels will be normal in some type 2B and 2M VWD patients), and abnormal VWF:Ag levels, although potentially consistent with VWD, do not identify VWD type (type 1 or type 2 VWD). Thus, testing for VWF activity is also required.

VWF: Activity by GPIb binding assays are also mandatory tests for VWD diagnosis/exclusion since they provide markers for a major VWF activity, being binding of VWF to its platelet receptor (GPIb). Functional tests are used to determine how well VWF binds to GpIbα. Previously, this was assessed using the VWF:RCo assay now there are three tests available for same—(1) VWF:RCo, (2) VWF:GPIbR, and (3) VWF:GPIbM.

The VWF:RCo has the advantage of being well established and is likely the cheapest of the VWF:GPIbB test; however, the main limitations are their high assay variability and poor low-level VWF sensitivity.[4,5]

The VWF:GPIbR or VWF:GPIbM assays represent more modern alternatives to VWF:RCo, primarily performed either by latex agglutination (automated hemostasis analyzer) or chemiluminescence and have the advantage of not being dependent on ristocetin and thus less likely to generate an associated false diagnosis. However, these are less well-established, less accessible, and perhaps more expensive than the classical VWF:RCo.

Second-line Tests for VWD

If abnormalities in the tests above are identified, specialized coagulation laboratories may also perform the following assays to determine the subtype of VWD:
- VWF multimer analysis—SDS-agarose electrophoresis is used to determine the complement of VWF oligomers in the plasma. Normal plasma contains VWF ranging from dimers to multimers comprising >40 dimers and molecular weight (MW) into gigadaltons. Multimers are classified as low (1–5-dimer), intermediate (6–10-dimer), and high (≥10-dimer) molecular weight (HMW). HMW multimers are decreased or missing in type 2A VWD and often in 2B VWD; intermediate MW may also be lost in type 2A VWD. Abnormalities in satellite ("triplet") band patterns can give clues as to pathogenesis and help to classify subtypes of type 2 VWD.[6-8]
- Ristocetin-induced platelet agglutination (RIPA)—platelet agglutination at a low concentration (~0.5–0.7 mg/mL) of ristocetin is abnormal and may indicate type 2B or platelet-type pseudo VWD (PT-VWD).
- VWF:FVIII binding assay—ability of VWF to bind FVIII can be used to identify type 2N VWD. It is a useful test, but not widely available and standardized.
- VWF:CB (collagen binding assay)—ability of VWF to bind to collagen can be used to help define functional VWF discordance (i.e., to help distinguish types 1 and 2 VWD)

Use of Test Ratio to Subtype VWD

Since the second line of tests is not available in most clinical settings especially in resource poor settings—some derived test ratios are good tools which come handy in subtyping VWD patients.

FVIII:C/VWF:Ag ratio provides context around the specific activity of FVIII:C, relative to the level of VWF. In healthy individuals and in those with types 1, 2A, 2B, 2M, and 3 VWD, levels of FVIII:C are relatively concordant (often a little higher) compared with those having VWF, so ratios approximate unity (or >0.7). This ratio is low in hemophilia A and type 2N VWD. Alternatively, a low ratio may potentially represent a preanalytical issue.

VWF:GPIbB/Ag ratio provides context around the specific VWF activity of platelet GPIb binding as compared to VWF antigen levels. These ratios will be normal (i.e., >0.7) in healthy individuals and in those with types 1 and 2N VWD. Ratios are not calculated in type 3 VWD, but levels would be expected to be concordant. These ratios will expectedly be low in types 2A, 2B, and most cases of 2M VWD. The low ratio in these cases is either due to low relative HMWM VWF (2A and 2B VWD) and/or presence of VWF variants expressing defective GPIb binding (2A or 2M VWD).

VWF:CB/Ag ratio provides context around the specific VWF activity of collagen binding, and will be normal (i.e., >0.7) in healthy individuals and in those with types 1 and 2N VWD. Ratios are not calculated in type 3 VWD but levels would be expected to be concordant. The ratio will expectedly be low in type 2A, 2B, and some cases of 2M VWD. The low ratio in these cases is either due to low relative HMWM VWF (2A and 2B VWD) and/or VWF variants expressing defective collagen binding (a proportion of type 2A and 2M VWD).

It is mandatory to perform at least three different tests as panel before VWD can be diagnosed effectively. These three tests are (1) the FVIII:C assay, (2) a VWF "antigen" (VWF:Ag) assay, and (3) a VWF GPIb binding (VWF:Rco) assay. Such three-test panels are recommended by the latest American Society of Hematology, International Society on Thrombosis and Haemostasis, National Hemophilia Foundation, and World Federation of Hemophilia 2021 guidelines.[1,2,7,8] Countries with resource rich setting can add VWF:CB tests to make it four tests panel for VWD.

Q5. What is the difference between type 1 and type 2 VWD?

Ans: VWD is an extremely heterogeneous disorder and can be due to a quantitative or qualitative deficiency of VWF. It is of three main subtypes mainly—type 1 defined as a partial deficiency of VWF, type 2 is qualitative defects of VWF, and type 3 resulting from an absolute deficiency of VWF. The clinical presentation and pathology are as per the **Table 1** below.

Q6. What is von Willebrand factor and what happens to VWF in von Willebrand disease? How is VWF levels assayed in laboratory?

Ans:

Von Willebrand Factor

It is glycoprotein crucial to both primary and secondary hemostasis. VWF is a multimeric glycoprotein synthesized in endothelial cells and megakaryocytes and then stored within Weibel–Palade bodies and alpha granules, respectively. It is cleared by macrophages in the liver and spleen. It is named after the physician Erik von Willebrand, who first identified and described a bleeding disorder later attributed to insufficient quantity or dysfunctional quality of this glycoprotein.

TABLE 1: ISTH classification of von Willebrand disease–2024.

	Type 1		Type 2				Type 3
	Classic	Type 1C	Type 2A	Type 2B	Type 2M	Type 2N	
Frequency	70% cases		25% cases				5% cases
Defect	Quantitative deficiency of VWF		Qualitative deficiency of VWF				Complete absence of VWF
Mechanism	Decrease synthesis of VWF	Increase clearance of VWF	Defects in VWF binding to GP1B	Increased clearance of HMW multimers of VWF	Defects in VWF binding to collagen binding	Defects in VWF binding to F8	Null synthesis of VWF
Inheritance	AD	AD	AD	AD	AD	AR	AR
Severity	Mild-to-moderate bleeding	Mild-to-moderate bleeding	Moderate bleeding	Moderate bleeding	Severe bleeding	Severe bleeding	Severe bleeding
Response to desmopressin	Good	ineffective	May show response	Contraindicated	May show response	May show response	Avoid

(AD: autosomal dominant; AR: autosomal recessive; HMW: high molecular weight; VWF: von Willebrand factor)

Von Willebrand Disease

It is an inherited bleeding disorder, is caused by decreased levels or activity of VWF activity in the blood. Within primary hemostasis, VWF binds extracellular matrix proteins such as subendothelial collagen, as well as platelets through the glycoprotein Ib receptor. In secondary hemostasis, VWF acts as a chaperone to factor VIII (FVIII) to prevent premature clearance and degradation. Therefore, quantitative or qualitative defects of VWF lead to defect in both primary and secondary phase of hemostasis leading to bleeding symptoms.[6-8]

VWF Antigen Assay

The VWF:Ag is most often an immuno-based assay that can be performed as an ELISA method or as an automated turbidimetric method using latex beads coated with antibody to VWF. If the VWF antigen is present in patient plasma, it will bind to the VWF antibody attached to the bottom of a microtiter plate in the ELISA assay or to the antibody-coated latex beads in the turbidimetric method. VWF is then quantified based on the amount of antigen/antibody binding that occurs. The normal range is 50–150 IU/dL but may vary with individual laboratories.[1,4,8] Limitation of assay includes that the assay measures the amount of protein that is present but does not assess the functional status of the protein, hence can be falsely normal in type 2 VWD.

Q7. What happens to factor VIII levels in VWD?

Ans: VWF acts as the transport protein/chaperone for FVIII circulating in the plasma, protecting it from proteolysis and prolonging its half-life (from 2 to 8 hours) in the circulation. This serves to colocalize FVIII to the site of vascular injury allowing it to interact with the proteins in the coagulation cascade.

If VWF is absent/reduced or defective in the body—this leads to short half-life of labile factor VIII and a secondary deficiency of factor VIII which could be moderate to severe depending upon the residual levels of VWF. This can lead to prolongation of aPTT. These features can lead to clinical confusion between VWD and hemophilia A in absence of complete work up especially type 2N which closely resembles it.[1-3]

Q8. How VWF and ADAMTS13 are linked and what happens If ADAMTS13 is deficient?

Ans: VWF is synthesized as a large pre-pro-VWF monomer composed of signal peptide (22aa), propeptide (741aa), and mature VWF protein (2050 aa). When the protein reaches the endoplasmic reticulum, the signal peptide is removed and the protein undergoes dimerization. As the protein passes to the Golgi apparatus glycosylation occurs, and the dimers undergo multimerization, increasing in size. The propeptide portion is cleaved by furin leaving a mature VWF molecule. Following cleavage, the mature VWF subunit is tightly coiled and packaged in the Weibel–Palade bodies.

The VWF is released from endothelial cells constitutively into the circulating plasma and the subendothelial matrix. In the plasma, these unusually high molecule large multimers of VWF have very high binding affinity to platelets which can consume platelets. These multimers are cleaved into smaller functional monomer units by a protease, ADAMTS13 (a disintegrin-like and metalloprotease with thrombospondin type 1 repeats, member 13), which is located on the endothelial cell surface. VWF monomer is the major circulating and functional form of VWF that binds platelets, collagen, and factor VIII.[6,8]

ADAMTS-13 deficiency may lead to persistence of high molecule multimers of VWF which bind platelets in circulation with high affinity, leading to formation of platelet thrombi which happens in thrombotic thrombocytopenic purpura (TTP).

Q9. Which type of VWD presents with thrombocytopenia and why?

Ans: Subtype 2B VWD can present with thrombocytopenia. This subtype accounts for about 5% of the cases of VWD and is inherited in an autosomal dominant mode. The causative mutation results in increased binding of the mutated VWF to the platelet GPIb receptor. This is referred to as a "gain-of-function" mutation and leads to spontaneous binding of VWF to platelets in the circulation leading to thrombocytopenia. This thrombocytopenia is secondary to increased binding of VWF to platelets leading to premature clearance.[1,5]

Interestingly, patients presenting with subtype 2B VWD demonstrate a rather vigorous agglutination response to low doses of ristocetin compared to normal individuals due to this gain of function mutation. Ristocetin-induced platelet aggregation (RIPA) has been used to differentiate between types 2A and 2B. Using an aggregometer, various concentrations of ristocetin are added, and platelet aggregation measured. Aggregation at concentrations < 0.5 mg/mL or less is consistent with increased VWF binding to GPIb. Pathogenic variants which cause type 2B are found in exon 28, so targeted genetic testing can also be used.

Q10. What is platelet-type VWD and what is its differential diagnosis?

Ans: A very close differential of type 2B VWD is platelet type VWD presenting with similar clinical and laboratory features. Platelet-type VWD is a GPIb gain-of-function platelet defect that causes hyperfunctional platelets and phenotypically mimics VWD with mucocutaneous bleeding, loss of higher VWF multimers, enhanced RIPA, and variable thrombocytopenia. It is critical to distinguish type 2B VWD from platelet-type VWD because platelet-type VWD is not responsive to VWF replacement therapy.[1-3]

The correct diagnosis can be established by:
- Specialized RIPA mixing tests that reconstitute separated patient blood components (plasma and platelets) with normal donor components (platelets and plasma) to determine if the gain-of-function RIPA abnormality is conferred by the patient's plasma (VWF) or platelets.
- Newer tests that use immobilized gain-of-function GPIb to measure VWF activity have also been reported to distinguish 2B VWD. However, these tests require specialty laboratories and are not widely available.
- The diagnosis of type 2B VWD can be made through genetic sequencing of VWF exon 28 which will identify the gain of function mutation in VWF.

Q11. What is the difference between VWF antigen levels and VWF activity levels? Which one should be assayed for diagnosing VWD?

Ans: A correct diagnosis and subclassification of VWD require both VWF antigen levels (which measures quantitative levels of VWF Ag in plasma) and VWF activity levels (which measures functional status of the available VWF in plasma with various binding proteins).

VWF: Ag levels—quantity of VWF protein (antigen) in the plasma, measured antigenically using ELISA or by LIA will establish the quantitative deficiency of VWF (subtype VWD 1 and 3) and should be performed even if the screening tests are normal in an individual in whom VWD is suspected. Normal ranges are determined by the individual laboratory. There are many preanalytical/analytical factors which may affect this level. Also, the quantitative levels are not true indicator of functional VWF in body.

VWF: Activity by GPIb binding assays are tests which measure the functional status of available VWF. These tests are used to determine how well VWF binds to GpIbα. The VWF:RCo assay is the most commonly used platelet binding assay and exploits the ristocetin-induced interaction between VWF and GPIbM, which results in platelet agglutination. Although widely available, the VWF:RCo assay is limited by poor reproducibility, high coefficient of variation, and low sensitivity at very low VWF levels.[1,3]

Ratio of VWF Activity to VWF Antigen

The VWF activity assay is a functional test that uses either the ristocetin cofactor assay or a monoclonal antibody that targets the region of the VWF molecule that binds to the glycoprotein Ib receptor as a measure of VWF activity. The VWF activity-to-antigen ratio helps distinguish quantitative versus qualitative deficiency of VWF (VWD type 1 vs. type 2). In type 1 VWD, there is a concordant decrease in both VWF activity and VWF antigen, leading to a ratio > 0.7. Type 2 VWD is characterized by a disproportionate reduction of VWF activity compared with VWF antigen levels, leading to a ratio < 0.7.[1,3]

Q12. What is the role of genetic testing in evaluation of VWD?

Ans: For most of the patients, phenotypic analysis yields sufficient information for VWD classification so that appropriate treatment can be started. However, certain circumstances, indicated below, may warrant additional genetic testing. This may help to clarify disease type, risk of disease inheritance, or to facilitate prenatal diagnosis.[2,4]

- Mild or moderate hemophilia A and 2N VWD can be challenging to discriminate, especially in the absence of a family history. The VWF:FVIIIB assay can discriminate between the two disorders, but is not widely available. Analysis of VWF exons 17–25 can identify missense VWF:FVIIIB mutations in patients that have type 2N VWD; individuals lacking these mutations should be investigated for sequence variation in the *F8* gene thereby differentiating the two disorders.
- Type 2B VWD and platelet type-VWD patients present with similar phenotypes and can be discriminated by plasma/platelet mixing studies or by genetic analysis. All 2B VWD mutations have been identified between amino acid residues 1266–1461 encoded by exon 28 of VWF whilst platelet type-VWD mutations affect either the beta hairpin or macroglycopeptide regions of GPIbα encoded by the central region of GP1BA exon 2. Discrimination using genetic analysis is straightforward and can help guide appropriate therapy.
- Prenatal diagnosis is occasionally requested by families with type 3 VWD, particularly where the parents already have one affected child. Mutation analysis of the index case can identify the familial mutation(s), which should be confirmed to be present in each parent and can subsequently be sought in a fetus using chorionic villus or amniocentesis samples. Both sequence and gene dosage analyses may be required to identify the two VWF mutations although mutations are not yet identified in all cases.
- For those patients where phenotypic analysis does not clarify VWD type, genetic analysis can be used to try and identify explanatory mutation(s), e.g., some patients with D3 domain missense mutations may have pleiotropic presentation.

CHAPTER 9: Von Willebrand Disease

Limitations of genetic testing—as with all testing, genetic testing is not without flaws. One drawback is the considerable variability seen in the *VWF* gene even within healthy cohorts. For type 1, the most common subtype, there is weak correlation between sequence variants and disease. A number of variants outside the VWF locus have also been implicated as modifiers of VWF levels including ABO blood group.

Q13. What are the challenges in the diagnosis of VWD ?

Ans: The challenges faced in the diagnosis of VWD include:
- Despite being the most common bleeding disorder, it is under recognized as the clinical symptoms can be heterogeneous.[5,7] Only a small percentage of patient receive a formal diagnosis, rest remain undetected.
- It is difficult to ascertain normal VWF levels/cut offs to call VWD, for populations as many factors affects its level.
- Low VWF levels does not proportionately cause symptoms—the diagnosis needs revision in long term to rule out transient causes.
- Confirmation of diagnosis requires a panel of tests—diagnostic approach is not standardized across the clinical practice.
- Limited availability and expertise of specialized laboratory testing is a big challenge.
- VWF levels/activity assays are affected by a number of preanalytical factors.
- Few subtypes require genetic testing to differentiate from close mimics.

Q14. What is acquired von Willebrand syndrome (AVWS)?

Ans: Acquired von Willebrand syndrome is the term used to describe an acquired loss of VWF function.[1-3] This acquired loss of VWF could be quantitative loss or functional impairment by various mechanism. Its exact incidence is unknown, but it has been associated with several disease states, including autoimmune diseases, hematologic malignancies, solid tumors, metallic heart valves, and high-vascular flow states, such as in patients with ventricular assist devices or receiving extracorporeal membrane oxygenation.

These patients do not have a positive family history of bleeding tendencies. Several mechanisms exist, including decreased production of VWF (e.g., in hypothyroidism), increased adsorption onto circulating cells (e.g., in chronic lymphocytic leukemia), increased antibody-mediated clearance (e.g., in lupus), high-flow states leading to increased circulatory clearance of VWF (e.g., in patients on left ventricular assist devices), formation of complexes with circulating proteins (e.g., in monoclonal gammopathies), and shear destruction (e.g., in aortic stenosis) which has been implicated in AVWS.

Heyde syndrome is a rare form of acquired von Willebrand syndrome consisting of a triad of aortic stenosis, recurrent gastrointestinal bleeding, and acquired VWF deficiency resulting from destruction of high-molecular-weight multimers of VWF under shear stress due to aortic stenosis.

REFERENCES

1. James PD, Connell NT, Ameer B, Di Paola J, Eikenboom J, Giraud N, et al. ASH ISTH NHF WFH 2021 guidelines on the diagnosis of von Willebrand disease. Blood Adv. 2021;5(1):280-300.
2. Weyand AC, Flood VH. Von Willebrand Disease: Current Status of Diagnosis and Management. Hematol Oncol Clin North Am. 2021;35(6):1085-101.

3. Roberts JC, Flood VH. Laboratory diagnosis of von Willebrand disease. Int J Lab Hematol. 2015;37:11-7.
4. Kaur V, Elghawy O, Deshpande S, Riley D. von Willebrand disease: A guide for the internist. Cleve Clin J Med. 2024;91(2):119-27.
5. Favaloro EJ, Pasalic L. Laboratory diagnosis of von Willebrand disease in the age of the new guidelines: considerations based on geography and resources. Res Pract Thromb Haemost. 2023;7(5):102143.
6. Ziemba YC, Abdulrehman J, Hollestelle MJ, Meijer P, Plumhoff E, Hsu P, et al. Diagnostic Testing for von Willebrand Disease: Trends and Insights from North American Laboratories over the Last Decade. Semin Thromb Hemost. 2022;48(6):700-10.
7. Salazar E, Long TA, Smock KJ, Wool GD, Rollins-Raval M, Chen D, et al. Analysis of College of American Pathologists von Willebrand Factor Proficiency Testing Program. Semin Thromb Hemost. 2022;48(6):690-9.
8. Hayward CP, Moffat KA, Graf L. Technological advances in diagnostic testing for von Willebrand disease: new approaches and challenges. Int J Lab Hematol. 2014;36(3):334-40.

10. Hemophilia

Kanwaljeet Kaur Chopra

Q1. What is hemophilia?

Ans: Hemophilia is an inherited disorder of coagulation. Hemophilia A and B, the common hemophilia are X-linked recessive disorders and therefore affects males. Females are carriers and are usually asymptomatic but rarely can suffer from mild hemophilia. The incidence of hemophilia A is 1/5,000 males and hemophilia B is 1/30,000 males.[1] Positive family history is documented only in two-thirds cases, whereas de novo mutations occur in one-third of cases and hence cannot be eliminated by genetic counseling and antenatal screening.

Q2. What are various types of hemophilia?

Ans: Hemophilia can be classified on the basis of various criteria as follows:

It is classified as hemophilia A, B, or C depending on the factor involved, i.e., VIII, IX, and XI, respectively. Hemophilia can be classified as inherited versus acquired depending upon the etiology of deficiency of factor VIII. On the basis of severity as it can be classified as mild, moderate, or severe.

Q3. How do you clinically differentiate between platelet and coagulation disorders?

Ans: When a patient presents with bleeding manifestations it is important to differentiate whether it is platelet or clotting system disorder **(Table 1)**. This further helps in determining the underlying cause and helps in management as well.

TABLE 1: Differences between platelet disorders and coagulation disorders.

Characteristics	Platelet disorders	Coagulation disorders
Site of bleeding	Skin, mucous membrane	Deep muscles, joints
Bleeding after minor cuts	Yes	No
Onset of bleed	Immediate post-trauma	Delayed
Type of skin bleed	Petechiae	Ecchymoses
Hemarthrosis	Absent	Present
History	Usually, acute	Chronic

Q4. A physician commonly sees patients with bleeding from nose or with menorrhagia. What factors decide whether to investigate for an underlying bleeding or clotting disorder?

Ans: Significant bleeding that requires further evaluation of an underlying bleeding disorder can be identified by any one of the following criteria:
- More than 1 site of bleeding.
- Single site but >3 episodes of bleeding on separate occasions, bleeding severe enough to require medical attention or transfusion.
- Family history of bleeding.
- Certain bleeding questionnaires such as pediatric bleeding questionnaire (PBQ) score. PBQ was developed for screening of von Willebrand disease.[2] Besides, the International Society on Thrombosis and Haemostasis Bleeding Assessment Tool (ISTH BAT) has questions pertaining to newborns and infancy.[3]

Q5. What is the clinical history of hemophilia patients?

Ans: The common clinical presentation is a male child or an older male with delayed and prolonged bleeding at the site of minor trauma. At birth there may be a history of prolonged umbilical cord bleeding or large cephalohematoma. In infancy and toddler stage, there is a history of frequent bruising and swelling of knee or ankle joints. There may also be hematoma formation after intramuscular vaccination, excessive bleeding during tooth eruption or postcircumcision. Mild hemophilia presents later.[4] Often there is positive family in males from the maternal side.

Q6. What is the pathophysiology of coagulation disorders?

Ans: A breach in the endothelium attracts the platelets to the site of injury to form a plug. However, this gives only a brief period of hemostasis as it is fragile. The activation of coagulation cascade results ultimately in conversion of fibrinogen to fibrin monomer which polymerizes to give rise to fibrin strands which strengthens the platelet plug. The intrinsic pathway is activated when the circulating factor XII comes in contact with endothelial collagen and it involves factors XII, XI, IX, and VIII. The extrinsic pathway of coagulation is triggered by external trauma which causes release of tissue factor from endothelial cells. It interacts with small amounts of circulating factor VIIa.[5] The complex activates factor X–Xa. When any coagulation factor is decreased, the coagulation cascade is affected resulting in decreased formation of fibrin polymer. The platelet plug, which is not stabilized by fibrin, is easily dislodged leading to typical delayed and prolonged bleeding.

Q7. How is hemophilia diagnosed?

Ans: The diagnosis of any bleeding disorder requires evaluation of platelet count and examination of peripheral smear to confirm platelet count and morphology. Prothrombin time (PT) APTT if prolonged raise suspicion of a coagulation disorder. PT measures extrinsic clotting system and the common pathway. PT is prolonged in deficiencies of plasma factors VII, X, V, II, and fibrinogen, and inhibitors of these factors. Prolongation of the PT requires factor levels < 30% or until fibrinogen is <100 mg/dL. However, if APTT only is prolonged then low levels of prekallikrein, kininogen, factor XII, XI, IX, and VIII, fibrinogen, prothrombin, and factor X and V levels or inhibitors may be the underlying cause.[6]

If PT is normal and APTT is prolonged, then we should suspect hemophilia in a male child with bleeding diathesis.[6] The APTT is usually not affected until the amount of factor VIII is <30%.[7] The reference range of APTT is 20–35 seconds for children and adults but longer (30–54 seconds) in term infants and even longer in premature infants.[8]

The following precautions need to be taken while doing tests for clotting disorders.[9] Improper sample collection is one of the most common reasons for abnormal coagulation test.

- Clean venous puncture with free flow thus avoiding release of tissue factor without air bubbles and without contamination by tissue fluids.
- Proper proportion of anticoagulant to blood, hence, fills the tube up to mark.
- Rapid processing and platelet poor plasma separation and storage. It should contain < 10,000 platelets/μL.
- Avoid testing in stressful situations such as pregnancy, vigorous exercise, and various drugs as they may affect the results.
- Drawing of samples from catheter often results in sample contamination with intravenous fluids or heparin-flush which may give spuriously abnormal values.
- Samples should be tested within 2 hours of collection if maintained at room temperature or within 4 hours if kept in cold.
- Plasma samples must be frozen if not tested within this time frame. When they are to be analyzed, frozen samples should be rapidly thawed at 37°C and tested immediately.

If APTT is prolonged, then the next step in making a definitive diagnosis is mixing study. The patient's plasma is mixed in 1:1 ratio with normal pooled plasma which is assumed to have 100% clotting factor. The mix is incubated at 37°C for 1–2 hours. This is followed by a repetition of APTT test. If APTT corrects then factor deficiency is likely and if it does not correct, then likely inhibitors are present. In the presence of suspected inhibitors, the sample is tested for lupus anticoagulant.

In the absence of lupus anticoagulant test, assay of VIII and IX level are done.

Simultaneous testing for von Willebrand antigen (vWAg) and activity is done to rule out von Willebrand disease (vWD). It is the most common coagulation disorder affecting 1% of the population. It is an autosomal dominant disorder. However, it presents commonly in females as menorrhagia which is the most common presenting symptoms in vWD.

Q8. How is the severity of hemophilia graded?

Ans: The hemophilia can be classified as mild, moderate, and severe **(Table 2)**.[10]

TABLE 2: Classification of severity of hemophilia.

Severity	Clotting factor level	Bleeding episode
Severe	<1%	Spontaneous bleed into muscles and joints
Moderate	1–5%	Occasional spontaneous bleed or after surgery
Mild	5–40%	Bleeding following major surgery

Q9. How inherited hemophilia is different from acquired hemophilia?

Ans: There are many features which can help in differentiating acquired from inherited hemophilia **(Table 3)**. This is important from management point of view.

TABLE 3: Characteristics of inherited and acquired hemophilia.

Clinical characteristics	Inherited defects (hemophilia, von Willebrand disease)	Acquired defects (sepsis, leukemia)
Age of onset	• Early, usually infancy • Umbilical stump • Cephalhematoma • Circumcision • Tooth eruption/fall	Variable, late age
Family history	Often present	Absent
Clinical setting	Well looking	Unwell

Q10. How are factor assays done?

Ans: The factors are assayed by two methods, one is bioassay of clotting activity and another is assessment of cross reacting material (CRM) by ELISA. Bioassay correlates better with disease activity than CRM assay. There are two bioassays available: (1) One-stage clotting assay, (2) two-stage chromogenic clotting assay.
- One-stage assay is based on measuring APTT and estimation factor level from the graph based on APTT.
- Two-stage assay involves two steps.[11] First step involves activation of X to Xa and this step is accelerated by FVIIIa. FXa hydrolyses an FXa-specific chromogenic substrate, resulting in the release of the chromophoric group para-nitro aniline (pNA). The extinction can be read in a photometer at 405 nm and is directly proportional to the FVIII concentration. The assay is not influenced by the presence of lupus anticoagulants and thus can be used to distinguish between FVIII inhibitors and lupus anticoagulants in patients with acquired deficiency of FVIII.[12] Additionally, it has a lower analytical variation and is more accurate especially in the lower range. It is recommended to use both the one-stage FVIII assay and the chromogenic FVIII:C assay in the initial diagnostic workup. Both assays should be performed even if the result of one of the two assays shows FVIII activity within the normal range.

For laboratory investigation of patients being assessed due to clinical suspicion of hemophilia B, the use of the one-stage FIX assay in the initial diagnostic workup is required.

Factor assay helps in determining diagnosis and identifying severity of disease. Besides factor VIII assay, von Willebrand factor (vWF) antigen, and activity are also tested as vWF acts as chaperone to factor VIII and any deficiency in vWF leads to low factor VIII level.

Q11. How carriers of hemophilia are identified?

Ans: Hemophilia carriers can be "At risk" or "Obligate" carriers. At risk carriers are diagnosed by using mutation studies of the proband case[13,14] whereas obligate carriers are diagnosed clinically. Obligate carriers are either of the following:
- Daughters of a person with hemophilia.
- Mothers of one son with hemophilia and who have at least one other family member with hemophilia.
- Mothers of one son with hemophilia and who have a family member who is a known carrier of the hemophilia gene.
- Mothers of two or more sons with hemophilia.

Identifying a carrier requires assessment of ratio of factor VIII:C and vWAg. If the ratio is <0.81 then the sensitivity and specificity of the test for identifying a carrier is 82.8% and 96.6%, respectively.[14]

All female carriers in the family should get their factor level tested specially prior to invasive procedure as they can have levels ranging from normal to borderline (40–60%). Those with borderline levels can have increased bleeding tendency, especially during pregnancy, invasive procedures, and trauma.[15] They might also require factor replacement during such conditions. Menorrhagia may be noted in such carriers, which may respond to antifibrinolytics or oral contraceptives.

Q12. How are rare inherited factor deficiencies diagnosed?

Ans: Factors deficiencies other than factors FVIII, FIX, and vWF are classified as rare coagulation factor disorders. Rare coagulation factor (deficiencies) disorders include fibrinogen, FII, FV (parahemophilia), FV+FVIII, FVII, FX, FXI, and FXIII deficiencies.[16] These disorders are largely inherited as autosomal recessive. As these are not well characterized clinically in comparison to common bleeding disorders, they do not have well-established treatment strategies. High index of suspicion is required to diagnose rare coagulation disorders. Rare factor deficiencies are suspected clinically and using baseline coagulation profile. They are diagnosed by factor assays and confirmed by mutation studies.[14]

Q13. What are the acquired causes of hemophilia?

Ans: Acquired hemophilia results from the development of antibodies [mostly of the immunoglobulin (Ig)G1 and IgG4 subclasses] directed against various clotting factors.[17] Numerous conditions that have been associated with acquired inhibitors to FVIII.[18,19]
- Frequent blood transfusions (as in hemolytic anemias)
- Pregnancy
- Autoimmune disorders
- Inflammatory bowel disease
- Dermatologic disorders, e.g., psoriasis, pemphigus
- Respiratory diseases, e.g., asthma
- Diabetes mellitus
- Infections
- Malignancies
- Rarely, FVIII antibodies arise as an idiosyncratic reaction to medications,[19] e.g., Penicillin and its derivatives, sulfonamides, phenytoin, chloramphenicol, methyldopa, and interferon-alpha. However, in approximately 50% of cases, no underlying or precipitating factor is found.[14]

Q14. What is the management of pain in a hemophilia patient?

Ans: Management of hemophilia patient involves:
- Protection/pain control using either or combination of paracetamol, tramadol, codeine, and morphine.[15]
- Rest of limb initially and as pain subsides. Optimal loading of the muscles and joints to prevent disuse atrophy.

- Ice application/immobilization—data from sports medicine and experimental studies have shown that cryotherapy help to decrease edema by decreasing leukocyte endothelial interactions and edema. Ice must be applied over a wet towel intermittently for periods of 10 minutes to achieve a 10-15°C lowering of temperature in the deeper tissues. A dose of FVIII or factor IX (10 U/kg) may be adequate to control pain and bleeding in most patients.[20]
  - Compression
  - Elevation

Q15. What products can be used when coagulation disorder is suspected and diagnosis is not confirmed?

Ans: Till the diagnosis of a specific factor deficiency is confirmed we can use fresh frozen plasma (FFP) or cryoprecipitate **(Table 4)**. Other pharmacological options include tranexamic acid and epsilon aminocaproic acid.[20]

TABLE 4: Features of fresh frozen plasma (FFP) and cryoprecipitate.

Component	FFP	Cryoprecipitate
Volume required	150–220 mL	15–20 mL
Content	Normal levels of stable factors	Factor I, VIII, XIII, vWF
Factor VIII	1 mL = 1U	1 mL = 3–5 IU
Factor IX	Present	Absent

Q16. How to dose the factor replacement?

Ans: Dose of factor VIII (IU) = % Desired FVIII × body weight (kg) × 0.5

Dose of factor IX (IU) = % Desired FIX × body weight (kg) This dose is given stat and is followed by half the dose at 12 hourly intervals as required, as the biological half-life of factor VIII is 8–12 hours, and at 24 hourly for factor IX as its half-life is 18–24 hours. The factors are given by slow intravenous bolus after reconstitution of lyophilized powder. Because recovery of recombinant factor IX activity is less than that of therapeutic plasma-derived factor IX, 1.2–1.5 times the dose should be administered if using recombinant factor IX.

Q17. What is the role of factor prophylaxis in hemophilia A and B?

Ans: The concept of factor prophylaxis was given by Inge Marie Nilsson.[21] It was observed that people with moderate hemophilia seldom experience spontaneous bleeding. It converts a person with severe hemophilia to a phenotype of moderate or mild hemophilia by maintaining factor levels above 1 IU/dL (1%).
- Primary prophylaxis—after first joint bleed, usually started at <3 years age.
- Secondary prophylaxis—after two or more bleeds, but before joint damage gets established, usually > 3 years age.
- Tertiary prophylaxis—after the setting of joint disease.

Doses:
- Doses of factors VIII and IX for various types of prophylaxis.
- Doses for prophylaxis have been studied such as Malmo protocol (25–40 IU/kg/dose) and Utrecht protocol (15–30 IU/kg/dose) **(Table 5)**.[21,22]

TABLE 5: Various protocols for hemophilia treatment.

	Malmo protocol	Utrecht protocol	Low dose protocol
Hemophilia A	25–40 IU/kg/dose three times a week	15–25 IU/kg/dose three times a week	10–15 IU/kg/dose 2–3 times per week
Hemophilia B	25–40 IU/kg/dose twice a week	15–25 IU/kg/dose twice a week	10–15 IU/kg/dose twice a week

Q18. What are extended half-life (EHL) factors?

Ans: A factor molecule can be fused with another moiety with extended half-life. Various moieties used for this purpose include polyethylene glycol, Fc portion of immunoglobulin G (IgG), and recombinant human albumin. PEGylation increases the half-life by reducing proteolytic cleavage and inhibiting receptor mediated clearance. Fusion with the Fc receptor helps to salvage and recycle factor proteins.

Q19. What are nonfactor therapies?

Ans: Treatment of hemophilia using drugs other than factor VIII or IX. There are two types of nonfactor therapies:[23]
- *Mimetics*—the drugs which mimic the action of factor VIII, e.g., emicizumab and Mim8 (denecimig).
- *Rebalancing agents*—the drugs which decrease the inhibitors of coagulation, e.g., fitusiran, concizumab, and marstacimab.

Q20. What is the mechanism of action of emicizumab? What makes it popular with patients?

Ans: Emicizumab is a factor VIII mimetic. It is a bispecific antibody that bridges FIXa and FX to allow the clotting cascade to continue. It does not replace the missing factor. There are no peak and trough curves of protection. Biggest advantage is that it can be administered subcutaneously in a dose of 1.5 mg/kg/week or 3 mg/kg/fortnightly or 6 mg/kg/4 weekly.[24,25] It is useful in the presence of inhibitors of factor VIII. However, it is not useful for breakthrough bleeding as its mean onset of action is 1.6±1 days.[26]

Q21. What are the various complications of hemophilia?

Ans: Various complications of hemophilia are as follows:
- *Life-threatening bleeds:* Intracranial bleed, intraperitoneal hemorrhage, musculoskeletal complications—chronic hemophilic arthropathy and osteoporosis, fractures, pseudotumor, compartment syndromes.
- *Tranfusion transmitted infection:* Human immunodeficiency virus (HIV)/hepatitis B surface antigen (HBsAg)/hepatitis C virus (HCV).
- Inhibitor formation

Q22. What is a target joint?

Ans: Target joint is a particular joint in which three or more spontaneous bleeds have occurred within a consecutive 6-month period. Knees and ankles are commonly affected. Flexion is usually the most comfortable position. The joint is boggy, with decreased range of motion and muscle wasting. There may be some warmth and pain.

Q23. What is annual joint bleed rate/annual bleed rate (ABR)?

Ans: The total number of spontaneous bleeds in any joint in last 1 year is termed as annual joint bleed rate (AJBR). Similarly, the number of spontaneous bleeds anywhere in muscle or joints in last 1 year is termed (ABR). Target is to keep the number of bleeds < 3 per year.

Q24. What is the role of self-care in hemophilia?

Ans: Self-management improves short-term and long-term outcomes.
Key components of self-management in hemophilia include:
- Bleed recognition, timely reporting aura associated with acute bleed may help prevent joint damage.
- Record keeping of bleeds and treatment.
- Self-administration of hemostasis products.
- Self-care (i.e., nutrition and physical fitness) and medicines management (i.e., record-keeping, treatment routines, maintenance of adequate treatment supply, proper storage, reconstitution, and administration of treatment products, compliance).
- Pain management
- Risk management

A hemophilia patient should always carry an identity card containing information about his diagnosis, severity, prophylaxis regimen, inhibitor status, and emergency contact details.

Q25. What are the causes of inhibitor development in hemophilia?

Ans: Inhibitors in hemophilia are neutralizing IgG alloantibodies to exogenous FVIII or FIX. A level of 0.6% Bethesda unit is considered significant. Prevalence of inhibitors in severe hemophilia A is about 30% in contrast to mild-to-moderate hemophilia A (3–13%). It is less common in severe hemophilia B (2%).[27] Inhibitors develop from a multicausal immune response involving both genetic (unmodifiable) and environmental (modifiable) factors. *F8* gene mutations are the most important genetic risk factor, with null mutations being associated with the highest risk of inhibitor development.[28] Regular factor prophylaxis decreases the risk of inhibitors. Factors that increase the risk of inhibitors include African race, history of inhibitors in family, severity of disease, and presence of high-risk genotype.

Q26. What is Bethesda assay?

Ans: It is an assay for inhibitor detection in hemophilia patient. It is usually suspected when a patient does not respond to usual doses of factor supplementation. Positive inhibitor is a Bethesda titer of >0.6 BU for FVIII and ≥0.3 BU for FIX respectively.[29,30]
- A low-responding inhibitor is <5.0 BU, with less risk of anamnestic response after rechallenge and tends to be transient (<6 months).
- High-responding inhibitor is ≥5.0 BU and tend to be persistent and may fall. However, they increase 3–5 days after rechallenge with factors (anamnestic response).

Q27. When should a patient be checked for inhibitors?

Ans: One should look for inhibitors in following situations:[31]
- After initial factor exposure with 5th–20th dose.
- Suboptimal clinical and laboratory response.

- Before and after elective surgical procedure.
- Once or twice yearly even when not suspected clinically (especially in high-risk patients).
- Positive family history of inhibitor.
- 2–4 weeks after intensive treatment (daily exposure for > 5 days).
- If a patient develops features of anaphylaxis or nephrotic syndrome specially in hemophilia B.
- Before and after switch of type of factor concentrate.

Q28. How will you manage acute bleed in patients with hemophilia with inhibitors?

Ans: In case of hemophilia A with inhibitors, acute bleed is managed as follows:[31]
- *For low-responding inhibitors:* FVIII clotting factor concentrates.
- *For high-responding inhibitors:* Bypassing agents, i.e., recombinant FVII, activated prothrombin complex concentrate (aPCC), or factor eight inhibitor bypassing activity (FEIBA).

In case of hemophilia B with inhibitors, acute bleed is managed as follows:
- *If low-responding FIX inhibitors:* FIX is given to treat acute bleeds as long as there is no allergic reaction to FIX.
- *High responding inhibitors:* Recombinant FVII preferred as aPCC has factor IX—hence risk of anaphylaxis.

Q29. What prophylaxis is used in hemophilia patients with inhibitors?

Ans: In patients with hemophilia A and low-responding inhibitors, immune tolerance induction[31] (ITI) with vWF containing FVIII alone or in combination with emicizumab/rituximab is indicated. If ITI fails, then the option is emicizumab. For those with hemophilia A and high-responding inhibitors the drug available is emicizumab. Emicizumab is a bispecific antibody binding both the enzyme factor IXa and the substrate factor X, thereby mimicking the actions of factor VIII.

In patients with hemophilia B with inhibitors, ITI can result in anaphylaxis, so immunosuppression is indicated as emicizumab is ineffective.

Q30. What are various disorders that can result in acquired causes of bleeding/coagulation that may affect hemostasis?

Ans: The following acquired disorders can result in bleeding/coagulation:[32]
- Hepatic disorders and malabsorption syndrome may be associated with vitamin K dependent coagulation factors deficiencies.
- *Renal disease:* Uremia can interfere with platelet function. Low-molecular-weight coagulation proteins (factors IX and XI) are lost through the kidney in children with nephrotic syndrome.
- Cyanotic congenital heart disease with polycythemia may have thrombocytopenia and hypofibrinogenemia with risk of bleeding and/or thrombosis.
- *Infections:* Meningococcemia and other infections can result in disseminated intravascular coagulation (DIC).
- Aspirin and other nonsteroidal anti-inflammatory agents affect platelet aggregation.
- Prolonged use of antibiotics can lead to decreased levels of vitamin K leading to decreased production of liver dependent coagulation factors.

CASE STUDY

A 6-year-old male child presented with swelling, pain, and restriction of right knee joint. He has history of multiple episodes of ecchymotic patches following trivial trauma. The maternal uncle had similar complaints.

His platelet counts were 2.6×10^9/L, PT 13 seconds, and APTT 70 seconds.
(a) How will you investigate this child further?
(b) How will you manage him till the diagnosis is confirmed?
(c) How will you treat him if the diagnosis is confirmed as hemophilia A or B?

Ans: On mixing study correction of APTT with pooled plasma was seen at 0, 1, and 2 hours, suggesting that there is factor deficiency and not inhibitors.

FVIII levels were found to be: <1% (severe hemophilia A), whereas factor IX levels were 86% (range 50–150%). The vWF: Ag and function tests were normal.

Till we have the final diagnosis FFP can be used to manage the joint bleed as it has both factors VIII and IX. Once the diagnosis is confirmed factor VIII or IX as per the diagnosis can be used. The family should be educated about the disease and need for lifelong prophylaxis with factor VIII.

REFERENCES

1. Mannucci PM, Tuddenham EG. The hemophilias–from royal genes to gene therapy. N Engl J Med. 2001;344(23):1773-9.
2. Bowman M, Riddel J, Rand ML, Tosetto A, Silva M, James PD. Evaluation of the diagnostic utility for von Willebrand disease of a pediatric bleeding questionnaire. J Thromb Haemost. 2009;7(8):1418-21.
3. Elbatarny M, Mollah S, Grabell J, Bae S, Deforest M, Tuttle A, et al. Normal range of bleeding scores for the ISTH-BAT: adult and pediatric data from the merging project. Haemophilia. 2014;20(6):831-5.
4. Aronstam A, Rainsford SG, Painter MJ. Patterns of bleeding in adolescents with severe haemophilia A. Br Med J. 1979;1(6161):469-70.
5. Chaudhry R, Usama SM, Babiker HM. Physiology, Coagulation Pathways. [Updated 2023 Aug 28]. In: StatPearls [Internet]. Treasure Island (FL): StatPearls Publishing; 2025 Jan. Available from: https://www.ncbi.nlm.nih.gov/books/NBK482253.
6. Kamal AH, Tefferi A, Pruthi RK. How to interpret and pursue an abnormal prothrombin time, activated partial thromboplastin time, and bleeding time in adults. Mayo Clin Proc. 2007;82(7):864-73.
7. Margaret C Mudge. Hemostasis, Surgical Bleeding, and Transfusion, Editor(s): Jörg A. Auer, John A. Stick. Equine Surgery (Fourth Edition), W.B. Saunders, 2012;35-47.
8. Davenport P and Sola-Visner M. Hemostatic Challenges in Neonates. Front Pediatr. 2021;9:627715.
9. Lippi G, Salvagno GL, Montagnana M, Lima-Oliveira G, Guidi GC, Favaloro EJ. Quality standards for sample collection in coagulation testing. Semin hromb Hemost. 2012;38(6):565-75.
10. White GC, Rosendaal F, Aledort LM, Lusher JM, Rothschild C, Ingerslev J; Factor VIII and Factor IX Subcommittee. Definitions in hemophilia: recommendation of the Scientific Subcommittee on Factor VIII and Factor IX of the Scientific and Standardization Committee of the International Society on thrombosis and Haemostasis. Thromb Haemost. 2001;85(3):560.
11. Verbruggen B, Meijer P, Nováková I, Van Heerde W. Diagnosis of factor VIII deficiency. Haemophilia. 2008;14(Suppl 3):76-82.
12. Blanco AN, Alcira Peirano A, Grosso SH, Gennari LC, Pérez Bianco R, Lazzari MA. A chromogenic substrate method for detecting and titrating anti-factor VIII antibodies in the presence of lupus anticoagulant. Haematologica. 2002;87(3):271-8.
13. Shetty S, Colah R, Gorakshakar A, Bhide A. Prenatal diagnosis of Hemophilia—A preliminary report. Nat Med J India. 1998;11(5):218 9.

14. Mohanty D, Shetty S, Ghosh K, Pathare A. Comparison of conventional coagulation parameters with DNA analysis in carrier detection in Indian hemophilia A families. Proceedings of the Sixteenth Congress of the International Society on Thrombosis and Haemostasis; 1997:979.
15. Paroskie A, Gailani D, DeBaun MR, Sidonio RF Jr. A cross-sectional study of bleeding phenotype in haemophilia A carriers. Br J Haematol. 2015;170(2):223-8.
16. Sharma SK, Kumar S, Seth T, Mishra P, Agrawal N, Singh G, et al. Clinical profile of patients with rare inherited coagulation disorders: a retrospective analysis of 67 patients from northern India. Mediterr J Hematol Infect Dis. 2012;4(1):e2012057.
17. Patrick Ellsworth, Sheh-Li Chen, Lee Ann Jones, Alice D Ma, Nigel S. Key, Acquired hemophilia A: a narrative review and management approach in the emicizumab era. Journal of Thrombosis and Haemostasis. 2025;23(3):824-35.
18. Lehoczki A, Fekete M, Mikala G, Bodó I. Acquired hemophilia A as a disease of the elderly: A comprehensive review of epidemiology, pathogenesis, and novel therapy. Geroscience. 2025;47(1):503-14.
19. Franchini M, Capra F, Nicolini N, Veneri D, Manzato F, Baudo F, et al. Drug-induced anti-factor VIII antibodies: a systematic review. Med Sci Monit. 2007;13(4):RA55-61.
20. Srivastava A, Santagostino E, Dougall A, Kitchen S, Sutherland M, Pipe SW, et al. WFH Guidelines for the Management of Hemophilia, 3rd edition. Haemophilia. 2020;26(Suppl 6):1-158.
21. Blanchette VS. Prophylaxis in the haemophilia population. Haemophilia. 2010;16(Suppl 5):181-8.
22. Srivastava, A. Dose and response in haemophilia—Optimization of factor replacement therapy. Br J Haematol. 2004;127(1):12-25.
23. Young G. Nonfactor therapies for hemophilia. Hemasphere. 2023;7(6):e911.
24. Mahlangu J, Oldenburg J, Paz-Priel I, Negrier C, Niggli M, Mancuso CE, et al. Emicizumab prophylaxis in patients who have hemophilia A without inhibitors. N Engl J Med. 2018;379:811-22.
25. Jimenez-Yuste V, Shima M, Fukutake K. Emicizumab subcutaneous dosing every 4 weeks for the management of hemophilia A: preliminary data from the pharmacokinetic run-in cohort of a multicenter, open-label, phase 3 study (HAVEN 4). Blood. 2017;130(Suppl 1):86.
26. Parisi K, Kumar A. Emicizumab. [Updated 2023 Jul 4]. In: StatPearls [Internet]. Treasure Island (FL): StatPearls Publishing; 2025 Jan. Available from: https://www.ncbi.nlm.nih.gov/books/NBK559180/
27. Meeks SL, Batsuli G. Hemophilia and inhibitors: current treatment options and potential new therapeutic approaches. Hematology Am Soc Hematol Educ Program. 2016;2(1):657-62.
28. Garagiola I, Palla R, Peyvandi F. Risk factors for inhibitor development in severe hemophilia a. Thromb Res. 2018;168:20-7.
29. Blanchette VS, Key NS, Ljung LR, Manco-Johnson MJ, van den Berg HM, Srivastava A, et al. Definitions in hemophilia: communication from the SSC of the ISTH. J Thromb Haemost. 2014;12(11):1935-9.
30. Miller CH. Laboratory testing for factor VIII and IX inhibitors in haemophilia: A review. Haemophilia. 2018;24(2):186-97.
31. Ragni MV, Berntorp E, Carcao M. Inhibitors to clotting factors. WFH guidelines for management of Hemophilia. 3rd edition.
32. Rydz Nt, James PD. Why Is My Patient Bleeding Or Bruising? Hematol Oncol Clin North Am. 2012;26(2):321-44, viii.

11
Thrombotic Thrombocytopenic Purpura

Monica Sharma

Q1. What is the pathophysiology of thrombotic thrombocytopenic purpura?

Ans: The pathophysiology of thrombotic thrombocytopenic purpura (TTP) is a severe deficiency of the activity of a disintegrin and metalloproteinase with thrombospondin motifs 13 (ADAMTS13), the protease that cleaves von Willebrand factor (vWF) multimeric strings.[1] Ultra-large vWF strings remain uncleaved after endothelial cell secretion and anchorage, bind to platelets, and form microthrombi. Mechanical fragmentation of erythrocytes during flow through partially occluded, high-shear small vessels cause a microangiopathic hemolytic anemia (MAHA). Median hemoglobin levels on admission are typically 8–10 g/dL. The combination of hemolysis and tissue ischemia produces elevated lactate dehydrogenase (LDH) values. Consumption of platelets in platelet-rich thrombi results in thrombocytopenia, with a median platelet count typically $10–30 \times 10^9$/L at presentation.

Q2. What is PLASMIC score?

Ans: ADAMTS13 activity testing typically requires prolonged turnaround times and might be unavailable in resource-poor settings, hence a method is needed to rapidly assess the likelihood of severe ADAMTS13 deficiency.

The word PLASMIC uses the seven features of the score [platelets, lysis, active cancer, stem cell or solid organ transplant, mean corpuscular volume (MCV), prothrombin time and international normalized ratio (PT-INR), and creatinine]. It is a simple, validated clinical scoring system, which can assist in the early diagnosis of TTP by identifying cases with a high probability of having severe ADAMTS13 deficiency.[2] The PLASMIC score—stratifies patients with thrombotic microangiopathy according to the severity of ADAMTS13 deficiency. Its use, together with clinical assessment, may facilitate treatment decisions in patients for whom timely results of ADAMTS13 activity testing are unavailable. PLASMIC score was designed for adult populations with no comorbid conditions (e.g., pregnancy, cancer, sepsis, organ/tissue transplantation, etc.), which may not be reliable in assessing children and patients with other comorbidities.

Q3. What is the difference between primary and secondary TTP?

Ans: Primary or congenital or hereditary TTP (Upshaw–Schulman syndrome) is the result of homozygous or compound heterozygous mutations in ADAMTS13, whereas acquired or secondary or idiopathic TTP (iTTP) is usually idiopathic, or associated with autoimmune disease, pregnancy, drugs, or infection, particularly human immunodeficiency virus (HIV) and is caused by circulating anti-ADAMTS13 autoantibodies, which inhibit the enzyme or increase its clearance. In contrast to patients with secondary TTP or hemolytic uremic syndrome (HUS), those with primary TTP have a higher refractory and relapse rate, but are also more likely to achieve remission and survive.

Q4. How is laboratory diagnosis of TTP made?

Ans: In addition to the MAHA and consumption thrombocytopenia, classical parameters for hemolysis show a high reticulocyte count, absent serum haptoglobin concentration, and an elevated LDH level, a marker for tissue damage.

The presence of schistocytes on the blood smear (helmet cells; small, irregular triangular, or crescent-shaped cells; pointed projections; and lack of central pallor) with a confident threshold value of 1% is the morphological hallmark of the disease. Coombs' test is negative. These standard investigations are not specific for TTP and may be present in the miscellaneous differential diagnosis for TTP, they should be complemented by assays for ADAMTS13 to confirm the diagnosis. Screening for ADAMTS13 activity is the first test to be performed.[3] If ADAMTS13 activity is <10%, TTP diagnosis is confirmed.

Subsequent investigations are aimed at documenting the mechanism for ADAMTS13 severe deficiency. These include assays for ADAMTS13 autoantibodies, searching for an ADAMTS13 inhibitor, and in selected cases, *ADAMTS13* gene sequencing.

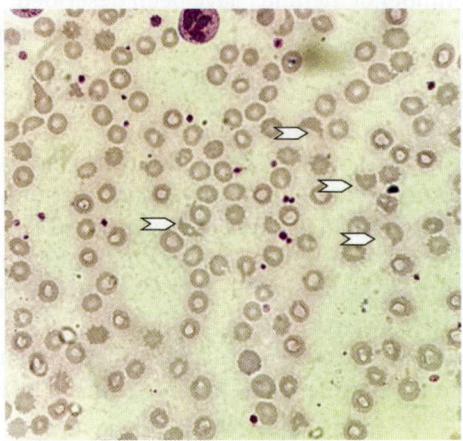

FIG. 1: Peripheral smear (100×): Schistocytes—fragmented RBCs (arrowhead).
Courtesy: Dr Abhishek Purohit.

Q5. What is ADAMTS13?

Ans: ADAMTS13 is a metalloproteinase—a disintegrin with a thrombospondin type 1 motif, member 13, also known as vWF protease, its main function is to cleave vWF into smaller multimers, thus modulating vWF level and activity.

ADAMTS13 has 14 domains and is synthesized principally in the liver and cleaves vWF at Tyr1605-Met1606 within the A2 domain. The ADAMTS13 cleavage site of vWF is exposed under conditions of shear stress facilitating clearance of high molecular weight vWF multimers, which would otherwise spontaneously bind platelets and cause widespread microthrombi.[4,5]

Q6. How is ADAMTS13 level assayed and what is the cutoff for diagnosis of TTP?

Ans: ADAMTS13 assays are essential in confirming the diagnosis of TTP, samples should be taken prior to treatment but treatment should not be delayed due to pending results.

ADAMTS13 activity <10 IU/dL ± presence of immunoglobulin (Ig)G antibodies or an inhibitor, confirms the diagnosis of TTP. ADAMTS13 activity <10 IU/dL has a high sensitivity (97%) and specificity (100%) in distinguishing TTP from other thrombotic microangiopathies (TMAs). Decreased ADAMTS13 activity can be seen in various conditions including metastatic cancer, sepsis, disseminated intravascular coagulation (DIC), liver disease, and pregnancy.

In general, measurement of ADAMTS13 activity is considered more clinically useful than assays, which measure only the amount of ADAMTS13 present, i.e., ADAMTS13 antigen.[6,7]

- *ADAMTS13 antigen assays*—a number of immunoassays employing varying principles, exist for the measurement of ADAMTS13 antigen but they vary in their ability to detect full-length, mutant, and truncated forms of ADAMTS13.

    ADAMTS13 antigen may be normal in TTP due to the presence of immune complexes, or reduced due to accelerated clearance. Assays of ADAMTS13 antigen are, therefore, generally unhelpful in the absence of a functional ADAMTS13 assay.

- *ADAMTS13 activity assays*—involve the detection of cleavage of products either of a full-length vWF molecule or a vWF fragment that encompasses the ADAMTS13 cleavage site (Tyr1605-Met1606). A number of methods have been described.
    - Sodium dodecyl sulfate–polyacrylamide gel electrophoresis (SDS-PAGE) and western blotting
    - Collagen binding assays
    - Fluorescence resonance energy transfer (FRET) assay
    - Chromogenic enzyme-linked immunoassays (ELISA) activity assay
    - *Anti-ADAMTS13 autoantibody (inhibitor) assays*—two types of anti-ADAMTS13 antibodies have been reported in patients with acquired TTP:
        - *Neutralizing antibodies* (two-thirds of cases) that inhibit the action of ADAMTS13. These are classically detected by performing a 1:1 mix of test:normal plasma and then measuring ADAMTS13 activity.
        - *Non-neutralizing antibodies* (one-third of cases) that bind and accelerate the clearance of ADAMTS13 from the plasma. These can be detected by western blotting but more conveniently by ELISA.

A chromogenic assay for the determination of antibodies directed against ADAMTS13 is available.

The ELISA assays for the detection of anti-ADAMTS13 antibodies have been developed and which can detect both inhibitory and noninhibitory antibodies.

Bethesda assay for the detection of inhibitory antibodies in immune-mediated TTP. A Bethesda assay for quantifying inhibitory antibodies to ADAMTS13. The assay can only detect anti-ADAMTS13 antibodies that functionally inhibit ADAMTS13.

Q7. What is the significance of ADAMTS13 functional inhibitor assay and anti-ADAMTS13 autoantibody assay?

Ans: ADAMTS13 functional inhibitor assay measures the residual activity in a mixture of patient plasma and normal plasma to detect ADAMTS13 neutralizing autoantibodies that inhibit the function of ADAMTS13 whereas, anti-ADAMTS13 autoantibody assay detects non-neutralizing antibodies which do not affect the function but increase the clearance of anti-ADAMTS13.

Q8. What diseases are associated with TTP?

Ans: The following diseases are associated with TTP:
- Idiopathic
- Familial
- Infection (*Escherichia coli* O157:H7, HIV)
- Autoimmune disorders (systemic lupus erythematosus)
- Pregnancy and postpartum period
- Malignancy
- Chemotherapy (mitomycin, cisplatin, and gemcitabine)
- Drugs (ticlopidine, clopidogrel, quinidine, and cyclosporine)
- Bone marrow transplantation (total body irradiation, cyclophosphamide)

Q9. How immune-mediated TTP is distinguished from congenital TTP?

Ans: More than 95% of all TTP cases are idiopathic TTP, whereas congenital TTP accounts for <5% of cases. Congenital TTP, also known as Upshaw–Schulman syndrome, is defined by ADAMTS13 activity <10 IU/dL, no anti-ADAMTS13 autoantibodies and is due to homozygous or compound heterozygous mutations in *ADAMTS13* gene, whereas acquired TTP is an autoimmune disorder caused by circulating anti-ADAMTS13 autoantibodies, which inhibit the enzyme or increase its clearance.[8]

Q10. How is TTP different from HUS? How are both differentiated?

Ans: Thrombotic thrombocytopenic purpura and HUS are both defined by a constellation of clinical manifestations.[9,10] HUS is characterized by thrombocytopenia, anemia, and renal insufficiency, whereas the pentad of signs and symptoms including thrombocytopenia, anemia, neurologic deficit, renal dysfunction, and fever is observed in TTP. HUS is observed more in pediatric group and can be associated with diarrheal disease. However, some overlap in clinical manifestations is observed, the distinction between the HUS and TTP may be difficult, especially in the adult presentations. Furthermore, platelet aggregation causing microvascular occlusion is an essential component of both disorders. The pathologic tissue abnormalities are similar; only the organ distribution is different. The probability of TTP can be calculated by the PLASMIC score but largely the distinction between TTP and HUS relies on the test of plasma ADAMTS13 activity. In general, the finding of severe ADAMTS13 deficiency (activity < 10%) is consistent with the diagnosis of TTP, and individuals with normal or moderately low activity (e.g., ≥10%) should have additional evaluation for the alternate causes, like HUS of their symptoms.

REFERENCES

1. Sukumar S, Lämmle B, Cataland SR. Thrombotic Thrombocytopenic Purpura: Pathophysiology, Diagnosis, and Management. J Clin Med. 2021;10(3):536.
2. Bendapudi PK, Hurwitz S, Fry A, Marques MB, Waldo SW, Li A, et al. Derivation and external validation of the PLASMIC score for rapid assessment of adults with thrombotic microangiopathies: a cohort study. Lancet Haematol. 2017;4(4):e157-64.

3. Favaloro EJ, Pasalic L, Henry B, Lippi G. Laboratory testing for ADAMTS13: Utility for TTP diagnosis/exclusion and beyond. Am J Hematol. 2021;96(8):1049-55.
4. Zheng X, Chung D, Takayama TK, Majerus EM, Sadler JE, Fujikawa K. Structure of von Willebrand factor-cleaving protease (ADAMTS13), a metalloprotease involved in thrombotic thrombocytopenic purpura. J Biol Chem. 2001;276(44):41059-63.
5. Gao W, Anderson PJ, Sadler JE. Extensive contacts between ADAMTS13 exosites and von Willebrand factor domain A2 contribute to substrate specificity. Blood. 2008;112(5):1713-9.
6. Peyvandi F, Palla R, Lotta LA, Mackie I, Scully MA, Machin SJ. ADAMTS-13 assays in thrombotic thrombocytopenic purpura. J Thromb Haemost. 2010;8(4):631-40.
7. Mackie I, Mancini I, Muia J, Kremer Hovinga J, Nair S, Machin S, et al. International Council for Standardization in Haematology (ICSH) recommendations for laboratory measurement of ADAMTS13. Int J Lab Hematol. 2020;42(6):685-96.
8. Kremer Hovinga JA, Vesely SK, Terrell DR, Lämmle B, George JN. Survival and relapse in patients with thrombotic thrombocytopenic purpura. Blood. 2010;115(8):1500-11
9. Scully M, Cataland S, Coppo P, de la Rubia J, Friedman KD, Kremer Hovinga J, et al. International Working Group for Thrombotic Thrombocytopenic Purpura. Consensus on the standardization of terminology in thrombotic thrombocytopenic purpura and related thrombotic microangiopathies. J Thromb Haemost. 2017;15(2):312-22.
10. Furlan M, Robles R, Galbusera M, Remuzzi G, Kyrle PA, Brenner B, et al. von Willebrand factor-cleaving protease in thrombotic thrombocytopenic purpura and the hemolytic-uremic syndrome. N Engl J Med. 1998;339(22):1578-84.

12 Thrombophilia

Sanjeev Kumar Sharma, Anamika Bakliwal

Q1. What is hereditary thrombophilia?

Ans: The term "hereditary" or "inherited" thrombophilia has most commonly been applied to conditions in which a genetic mutation affects the amount or function of a protein in the coagulation system. Loss of function mutations include those affecting antithrombin (AT), protein C (PC), and protein S (PS). Gain of function mutations include the factor V Leiden (FVL) and the prothrombin gene 20210 A/G (PGM) mutations.[1]

Q2. What are the tests for inherited thrombophilia?

Ans: Testing for thrombophilias should only be performed when results will be used to improve or modify management.[1] Test for acquired causes can also be done simultaneously to rule out other causes of thrombophilia. The following tests are routinely done for evaluation of inherited thrombophilia:
- Antithrombin (previously called antithrombin III)
- Protein C
- Protein S
- Lupus anticoagulant
- Factor V Leiden
- Prothrombin gene mutation
- Anti-β2-glycoprotein-1 antibodies
- Anticardiolipin antibodies

Q3. When should routine tests for thrombophilia be done?

Ans: Routine testing of coagulation factors to assess the risk of thrombosis is not currently recommended. When the decision has been made to test for deficiencies of physiological anticoagulants, this should be performed only after 3 months of anticoagulation for acute thrombosis, as there is uncertainty over the validity of the results obtained earlier.[2] Genotype-based tests (such as those for FVL and PGM 20210 A/G) and antibody titers (for cardiolipin and β-2 glycoprotein I) can be performed accurately at any point in the care of a patient.[1]

Q4. Should tests for thrombophilic risk factors be performed as screening of family members of deep vein thrombosis (DVT) patients?

Ans: Routine thrombophilia testing to first-degree relatives of people with a history of venous thromboembolism (VTE) is not recommended.[2] In selected cases testing of asymptomatic first-degree relatives of probands with protein C, protein S, and AT deficiency can be considered where this may influence the management and life choices depending on personal circumstances. Paroxysmal nocturnal hemoglobinuria (PNH) testing should be done in patients with thrombosis at unusual sites and abnormal hematological parameters.

Similarly, patients should be evaluated for myeloproliferative neoplasms (MPN) panel who develop thrombosis at unusual sites with full blood count abnormalities suggestive of MPN.[2] Patient should also be tested for antiphospholipid antibodies if there is thrombosis at unusual sites in the absence of clear provoking factors as the type and duration of anticoagulation are affected by the presence of these antibodies.

Q5. Which assays are used to measure protein S levels?

Ans: Plasma protein S exists in two forms: (i) Bound to C4b-binding protein (C4bBP); and (ii) free unbound protein S (FPS). Under normal circumstances FPS antigen concentration usually reflects functional protein S activity in plasma and can be measured by immunoassays. Latex-based immunoturbidimetric assays use either: Two monoclonal antibodies specific for FPS; or latex particles coated with C4bBP to capture FPS, then monoclonal antibody-coated particles, which agglutinate in the presence of captured FPS. Bound and free (total) protein S antigen (TPS) can be measured by immunoassay. Protein S activity assays measure the ability of protein S to inactivate FVIIIa and/or FVa in the presence of activated protein C (APC), detected using prothrombin time (PT), activated partial thromboplastin time (APTT), or Russell's viper venom (RVV)-based coagulation times. Coagulation-based protein S activity assays are not recommended for routine use, although type II protein S deficiency can only be detected in the clotting assay.[3]

Q6. How is protein C deficiency diagnosed and what is its relevance?

Ans: Protein C deficiency can be classified as quantitative (type 1) and functional PC (type 2) and subsequently subtyped as 2a and 2b. Inherited PC deficiency increases risk of VTE by 5- to 10-fold in thrombosis-prone families; however, heterozygous PC deficiency alone does not determine that a subject has thrombophilia.[4] Protein C deficient subjects, who lack additional inherited risk factors such as FVL or have no major acquired risk factors, may not suffer from VTE. In addition, PC deficiency may be acquired, often due to vitamin K antagonist treatment or liver disease. In contrast, homozygous or compound heterozygous PC deficiencies are rare and serious disorders, and affected infants are often in families with no history of PC deficiency or thrombosis. Laboratories commonly use the chromogenic PC assay to diagnose deficiency. Chromogenic assay is recommended due to its good specificity, but this assay fails to detect the rare type 2b deficiency where the defect is due to poor interaction with calcium ions, phospholipid, protein S, and factor Va, and factor VIIIa. The clotting-based assay of PC is capable of detecting type 2b deficiency, but it has reduced specificity.[4]

Q7. What is the role of D-dimer in the assessment of DVT?

Ans: D-dimer is a marker of endogenous fibrinolysis and should therefore be detectable in patients with DVT.[5] DVT can be ruled out in a patient who is judged clinically unlikely to have DVT and who has a negative D-dimer test. Ultrasound testing can be safely omitted in such patients.

Q8. What are the assays used for D-dimer measurement?

Ans: D-dimer molecules are generated through the degradation of cross-linked fibrin during fibrinolysis. D-dimer generation requires the activity of three enzymes: (i) Thrombin, (ii) activated factor XIII (factor XIIIa), and (iii) plasmin. Plasmin digestion of the fibrin clot results in the D-dimer molecule. D-dimer is detected and quantified in whole blood, plasma, or serum using monoclonal antibodies that recognize a specific epitope on cross-linked D-dimer molecules that are otherwise absent on the D-domain of fibrinogen and fibrin monomers that are noncross-linked. The commonly used assays are—enzyme-linked immunosorbent assays (ELISA), immunofluorescent assays, and latex agglutination assays.[6]

REFERENCES

1. Stevens SM, Woller SC, Bauer KA, Kasthuri R, Cushman M, Streiff M, et al. Guidance for the evaluation and treatment of hereditary and acquired thrombophilia. J Thromb Thrombolysis. 2016;41(1):154-64.
2. Arachchillage DJ, Mackillop L, Chandratheva A, Motawani J, MacCallum P, Laffan M. Guidelines for thrombophilia testing: A British Society for Haematology guideline. Br J Haematol. 2022;198(3):443-58.
3. Baker P, Platton S, Gibson C, Gray E, Jennings I, Murphy P, et al.; British Society for Haematology, Haemostasis and Thrombosis Task Force. Guidelines on the laboratory aspects of assays used in haemostasis and thrombosis. Br J Haematol. 2020;191(3):347-62.
4. Cooper PC, Pavlova A, Moore GW, Hickey KP, Marlar RA. Recommendations for clinical laboratory testing for protein C deficiency, for the subcommittee on plasma coagulation inhibitors of the ISTH. J Thromb Haemost. 2020;18(2):271-7.
5. Wells PS, Anderson DR, Rodger M, Forgie M, Kearon C, Dreyer J, et al. Evaluation of d-Dimer in the Diagnosis of Suspected Deep-Vein Thrombosis. N Engl J Med. 2003;349(13):1227-35.
6. Johnson ED, Schell JC, Rodgers GM. The D-dimer assay. Am J Hematol. 2019;94(7):833-9.

13 Inborn Errors of Immunity

Vipin Khandelwal

Q1. What are inborn errors of immunity?

Ans: Our immune system is made up of cells which continuously keep on patrolling the humoral system and tissues from where the foreign agents can invade the body. This defensive immune system is divided into innate and adaptive immune system. Neutrophils, macrophages, and eosinophils are primarily involved in adaptive immune system whereas T and B lymphocytes form the adaptive immune system.[1,2] Any genetic or inherited defect in the immune system can lead to inborn errors of immunity (IEI), also termed primary immunodeficiency diseases (PIDs).

Q2. When do you suspect inborn errors of immunity or primary immunodeficiency diseases?

Ans: Inborn errors of immunity or PIDs should be suspected in children if they exhibit any of the following:[3]
- Recurrent infections—recurrent, severe, or unusual infections that do not respond well to standard treatments.
- Infections with unusual pathogens—infections caused by uncommon or opportunistic pathogens, or infections that occur in an otherwise healthy child.
- Failure to thrive—poor growth or failure to gain weight despite adequate nutrition.
- Autoimmune symptoms—the presence of autoimmune conditions or symptoms, such as recurrent rashes, arthritis, or other inflammatory issues.
- Family history—a family history of immunodeficiency disorders, which might suggest a hereditary condition.

The Jeffrey Modell Foundation has given 10 warning signs of primary immune deficiency which are easy to remember and are a great help for primary doctors when to suspect PID **(Table 1)**.[4]

Q3. How are primary immunodeficiency diseases classified?

Ans: Primary immunodeficiency disorders comprise > 150 different disorders that affect the development, function, or both of the immune system.[5]

The PIDs are classified into eight major categories according to the component of the immune system primarily involved:
1. Combined T-cell and B-cell immunodeficiencies—severe combined immunodeficiency disease (SCID) is most common.

TABLE 1: Warning signs in children and adult.	
Warning signs in children	**Warning signs in adults**
≥ 4 new ear infections within 1 year	≥ 2 new ear infections within 1 year
≥ 2 serious sinus infections within 1 year	≥ 2 new sinus infections within 1 year, in the absence of allergy
≥ 2 months on antibiotics with little effect	One pneumonia per year for > 1 year
≥ 2 pneumonias within 1 year	Chronic diarrhea with weight loss
Failure of an infant to gain weight or grow normally	Recurrent viral infections (colds, herpes, warts, and condyloma)
Recurrent, deep skin, or organ abscesses	Recurrent need for IV antibiotics to clear infections
Persistent thrush in mouth or fungal infection on skin	Recurrent, deep abscesses of the skin, or internal organs
Need for intravenous (IV) antibiotics to clear infections	Persistent thrush or fungal infection on skin or elsewhere
≥ 2 deep-seated infections including septicemia	Infection with normally harmless tuberculosis-like bacteria
A family history of PID	A family history of PID

2. Predominantly antibody deficiencies—selective immunoglobulin (Ig)A deficiency, X-linked agammaglobulinemia (XLA), and common variable immunodeficiency disease (CVID) are most common.
3. Other well-defined immunodeficiency syndromes—Wiskott–Aldrich syndrome (WAS), hyper-IgE syndrome (Job Syndrome)
4. Diseases of immune dysregulation—familial hemophagocytic lymphohistiocytosis (FHL)
5. Congenital defects of phagocyte number and function—chronic granulomatous disease (CGD), leukocyte adhesion deficiency (LAD)
6. Defects in innate immunity
7. Autoinflammatory disorders
8. Complement deficiencies

The PIDs can also be classified based on various other criteria also:
- *By genetic basis:*
  - *Monogenic disorders*: Caused by mutations in a single gene. Examples include:
    - X-linked SCID (caused by mutations in the *IL2RG* gene)
    - Wiskott–Aldrich syndrome (caused by mutations in the *WAS* gene)
  - *Polygenic disorders*: Involving mutations in multiple genes. These are less common and often result from complex interactions among several genetic factors.
- *By mode of inheritance:*
  - *Autosomal dominant*: Only one copy of the mutated gene is required for the disorder to manifest. Example: Hyper-IgE syndrome.
  - *Autosomal recessive*: Requires two copies of the mutated gene (one from each parent). Example: SCID.
  - *X-linked*: The gene mutation is located on the X chromosome. Example: XLA.
- *By age of onset:*
  - *Early onset*: Symptoms appear in infancy or early childhood, such as SCID.
  - *Late onset*: Symptoms may appear later in life, such as CVID.

Classification helps guide diagnosis and treatment strategies and is essential for managing these complex disorders effectively.

Q4. What are the common inborn errors of immunity?

Ans: Inborn errors of immunity are genetic disorders that lead to defects in the immune system. Here are some common and notable examples:[3,6]

- *Severe combined immunodeficiency:*
  - *Characteristics*: Severe deficiency in both T and B lymphocytes, leading to very weak or absent immune responses.[1,2]
  - *Causes*: Various genetic mutations, including those in the *IL2RG* gene (X-linked SCID), adenosine deaminase (ADA) gene deficiency, and others.
- *Common variable immunodeficiency:*
  - *Characteristics*: Low levels of immunoglobulins (antibodies) and increased susceptibility to infections.
  - *Causes*: Can be due to a variety of genetic mutations or, in some cases, may be acquired.
- *X-linked agammaglobulinemia [Bruton's tyrosine kinase (BTK) deficiency]:*
  - *Characteristics*: Absence of B cells and very low levels of immunoglobulins, leading to recurrent bacterial infections.
  - *Causes*: Mutation in the *BTK* gene, which is X-linked.
- *Hyper-IgE syndrome (Job syndrome):*
  - *Characteristics*: High levels of IgE antibodies, recurrent skin, and lung infections, and eczema.
  - *Causes*: Mutations in the *STAT3* gene (autosomal dominant) or other genes.
- *Chronic granulomatous disease:*
  - *Characteristics*: Defects in phagocytes' ability to kill certain bacteria and fungi, leading to recurrent infections and granuloma formation.
  - *Causes*: Mutations in genes encoding components of the NADPH oxidase complex.
- *Leukocyte adhesion deficiency:*
  - *Characteristics*: Defects in the ability of white blood cells to adhere to blood vessel walls, leading to recurrent bacterial infections and impaired wound healing.
  - *Causes*: Mutations in genes such as *ITGB2*, affecting integrins.
- *Selective IgA deficiency:*
  - *Characteristics*: Low levels of IgA antibodies, often asymptomatic but can lead to increased susceptibility to infections, particularly mucosal infections.
  - *Causes*: The exact genetic cause is often unknown, but it is one of the most common antibody deficiencies.
- *Wiskott–Aldrich syndrome:*
  - *Characteristics*: A triad of symptoms including eczema, recurrent infections, and thrombocytopenia (low platelet count).
  - *Causes*: Mutations in the *WAS* gene, X-linked recessive.
- *DiGeorge syndrome (22q11.2 deletion syndrome):*
  - *Characteristics*: Thymic hypoplasia leading to T cell deficiencies, heart defects, and hypoparathyroidism.
  - *Causes*: Deletion of a segment on chromosome 22 (22q11.2).

- *Autosomal recessive hyper-IgM syndrome:*
  - *Characteristics*: Elevated levels of IgM and low levels of other immunoglobulins (IgG, IgA, and IgE), leading to increased susceptibility to infections.
  - *Causes*: Mutations in genes such as *CD40L*, affecting class switching of antibodies.
- *Chediak–Higashi syndrome:*
  - *Characteristics*: Defects in lysosomal trafficking (LYST), leading to immunodeficiency, partial oculocutaneous albinism, and neurological issues.
  - *Causes*: Mutations in the *LYST* gene.
- *Hyper-IgM syndrome:*
  - *Characteristics*: Characterized by normal or elevated IgM levels and low levels of IgG, IgA, and IgE, leading to recurrent infections.
  - *Causes*: Mutations in the *CD40L* gene (X-linked) or other genes affecting class-switch recombination.
- *Bloom syndrome:*
  - *Characteristics*: Increased susceptibility to infections, short stature, and a high incidence of cancer.
  - *Causes*: Mutations in the *BLM* gene, leading to defective deoxyribonucleic acid (DNA) repair mechanisms.
- *Ataxia telangiectasia (AT):*
  - *Characteristics*: A disorder involving immune deficiency, neurological problems (ataxia), and telangiectasias (small, dilated blood vessels).
  - *Causes*: Mutations in the *ATM* gene, affecting DNA repair and cellular responses to damage.

Q5. How should a child with suspected inborn errors of immunity be evaluated?

Ans: Evaluating a child with suspected IEI (PIDs) involves a systematic approach to diagnose and characterize the condition accurately.[7,8] Here is a comprehensive overview of the evaluation process.

Detailed Medical History and Physical Examination

Information on the child's infection history, including frequency, severity, and types of infections (e.g., recurrent ear infections, pneumonia). History of any autoimmune symptoms, failure to thrive, and family history of immunodeficiency or autoimmune diseases is very important.

Severe combined immunodeficiencies patients usually present within the first 6 months of life with failure to thrive, chronic diarrhea, persistent oral thrush, skin rash, pneumonia, and sepsis. Disseminated bacillus Calmette–Guérin (BCG) infection is commonly seen in patients with SCID. Similarly, presence of cytomegalovirus or *Pneumocystis jirovecii* is also common in patients with combined immunodeficiency.

Patients with antibody deficiencies like *XLA* typically present after 6–9 months of age when the level of protective maternal IgG starts going down. They have history of recurrent sinopulmonary infections due to *Streptococcus pneumoniae* or *Haemophilus influenzae*, otitis media, and sometimes septicemia. Less common manifestations include enteroviral infections with resultant chronic meningitis, dermatomyositis, and rheumatoid arthritis.

Patients of CVID usually present later in life that is after 5 years.

Patients with phagocytic defects, leukocyte adhesion deficiency-I (LAD-I), CGD, and severe congenital neutropenia (SCN) are some of the common diseases usually present in neonatal period. Delayed separation of umbilical cord beyond 2 weeks along with omphalitis is suggestive of a neutrophil disorder like LAD-I. Eczematous rash with deep seated abscesses is associated with CGD. Infections due to *Staphylococcus aureus, Burkholderia cepacia*, and fungal infections (mainly *Aspergillus*) are common in CGD.

Patients with AT can present at the age of 6 months to 5 years with gait abnormalities or neurodevelopmental delay. Progressive cerebellar ataxia with discrete or pronounced telangiectasia involving the conjunctiva ears and sometimes face are the classical findings in AT.

Patients with DiGeorge syndrome present in neonatal period. This defect should be suspected in patients with cardiac defects with hypoplastic thymus, hypocalcemia, and facial dysmorphism.

Eczema in infancy and recurrent staphylococcal skin boils and pneumonia with pneumatocele formation are the most common presenting manifestations of hyper IgE syndromes (HIES) due to STAT3 defect. Patients with HIES due to DOCK8 deficiency usually present with disseminated molluscum contagiosum or disseminated viral warts. Autosomal dominant HIES is commonly associated with multiple connective tissue and skeletal abnormalities including scoliosis, hyperextensibility, pathologic fractures, retained primary dentition, craniosynostosis, and vascular abnormalities. WAS patients present with eczema, petechiae, and recurrent sinopulmonary manifestations.

Patients with autoimmune lymphoproliferative syndrome (*ALPS*) present at the median age of around 2 years with chronic nonmalignant lymphadenopathy, splenomegaly, and immune cytopenias.

Mucocutaneous albinism is seen with patients with *Griscelli* syndrome and *Chediak–Higashi* syndrome.

Patients with complement deficiency present later in life, usually after 5 years of age. Autoimmune disease and pyogenic infections are often associated with a deficiency of early components (complements 1-4) of the classic pathway. Terminal complement component deficiencies (complements 5-9) have increased susceptibility to serious infections from *Neisseria* species.

Detailed skin examination is important. It can provide clue toward diagnosis **(Table 2)**.

TABLE 2: Skin findings and their associated immune defects.	
Skin findings	**Associated immune defect**
Eczema and petechiae	Wiskott–Aldrich syndrome
Telangiectasia	Ataxia-telangiectasia syndrome
Generalized molluscum contagiosum	T-cell deficiency
Extensive warts	T-cell deficiency
Candidiasis	T-cell deficiency
Oculocutaneous albinism	Chediak–Higashi syndrome

Initial Laboratory Tests

Complete blood count (CBC): To assess white blood cell count, hemoglobin levels, and platelet count. Look for abnormalities such as low levels of lymphocytes, neutrophils, or elevated eosinophils.

Lymphopenia is commonly seen with patients with SCID and requires further evaluation for specific diagnosis. However, normal absolute lymphocyte count does not rule out combined immunodeficiency, thus further laboratory evaluation is required in case of strong clinical suspicion.

Neutropenia is seen in many PIDs including CD40L deficiency.

In severe congenital neutropenia child has persistently low absolute neutrophil counts (ANC) with elevated monocytes and eosinophils counts.

Cyclic neutropenia patients present with drop in ANC every 3-4 weeks with fever, infections, and mouth ulcers.

Thrombocytopenia with low mean platelet volume gives important clue for diagnosis of WAS.

Autoimmune cytopenias are also commonly seen in patients with immune dysregulation, polyendocrinopathy, enteropathy, or X-linked (IPEX) syndrome.

Persistent neutrophilia even in the absence of active infection is a common feature of LAD-I.

Patients with ALPS generally have elevated ALC.

Bone marrow aspiration and biopsy: Patients with hemophagocytic lymphohistiocytosis (HLH) (either familial or associated with Chediak–Higashi or Griscelli syndrome-II, X-linked lymphoproliferative syndrome) are associated with varying degrees of cytopenias with hemophagocytosis seen in the bone marrow.

Immunoglobulin levels: Measure serum levels of IgG, IgA, IgM, and sometimes IgE to assess antibody production.

Flowcytometry

Lymphocyte subset analysis: Flowcytometry can determine the proportions of different T, B, and natural killer (NK) cell subsets, helping identify deficiencies or abnormal distributions. It is very important to note that the total lymphocyte numbers and T-lymphocyte subsets are age-dependent, being markedly increased in newborns and young infants and decreasing with age. In infants below 4 months of age, a CD4 count of <1,000/mm^3 is generally associated with impaired cellular immunity, whereas the corresponding value is <500/mm^3 in children over 2 years of age and in adults. Immunosuppressive therapies like steroids also significantly alter the values of T and B cell subsets and should be interpreted carefully.

The SCID children are categorized broadly as T+ SCID and T-SCID depending on presence or absence of the T cells.[2] T-SCID can be further evaluated by lymphocyte subset analysis.

Flowcytometric analysis of *CD18, CD11a, CD11b, and CD11c* expression on peripheral blood leukocytes is helpful in patients with LAD-I.

Flowcytometric analysis is helpful If ALPS is suspected based on clinical findings. The recommended percentage of CD3+TCRαβ+CD4–CD8– DNT cells required for a diagnosis is ≥1.5% of total lymphocytes or 2.5% of T lymphocytes in the setting of normal or elevated lymphocyte counts. The presence of elevated double-negative T (DNT) cells coupled with high serum or plasma levels of either interleukin (IL)-10, IL-18, (sFASL), or vitamin B12 can accurately predict the presence of germ line or somatic *FAS* mutations.

Specific Immune Function Tests

- *Quantitative immunoglobulins*: Confirm levels of specific antibodies (IgG subclasses) and assess responses to vaccinations.
- *T-cell function tests*: Evaluate T-cell proliferation and function using assays like mitogen stimulation tests or lymphocyte proliferation assays. Patients with normal T-cell numbers can still have CID. This is usually seen with patients with Omenn syndrome, MHC-I or MHC-II deficiency, ZAP70 deficiency, etc. These patients can be evaluated by doing T-cell proliferation assays (for evaluation of T-cell function), expression of HLA-DR on T and B cells (for MHC class-II expression) and T-cell receptor (TCR) V-β repertoire analysis (for assessment of diversity of immune response).
- *Phagocyte function tests*: Assess the ability of neutrophils and other phagocytes to kill bacteria, using tests like the nitroblue tetrazolium (NBT) test or dihydrorhodamine (DHR) assay.
- Specific component assays for complement deficiency.

Genetic Testing

- *Genetic analysis*: Identify specific genetic mutations associated with PIDs. This may include targeted gene panels, clinical exome sequencing, or whole genome sequencing (WGS) depending on the suspected condition.
- *Family genetic testing*: May be useful for understanding inheritance patterns or identifying carrier status in relatives.

Q6. How is a child with inborn errors of immunity treated?

Ans: Treatment options available are:[9,10]
- *Immunoglobulin replacement therapy*: For conditions where antibody deficiency is there, like CVID, intravenous or subcutaneous Ig therapy to provide necessary antibodies.
- *Bone marrow or stem cell transplantation*: For severe cases, such as SCID and most of PIDs hematopoietic stem cell transplantation (HSCT) can be a curative treatment.
- *Gene therapy*: An emerging field where gene therapy may offer potential cures by correcting defective genes responsible for the immune deficiency.
- *Specialized medications*: Use of targeted therapies for specific conditions, such as enzyme replacement for ADA deficiency.
- *Other measures:*
  - Prophylactic antibiotics to prevent infections.
  - Prompt recognition of infection and aggressive treatment are essential to avoid life-threatening complications and improve prognosis and quality of life.
  - Regular monitoring for infections, growth, and development.
  - Live-attenuated vaccines, such as oral polio, varicella, and BCG should not be given to children with suspected or diagnosed antibody or T-cell defects, because vaccine-induced infection is a risk in these patients. Inactivated polio vaccine should be given to household members to prevent transmission of the virus that can occur by shedding of the attenuated virus in the stool.

- Only irradiated, leukocyte-poor, and virus-free (i.e., cytomegalovirus) products should be used in patients with T-cell defects to avoid graft-versus-host disease (GVHD) and cytomegalovirus infection.
- Genetic counseling is important not only for a child's parents but also for siblings.
- Prenatal diagnosis can be established by performing analyses on fetal blood samples, amniotic fluid cells, or chorionic villus biopsy specimens.

Each treatment plan is customized based on the specific type of IEI and the child's overall health, so a team of specialists including immunologists, infectious disease experts, and other healthcare professionals work together to provide comprehensive care.

Q7. **Can we cure patients with primary immunodeficiency disease? What is the role of allogeneic stem cell transplant?**

Ans: Yes, most of the patients with PIDs can be effectively treated or even cured, depending on the specific condition and its severity. Allogeneic stem cell transplantation (HSCT) plays a crucial role in the management of these disorders.[11,12]

Role of Allogeneic Stem Cell Transplantation

Curative Potential
- *Severe combined immunodeficiency*: HSCT can be curative, providing a new, functioning immune system if done early in life. This is often considered the standard treatment for SCID.
- *Other severe immunodeficiencies*: Conditions like Wiskott–Aldrich syndrome or hyper-IgM syndrome may also be treated with HSCT if they are severe and not manageable by other means.

Mechanism
- *Replacement of immune system*: The transplantation involves replacing the defective immune system with healthy stem cells from a donor. These stem cells can develop into a fully functional immune system.[13]
- *Donor matching*: Success depends on finding a compatible donor, typically a sibling or other related individual. Unrelated and haploidentical donors can also be used if a matched sibling is not available.

Timing and Outcome
- *Early intervention*: The sooner the transplant is done, the better the outcomes, especially before the child has significant infections or other complications.
- *Long-term monitoring*: Posttransplant, patients require ongoing monitoring for potential complications such as GVHD, infections, and other issues.

Limitations and Risks
- *Not suitable for all*: HSCT may not be suitable for all types of PIDs. Some conditions may not have a clear benefit from transplantation or may have high risks associated.

In summary, while not all PIDs can be cured, allogeneic stem cell transplantation offers a potential cure for several severe conditions and plays a pivotal role in improving outcomes and quality of life for many patients.

Q8. What is the role of gene therapy in inborn errors of immunity?

Ans: Gene therapy holds a significant promise for treating IEI by directly addressing the underlying genetic defects that cause these disorders. Here is a detailed look at its role and potential:

Correcting Genetic Defects

- *Direct correction*: Gene therapy aims to correct or replace defective genes responsible for the immune deficiency. For example, if a specific gene mutation is known to cause a particular IEI, gene therapy can introduce a normal copy of that gene into the patient's cells.
- *Gene editing*: Techniques such as CRISPR/Cas9 can be used to edit the genome, correcting mutations at specific locations in the DNA.

Treatment of Specific Conditions

- *Severe combined immunodeficiency*: Gene therapy has shown considerable success in treating SCID, particularly the ADA deficiency variant. In these cases, the patient's own hematopoietic stem cells are modified to include a functional copy of the defective gene and then reintroduced into the patient.
- *X-linked SCID*: This form has also been treated using gene therapy, where the functional gene is added to the patient's T cells, restoring their ability to function normally.
- *Wiskott–Aldrich syndrome*: Early clinical trials have shown promise in treating this condition by correcting the defective gene in the patient's stem cells.

Procedure

- *Cell collection*: The patient's stem cells are collected, usually from bone marrow or blood.
- *Gene modification*: The collected cells are then modified in the laboratory to correct the genetic defect.
- *Reinfusion*: The corrected cells are reintroduced into the patient's body, where they can generate a healthy immune system.

Advantages Over Traditional Treatments

- *Potential for cure*: Gene therapy has the potential to provide a long-term or permanent cure by directly addressing the root cause of the disease.
- *Reduced need for ongoing therapies*: For some conditions, successful gene therapy may reduce or eliminate the need for lifelong treatments such as immunoglobulin replacement or prophylactic antibiotics.

Challenges and Risks

- *Technical challenges*: Ensuring that the gene is inserted correctly and safely into the patient's cells can be technically complex.
- *Safety concerns*: There are risks of adverse effects, such as insertional mutagenesis (where the new gene insertion causes unintended effects), immune responses against the modified cells, or other unforeseen complications.
- *Cost and accessibility*: Gene therapy is often expensive and may not be accessible to all patients, though costs are expected to decrease as the technology matures.

Regulatory and Research Status

- *Clinical trials*: Many gene therapies are still undergoing clinical trials, and their long-term safety and efficacy are continually being evaluated.
- *Approval*: Some gene therapies have received regulatory approval for specific conditions, representing a significant milestone in the treatment of IEIs.

In summary, gene therapy represents a revolutionary approach to treating IEI, with the potential to offer cures for certain genetic conditions. While there are still challenges to overcome, ongoing research and clinical trials continue to advance the field and improve outcomes for patients.

REFERENCES

1. Sharma SK. What a clinical hematologist should know about B cells? Internat Blood Res Rev. 2022;13(1):8-22.
2. Sharma SK. What a clinical hematologist should know about T cells? Internat Blood Res Rev. 2020;11(4):20-32.
3. Tangye SG, Al-Herz W, Bousfiha A, Cunningham-Rundles C, Franco JL, Holland SM, et al. Human Inborn Errors of Immunity: 2022 Update on the Classification from the International Union of Immunological Societies Expert Committee. J Clin Immunol. 2022;42(7):1473-507.
4. Modell V, Orange JS, Quinn J, Modell F. Global Report on Primary Immunodeficiencies: Update from the Jeffrey Modell Centers Network on disease classification, regional trends, treatment modalities, and physician reported outcomes. Immunol Res. 2018;66(3):367-80.
5. Al-Herz W, Bousfiha A, Casanova JL, Chatila T, Conley ME, Cunningham-Rundles C, et al. Primary immunodeficiency diseases: an update on the classification from the international union of immunological societies expert committee for primary immunodeficiency. Front Immunol. 2014;5:162.
6. Akalu YT, Bogunovic D. Inborn errors of immunity: an expanding universe of disease and genetic architecture. Nat Rev Genet. 2024;25(3):184-95.
7. Bousfiha A, Jeddane L, Picard C, Al-Herz W, Ailal F, Chatila T, et al. Human Inborn Errors of Immunity: 2019 Update of the IUIS Phenotypical Classification. J Clin Immunol. 2020;40(1):66-81.
8. Grumach AS, Goudouris ES. Inborn Errors of Immunity: how to diagnose them? J Pediatr (Rio J). 2021;97 Suppl 1 (Suppl 1):S84-S90.
9. Perez E. Future of therapy for inborn errors of immunity. Clin Rev Allergy Immunol. 2022;63(1):75-89.
10. Paris K, Wall LA. The treatment of primary immune deficiencies: Lessons learned and future opportunities. Clin Rev Allergy Immunol. 2023;65(1):19-30.
11. Sung-Yun Pai. Treatment of primary immunodeficiency with allogeneic transplant and gene therapy. Hematology Am Soc Hematol Educ Program. 2019;2019(1):457-65.
12. Slatter M, Lum SH. Personalized hematopoietic stem cell transplantation for inborn errors of immunity. Front Immunol. 2023;14:1162605.
13. Sharma SK. Basics of hematopoietic stem cell transplant. Singapore: Springer Nature; 2023.

14. Bone Marrow Examination

Jyoti Bajaj Sawhney

Q1. What are the indications for bone marrow aspiration and biopsy?

Ans: *The indications of a bone marrow examination are:*[1]
- Packed marrow (acute leukemia)
- Dry marrow (aplastic anemia)
- Fibrotic marrow (myelofibrosis, metastasis, and lymphoma)
- Myelodysplasia (blasts, cellularity, and fibrosis)
- Myeloma evaluation
- Tumor staging
- Marrow aplasia, evaluation of cytopenias
- Post chemotherapy to determine aplasia/regeneration
- Evaluation of prolonged fever or fever of unknown origin

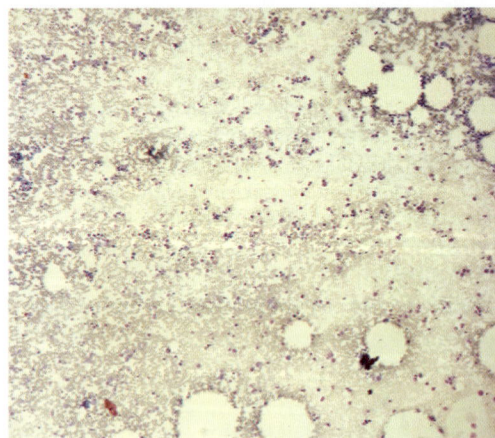

FIG. 1: Normal marrow at 10×.
Courtesy: Dr Jyoti Sawhney.

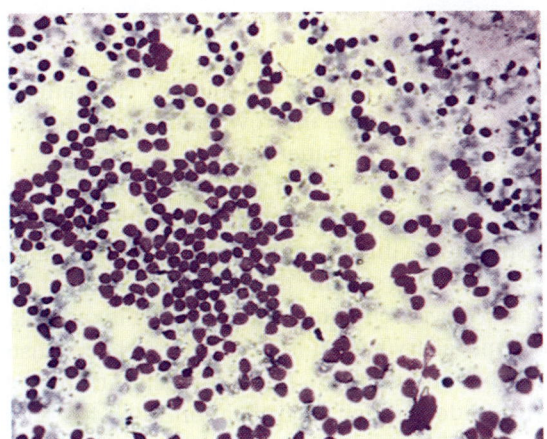

FIG. 2: Bone marrow aspirate (10×): Case of acute leukemia-blast replacing normal hematopoietic elements.
Courtesy: Dr Abhishek Purohit.

Q2. What are the processing and staining methods for bone marrow aspirate and biopsy?

Ans: The bone marrow aspirate should be drawn with a 10- or 20-mL plastic syringe, to provide adequate negative pressure, attached to the aspiration needle. To preserve morphology, the syringe should not contain anticoagulant. Approximately, 0.5 mL of the first draw of the aspirate should be collected to make bone marrow smears by the bedside. If sample for measurable residual disease (MRD) assessment has to be drawn, then it should be the first aspirated sample.

With increasing volumes of bone marrow aspirate drawn, there is progressive dilution of the aspirate with peripheral blood.[1]

A second syringe should be attached to the aspiration needle to draw additional samples for supplementary tests, such as flow cytometry, cytogenetic analysis and molecular genetic studies, microbiology, electron microscopy, or bone marrow aspirate culture. Bone marrow smears should be prepared immediately following aspiration. Smears are made with a glass spreader with beveled edges so that the width of the spreader is narrower than the width of the specimen slide. The spreader is placed in front of the drop of aspirate at an angle of approximately 30° and pulled back to make contact with the drop, to enable the drop to spread along the line of contact with the slide. The spreader is then pushed forward in a smooth action, in contact with the slide. A minimum of six smears should be made.

The glass slides should be frosted glass at one end so that details can be written with pencil.

Two air-dried smears and one squash slide should be fixed with fresh acetone-free absolute methanol and stained with a Romanowsky stain, such as May–Grünwald–Giemsa (MGG) or Wright–Giemsa stain. All bone marrow smears should be coverslipped using a mounting medium that hardens and dries rapidly.

Trephine sections are particularly useful for the assessment of overall marrow architecture and cellularity and provide greater sensitivity for the assessment of focal lesions and patchy infiltrates. The percentage cellularity may be obtained by estimating the proportion of cells occupying the total marrow cavity. Bone marrow cellularity varies with age and should be assessed with reference to the age of the patient.

Trephine biopsy sections should be stained with hematoxylin and eosin. One section may be stained for reticulin by the silver impregnation method. Other special stains such as periodic acid-Schiff (PAS) for dysplastic erythroid, micromegakaryocytes, and Masson trichrome for collagen may be used for supporting specific diagnosis.

Trephine sections should be viewed initially at low power for adequacy, pattern, cellularity, presence of focal lesions, megakaryocyte number, abnormal cell clusters and location, bone structure (trabecular number and thickness), and osteoclastic and osteoblastic activity. The sections are next viewed under higher magnification (200–400 X) to assess hemopoietic activity (e.g., erythroid, myeloid, megakaryocytic lineages, lymphoid cells, plasma cells, and macrophages) and cytological detail.

Two to four sections should be reviewed routinely. In lymphoma staging and in cases of suspected metastatic infiltrate, the chances of detecting a focal lesion are increased if more sections are reviewed. If immunohistochemistry (IHC) is performed, additional sections will have to be reviewed.

Q3. What parameters should be included in reporting the results of a bone marrow evaluation?

Ans: The bone marrow aspirate smear preparation should first be viewed under low power magnification to determine the number and cellularity of particles, the number of megakaryocytes, and to scan for clumps of abnormal cells and for abnormal cells of low incidence. Areas of well-spread marrow cells in the cellular trails of the bone marrow smear behind the particles are selected for assessment at higher magnification for morphological assessment of cells, including cytological details, parasites, or cell inclusions. Bone marrow smears are particularly useful for cellular detail and differential cell counts.[1] It is also useful for the assessment of cellularity, megakaryocyte numbers, focal disease (e.g., lymphoma, plasma cell myeloma, mast cells, metastatic carcinoma, storage histiocytes, and granulomas), fibrotic marrows, and the detection of abnormal tumor cells that have metastasized to the bone marrow **(Box 1)**.

BOX 1: The report should include the following parameters.

- Name of institution
- Unique specimen identifier (laboratory accession number)
- *Details of patient*: Surname, first name(s), identification number, age or date of birth, gender, and contact details (e.g., address and hospital location)
- Name of responsible physician
- Name of requesting doctor
- Date of procedure
- Significant clinical history including physical findings, recent chemo/radiotherapy, cytokine therapy, and pertinent lab results

Continued

Continued

Indication for bone marrow examination:
- Procedure performed (aspirate/trephine biopsy)
- Anatomic site of aspirate/biopsy
- Ease/difficulty of aspiration
- *Blood count*: Hemoglobin concentration, total and differential white cell count (neutrophils, eosinophils, basophils, monocytes, and lymphocytes) and platelet count
- Blood smear description and diagnostic conclusion cellularity of particles and cell trails
- Nucleated differential cell count
- Total number of cells counted
- *Myeloid*: Erythroid ratio erythropoiesis myelopoiesis megakaryocytes lymphocytes
- Plasma cells
- Other hemopoietic cells
- Abnormal cells (e.g., blast cells and metastatic infiltrates)
- Iron stain
- Cytochemistry
- Other investigations (e.g., cytogenetics, PCR, FISH, and microbiology)
- Summary of flow cytometry findings, if available
- Conclusion
- WHO classification (if relevant)
- Disease code
- Signature and date of report

(FISH: fluorescent in-situ hybridization; PCR: polymerase chain reaction; WHO: World Health Organization)

Trephine sections should be viewed initially at low power for adequacy, pattern, cellularity, presence of focal lesions, megakaryocyte number, abnormal cell clusters and location, bone structure (trabecular number and thickness), and osteoclastic and osteoblastic activity. The sections are next viewed under higher magnification to assess hematopoietic activity (e.g., erythroid, myeloid, megakaryocytic lineages, lymphoid cells, plasma cells, and macrophages) and cytological detail. Two to four sections should be reviewed routinely. In lymphoma staging and in cases of suspected metastatic infiltrate, the chances of detecting a focal lesion are increased if more sections are reviewed. If IHC is performed, additional sections will be reviewed.

Q4. **What cytochemical staining is done on bone marrow aspirates?**

Ans: Cytochemistry is the branch of cell biology dealing with the detection of cell constituents by means of biochemical analysis and visualization techniques.[1,2] The benefits of cytochemical stains are:
- *Diagnostic importance*: Useful in differentiating various types of leukemia. It is used in differentiating acute leukemia (e.g., acute lymphoblastic leukemia or acute myeloblastic leukemia). It is also helpful in differentiating of chronic myeloid leukemia (CML) chronic phase from leukemoid reaction. In lymphoid neoplasms, it has been used to diagnose hairy cell leukemia (HCL).
- Preliminary screening tool (in absence of advanced techniques)
- Cheap and cost effective, less time consuming
- Easy to perform

These stains include:
- Myeloperoxidase (MPO)
- Sudan Black B (SBB)
- PAS
- Nonspecific esterase (NSE)
- Iron staining/Perls' reaction/Prussian blue staining
- Leukocyte alkaline phosphatase (LAP)
- Tartrate-resistant acid phosphatase (TRAP)
- Toluidine blue

Myeloperoxidase

Myeloperoxidase is located in the primary and secondary granules of neutrophils and their precursors, in eosinophil granules and in the azurophilic granules of monocytes. MPO splits H_2O_2 and in the presence of a chromatic electron donor forms an insoluble reaction product. Various benzidine substitutes have been used, of which 3,3'-diaminobenzidine (DAB) is the preferred chromogen. The reaction product is stable, insoluble, and nondiffusible.

Results and interpretation: The reaction product is brown and granular. The most primitive myeloblasts are negative, with granular positivity appearing progressively as they mature toward the promyelocyte stage. The positivity may be localized to the Golgi region. Promyelocytes and myelocytes are the most strongest staining cells in the granulocyte series, with positive (primary) granules packing the cytoplasm.

Metamyelocytes and neutrophils have progressively fewer positive (secondary) granules. Monoblasts and monocytes may be negative or positive.

Sudan Black B

Sudan Black B is a lipophilic dye that binds irreversibly to an undefined granule component in granulocytes, eosinophils and some monocytes. It cannot be extracted from the stained granules by organic dye solvents and gives comparable information to that of MPO staining.

Results and interpretation: The reaction product is black and granular. The results are essentially similar to those seen with MPO staining, both in normal and leukemic cells.

MPO-negative neutrophils are also SBB negative.

Periodic Acid–Schiff Reaction

Periodic acid specifically oxidizes 1–2 glycol groups to produce stable dialdehydes. These dialdehydes give a red reaction product when exposed to Schiff reagent. Positive reactions occur with carbohydrates, principally glycogen, but also monosaccharides, polysaccharides, glycoproteins, and mucoproteins. In hemopoietic cells, the main source of positive reactions is glycogen.

Results and interpretation: The reaction product is reddish pink. The lymphoblasts show variable PAS-positive cytoplasmic granules or blocks on a clear background; it is block positivity on a clear background that is most characteristic of lymphoblasts rather than myeloblasts.

Nonspecific Esterases

Leukocyte esterases are a group of enzymes that hydrolyze acyl or chloroacyl esters of α-naphthol or naphthol AS.

The isoenzymes fell into two groups—bands 1, 2, 7, 8, and 9 corresponded to the "specific" esterase of neutrophils, staining specifically with naphthol AS-D chloroacetate esterase (CAE), whereas bands 3, 4, 5, and 6 corresponded to NSE, staining with α-naphthyl acetate esterase (ANAE) and α-naphthyl butyrate esterase, (ANBE). Naphthol AS acetate and naphthol AS-D acetate react with both specific and NSEs, but only the reaction with the NSEs is inhibited by NaF.

Results and interpretation: In ANBE, reaction product is brown and granular. The majority of monocytes (>80%) stain strongly, the remainder showing some weak staining. In the bone marrow, monocytes, monocyte precursors, and macrophages stain strongly. Alpha-naphthyl butyrate is more specific for identifying a monocytic component in acute myeloid leukemia (AML) than α-naphthyl acetate.

Iron Staining/Perl's Reaction/Prussian Blue Staining

Siderocytes are red cells containing granules of nonheme iron. The granules are formed by water-insoluble complex of ferric iron, lipid, protein, and carbohydrate. This siderotic material (or hemosiderin) reacts with potassium ferrocyanide to form a blue compound, ferri-ferrocyanide, this reaction is the basis of a positive Prussian blue (Perl's) reaction. It is used to measure the iron stores and for evaluation of ring-sideroblasts. Iron stores are reduced or absent in iron-deficiency anemia. They are increased when there is iron overload, in infections, dyserythropoietic anemias, sideroblastic anemias, and thalassemia. It is also used in MDS cases to identify pathological ring sideroblasts.

Leukocyte Alkaline Phosphatase

Alkaline phosphatase activity is found predominantly in mature neutrophils, with some activity in metamyelocytes.

Results and interpretation: The reaction product is blue and granular. The intensity of reaction product in neutrophils varies from negative to strongly positive, with coarse granules filling the cytoplasm and overlying the nucleus. An overall score is obtained by assessing the stain intensity in 100 consecutive neutrophils, with each neutrophil scored on a scale of 0–4 as follows:
- 0: Negative, no granules
- 1: Occasional granules scattered in the cytoplasm
- 2: Moderate numbers of granules
- 3: Numerous granules
- 4: Heavy positivity with numerous coarse granules crowding the cytoplasm, frequently overlying the nucleus

The overall possible score will range between 0 and 400 (assessed on 100 neutrophils). Reported normal ranges may range from 14 to 100 (mean 46).

In pathological states, the most significant diagnostic use of the LAP score has been in CML. In the chronic phase of the disease, the score is almost invariably low, usually zero. Transient increases may occur with intercurrent infection. In myeloid blast transformation or accelerated phase, the score rises. Low scores are also commonly found in paroxysmal nocturnal hemoglobinuria. A raised LAP score, notably in the neutrophilia of infection, polycythemia vera, leukemoid reactions, and Hodgkin lymphoma.

Acid Phosphatase Reaction, Including Tartrate-resistant Acid Phosphatase Reaction

Its main diagnostic use is in the diagnosis of T-cell ALL and HCL.

In T cells, acid phosphatase is an early differentiation feature. Almost all acute and chronic T-lineage leukemias show strong activity. In T lineage ALL, the activity is usually highly localized (polar). In HCL, the majority of leukemic cells react equally positively in the presence and absence of tartaric acid.

Toluidine Blue Stain

Toluidine blue staining is useful for the enumeration of basophils and mast cells. It binds strongly to the granules in these cells and is particularly useful in pathological states in which the cells may not be easily identifiable on Romanowsky stains.

In AML and in CML and other MPN, basophils may be dysplastic and poorly granular, as may the mast cells in systemic mastocytosis.

Q5. Which immunohistochemical staining is done on bone marrow trephine biopsy sections?

Ans: Immunohistochemical staining can be done for both acute and chronic hematolymphoid neoplasms.[1,2] All these markers can also be assessed by flow cytometry immunophenotyping **(Table 1)**. In cases where the disease is not found in the peripheral blood or the bone marrow aspirate is dilute without tumor cells then IHC can be done to identify the tumor cells if they are present in the bone marrow biopsy. IHC can be done for both immature and mature B and T cell (**Tables 1 and 2**, respectively). It can also be done to identify AML, myelodysplastic syndrome (MDS), and myeloproliferative neoplasm (MPN) **(Table 3)**.

TABLE 1: Immunohistochemical staining for immature and mature B cell malignancies.

	Immature B cells (B-ALL/B-LBL)	Mature B cells (B-cell NHL)
TdT	———————	
CD34	———————	
CD19	———————	———————
CD79a	———————	———————
PAX-5	———————	———————
CD10**	———————	———————
CD22	———————	———————
CD20		———————
BCL-6**		———————
Kappa-lambda*		———————

*Surface Kappa/Lambda on mature B-cells.
**CD10 and BCL-6 expression in B-NHL indicates germinal center cell origin.
(B-ALL: B-acute lymphoblastic leukemia; B-LBL: B-lymphoblastic lymphoma; NHL: non-Hodgkin lymphoma)

CHAPTER 14: Bone Marrow Examination

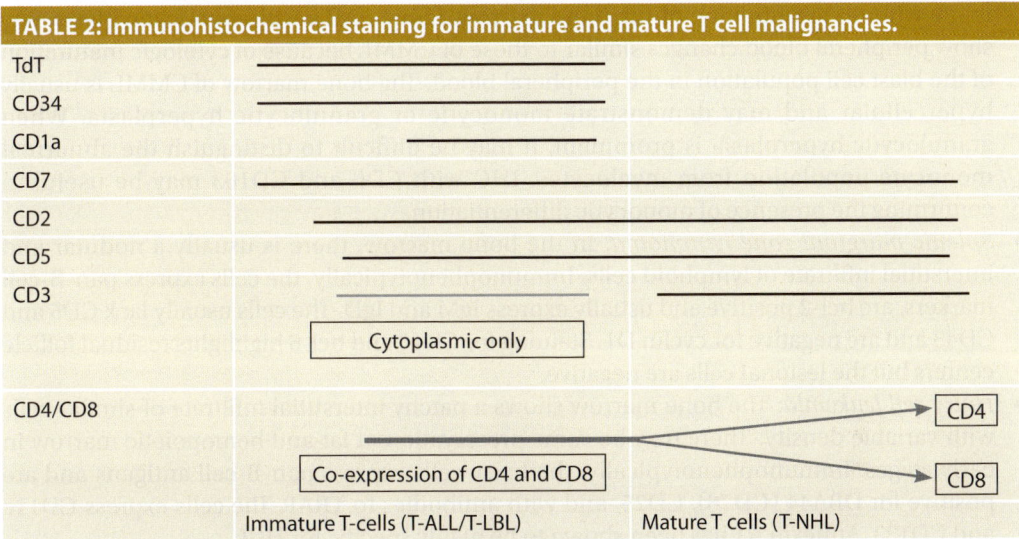

TABLE 2: Immunohistochemical staining for immature and mature T cell malignancies.

(T-ALL: T-acute lymphoblastic leukemia; T-LBL: T-lymphoblastic lymphoma; NHL: non-Hodgkin lymphoma)

TABLE 3: Immunohistochemical staining for myeloid malignancies.

Precursor	CD34 and CD117
Erythroid	Glycophorin A and hemoglobin A
Myeloid	Myeloperoxidase, CD13, CD33, HLA-DR, and CD117
Megakaryocytic	CD41, CD42b, CD61, and von Willebrand factor
Monocytic	CD14, CD68, and CD163

Q6. Which diseases can be diagnosed with immunohistochemical staining of bone marrow biopsy?

Ans: The diseases where IHC can be helpful include:
- *AML*: Cases of AML associated with marrow fibrosis represent a diagnostic challenge. Two subtypes which typically cause the diagnostic difficulties are acute megakaryoblastic leukemia (AMKL) and acute panmyelosis with myelofibrosis. Immunohistology can also be helpful in drawing the line between MDS-IB and AML by facilitating the detection of the blasts and the assessment of their distribution.[3,4]
- *Hypoplastic myelodysplastic syndrome*: The presence of easily identifiable megakaryocytes within an architecturally disorganized marrow and the presence of reticulin fibrosis favor MDS over aplastic anemia. IHC can help in distinguishing hypoplastic-MDS from acquired aplastic anemia, the former disorder being characterized by higher CD34 expression as compared to aplastic anemia. The distinction from aplastic anemia, however, is significant because the risk of progression to acute leukemia is much greater in hypoplastic-MDS.
- *Myelodysplastic/myeloproliferative disorders:* Although an elevated peripheral blood monocyte count is necessary for the diagnosis of CMML, such a diagnosis should never be

made without examination of the bone marrow. Some AMLs with monocytic blasts may show peripheral blood changes similar to those of CMML because of cytologic maturation of the blast cell population in the peripheral blood. The bone marrow of CMML is usually hypercellular and may demonstrate monocytic or granulocytic hyperplasia. When granulocytic hyperplasia is prominent, it may be difficult to distinguish the abnormal monocyte population from myelocytes. IHC with CD6 and CD163 may be useful in confirming the presence of monocytic differentiation.

- *Splenic marginal zone lymphoma*: In the bone marrow, there is usually a nodular and interstitial infiltrate of lymphoid cells. Immunophenotypically, the cells express pan-B-cell markers, are bcl-2 positive and usually express IgM and IgD. The cells usually lack CD5 and CD43 and are negative for cyclin D1. Staining for CD10 and bcl-6 highlights residual follicle centers but the lesional cells are negative.[5]
- *Hairy cell leukemia*: The bone marrow shows a patchy interstitial infiltrate of similar cells with variable density. There may be some preservation of fat and hemopoietic marrow in early stages. Immunophenotypically, the hairy cells express pan-B-cell antigens and are positive for DBA44 (CD76), CD25, and with antibodies to TRAP. The cells express CD11c and CD123. Annexin A1 has been shown to be highly specific for HCL.
- *Hairy cell leukemia variant*: In the bone marrow, the infiltrate is also strikingly intrasinusoidal. Immunophenotypically, the cells are positive for pan B-cell markers, usually positive for CD11c and DBA44 (CD76). Staining for CD5, CD23, CD25, and CD123 is usually negative. Annexin A1 is not present.

Thus immunohistochemical staining is a very helpful ancillary technique in supporting morphological diagnosis for both myeloid and lymphoid neoplasms.

Q7. What are the pitfalls in the interpretation of immunohistochemistry?

Ans: Although there has been a considerable progress in automation and standardization of IHC, there are still many things to be considered in proper optimization and appropriate interpretation **(Table 4)**.[2]

TABLE 4: Pitfalls in immunohistochemistry (IHC).

Pitfalls	Solution
Weak or absent staining	
Antigen levels are too low	Prolong incubation time of primary antibody. Use a higher sensitivity staining system
Incomplete fixation	Prevent under (>30 minutes) or over fixation (>48 hours)
Use of inappropriate fixative	Check manufacturer's specifications regarding recommended fixative
Insufficient dehydration	Operating regular reagent changes, (i.e., alcohol)
Paraffin too hot	Monitor temperature of paraffin (<60°C)
Embedding and defacing at high oven temperature	Oven temperature not to exceed 60°C
Heating for antigen retrieval	Optimize antigen retrieval time

Continued

Continued

Pitfalls	Solution
Reagents not working	Monitor expiration dates, storage parameters, and pH
Antibody too dilute, improper antibody dilution	Determine correct concentration check incubation time and temperature
Partial drying out of tissue during processing	• Immerse tissue immediately in fixative • Use a humidity or moist chamber during incubation steps. Avoid evaporation with humidity chamber
Chromogen not working	Add chromogen to labeling solution. Monitor for change in color
Background or artifactual staining	
Excessive incubation	Reduce incubation
Necrotic or otherwise damaged tissue	Avoid sampling of necrotic areas
Antigen diffusion before fixation leading to specific background	Avoid delays in fixation
Thick preparation	Cut sections at 4–6 mm
Inappropriately concentrated antibody	• Check titration and concentration • Decrease temperature of reaction
Presence of chromogen or undissolved counterstain deposits	• Filter the chromogen or counterstain • Insure that chromogen is completely dissolved
Incomplete inadequate rinsing of slides	• Follow protocol for proper slide rinsing • Mildly rinse slide with wash buffer bottle and place in wash bath in 5 minutes
Endogenous pigments	Check the negative control for the presence of these pigments. Use a chromogen of contrasting color

REFERENCES

1. Lee SH, Erber WN. ICSH guidelines for the standardization of bone marrow specimens and reports. Int Jnl Lab Hem. 2008;30:349-64.
2. Kim SW, Roh J, Park CS. Immunohistochemistry for Pathologists: Protocols, Pitfalls, and Tips. J Pathol Transl Med. 2016;50(6):411-8.
3. Olsen RJ, Chang C, Herrick JL, Zu Y, Ehsan A. Acute leukemia Immunohistochemistry: A Systematic Diagnostic Approach. Arch Pathol Lab Med. 2008;132(3):462-75.
4. Cruise MW. Immunohistochemistry in Acute Myeloid Leukemia. Methods Mol Biol. 2017;1633:33-49.
5. Wotherspoon AC. Extranodal and splenic small B-cell lymphoma. Mod Pathol. 2013;26:S29-41.

15. Flowcytometry

Gurleen Oberoi

Q1. What is flowcytometry?

Ans: Flowcytometry is a sophisticated technology that simultaneously measures and analyses multiple physical and chemical characteristics of single particles, usually cells, as they flow in a fluid stream through a beam of light/laser. It enables measurement of a particle's relative size, relative granularity or internal complexity, and relative fluorescence intensity. These characteristics are determined using an optical-to-electronic coupling system that records how the cell or particle scatters incident laser light and emits fluorescence. Flowcytometry is a powerful tool in both research and clinical settings, providing detailed insights into cell populations and their characteristics.

A flowcytometer is made up of three main systems: (1) fluidics, (2) optics, and (3) electronics.

1. *Fluidics system*:
   - The fluidics system directs cells or particles through a narrow, focused stream to ensure they pass through the detection area one at a time.
   - Includes a sample injector, sheath fluid, and flow cells.
2. *Optics system*:
   - It uses lasers to excite fluorescently labeled particles or cells and optical filters to direct the resulting light signals to the appropriate detectors.
   - Components: Lasers for excitation, filters, and detectors for measuring scattered and emitted light.
3. *Electronics system*: It converts the detected light signals into electronic signals that can be processed by the computer. For some instruments equipped with a sorting feature, the electronics system is also capable of initiating sorting decisions to charge and deflect particles.[1,2]

Advantages of Flowcytometry

- *Multiparametric analysis*: It can measure multiple characteristics of individual cells simultaneously.
- *High throughput*: It is capable of analyzing thousands of cells per second.
- *Quantitative data*: It provides quantitative information on cell populations.
- *Specificity*: It allows for the detection of specific cell markers using fluorescent antibodies.

Limitations of Flowcytometry
- *Complexity*: It requires specialized training for operation and data interpretation.
- *Cost*: It can be expensive due to the high cost of equipment and reagents.
- *Sample preparation*: Samples often need to be processed and stained, which can be time-consuming.

Q2. What is the principle of flowcytometry?

Ans: In the flow cytometer, particles are carried to the laser intercept in a fluid stream. Any suspended particle or cell from 0.2–150 µm in size is suitable for analysis. Cells from solid tissue must be disaggregated before analysis. The portion of the fluid stream where particles are located is called the sample core which is surrounded by a layer of sheath fluid. When particles pass on the particle fluoresce. The scattered and fluorescent light is collected by appropriately positioned lenses. A combination of beam splitters and filters steers the scattered and fluorescent light to the appropriate detectors. The detectors produce electronic signals proportional to the optical signals striking them. List mode data are collected on each particle or event. The characteristics or parameters of each event are based on its light scattering and fluorescent properties. The data are collected and stored in the computer. This data can be analyzed to provide information about subpopulations within the sample.

- *Fluidics*: Cells or particles of interest are suspended in a fluid (often saline solution) and injected into the flow cytometer. The sample flows in a narrow, single-file stream through the instrument.
- *Laser light source*: A laser beam (commonly a focused beam of coherent light, such as from a solid-state laser) is directed into the flow of cells. The laser typically emits light at a specific wavelength, such as blue (488 nm) or red (633 nm), depending on the fluorochromes used for labeling.
- *Scattered light and fluorescence detection*: As each cell or particle passes through the laser beam, it scatters light and emits fluorescence.
  - *Forward scatter (FSC)*: Light scattered in the direction of the laser beam, which correlates with cell size.
  - *Side scatter (SSC)*: Light scattered perpendicular to the laser beam, which correlates with internal complexity or granularity of the cell.
  - *Fluorescence emission*: Fluorescently labeled cells emit light at specific wavelengths when excited by the laser. Detectors in the flow cytometer capture this emitted light.
- *Optical filters and detectors*: They are used to separate and detect different wavelengths of emitted light corresponding to different fluorescent labels. Multiple detectors are often used to capture fluorescence emission from different fluorochromes simultaneously, allowing for multiparameter analysis.
- *Data acquisition and analysis*:
  - Data from each detected event is collected and analyzed by computer software. Parameters such as cell size (FSC), granularity (SSC), and fluorescence intensity are quantified for each cell.
  - Data can be displayed as histograms, dot plots, or other graphical formats to visualize and interpret cell populations.

Overall, flowcytometry enables quantitative analysis of cells based on their physical characteristics (size, granularity) and molecular properties (fluorescent labeling). It is a versatile tool used extensively in research, clinical diagnostics, and various applications in biology and medicine.[2,3]

Q3. What are the various methods of performing flowcytometry?

Ans: Various methods and technologies within flowcytometry enable researchers to gather different types of information. Common methods and approaches used:

- *Standard flowcytometry*: Cells are labeled with fluorescent dyes or antibodies. As cells pass through a laser beam, they emit fluorescence that is detected and analyzed. FSC measures cell size, while SSC provides information about granularity or internal complexity. Both are crucial for initial cell population characterization.[1,2]
- *Multicolor flowcytometry*: Uses different fluorescent dyes to label different cellular components or markers simultaneously. This allows for the simultaneous analysis of multiple parameters.[3]
- *Spectral flowcytometry*: Instead of using filters to detect specific wavelengths, spectral flowcytometry uses multiple detectors to capture a broad range of emission spectra. This allows for more parameters to be analyzed in a single sample.[4]
- *Imaging flowcytometry*: A technique that combines traditional flowcytometry with imaging to provide more detailed information about cells. While conventional flowcytometry analyzes cells based on their fluorescence and light scattering properties, image flowcytometry captures images of individual cells as they pass through a laser. This allows for the analysis of cellular morphology, size, and specific subcellular structures in addition to fluorescence intensity.[5]
- *Time-of-flight (ToF) flowcytometry*: Instead of using fluorescent markers, mass cytometry (CyTOF) uses heavy metal isotopes as tags and measures them using ToF mass spectrometry. It allows for the analysis of more parameters with minimal spectral overlap.[6]
- *Cell sorting [fluorescence-activated cell sorting (FACS)]*: In addition to analysis, flow cytometers equipped with sorting capabilities can physically separate and collect specific cell populations based on fluorescence and scatter properties.[3]
- *Acoustic-assisted flowcytometry*: Uses acoustic waves to focus cells in the fluid stream, improving precision and reducing sample loss. Applications requiring minimal sample volumes or higher precision in sorting. Acoustic flow cytometers are used in the study of multidrug-resistant bacteria in the blood and other samples.[7]
- *Microfluidic flowcytometry*: It integrates flowcytometry on a microchip using microfluidic channels for smaller sample volumes and enhanced portability. It can be used in point-of-care diagnostics and single-cell analyses.[8]
- *Functional flowcytometry*: Measures cellular functions, such as intracellular calcium levels, cytokine production, or cell cycle status, often through additional dyes or reporters.

Each method has its own advantages and applications, depending on the specific requirements of the analysis, such as the number of parameters to be studied, the type of cells or particles, and the desired resolution.[2]

Q4. What disease can be diagnosed with the help of flowcytometry?

Ans: Flowcytometry is a versatile tool used to diagnose and monitor a variety of diseases, particularly those involving blood cells and the immune system. Here are some diseases and conditions that can be diagnosed or managed using flowcytometry:

- *Hematological disorders*:
  - *Benign disorders:*
    - Diagnosis of paroxysmal nocturnal hemoglobinuria (PNH) by detecting and quantifying PNH clones on leukocytes and red blood cells (RBCs). Glycosylphosphatidylinositol (GPI)-linked antigens such as CD24, CD157, CD58, and CD59 along with FlAER are commonly used.
    - Platelet flowcytometry: Use of CD41, CD61 and Cd42a, and Cd42b helps in diagnosing disorders such as Bernard–Soulier syndrome and Glanzmann syndrome. Platelet aggregometry is also performed by flowcytometry.
    - Osmotic fragility test (OFT) and EMA binding test: OFT helps in indicating presence of hereditary spherocytosis (HS). While EMA binding test is one of the recommended tests for diagnosing HS by measuring binding of EMA by RBCs.
    - Immunodeficiencies:
      - Primary immunodeficiencies (PIDs): It helps diagnose congenital immunodeficiencies by analyzing specific immune cell populations, such as T cells, B cells, and NK cells. Primary immune deficiency orientation tube (PIDOT) with several markers to identify and quantify different subsets of T, B, and NK cells helps in diagnosing PIDs.
      - Acquired immunodeficiencies: Monitoring immune cell subsets in conditions like HIV/AIDS to evaluate immune system status.
    - Autoimmune diseases:
      - Systemic lupus erythematosus (SLE) and other autoimmune disorders: Flowcytometry can be used to assess immune cell populations and activation status, which may help in diagnosing and monitoring autoimmune conditions. HLA-b27 expression can be used for diagnosing ankylosing spondylitis.
    - Infections:
      - Viral infections: For example, monitoring T-cell subsets and activation status in HIV patients helps in assessing disease progression and response to antiretroviral therapy.
      - Fungal and bacterial infections: Flowcytometry can be used to identify and quantify pathogens and assess immune responses.
  - *Malignant disorders:*
    - Leukemias: Flowcytometry can identify and characterize different types of leukemia including acute lymphoblastic leukemia (ALL) and acute myeloid leukemia (AML) by detecting abnormal cell surface markers and patterns of expression.
    - Lymphomas: Differentiates reactive from malignant lymphadenopathy. Analysis of surface markers (e.g., CD19, CD5, and CD10) along with restriction pattern on kappa and lambda aids for concluding if the B lymphocytes are polyclonal (reactive) or monoclonal (malignant). In case of T lymphocytes, the clues comes from CD4, CD8, TCRab, TCRgd, and loss of expression/downregulation or presence of any aberrancies. Thus it helps in the diagnosis, classification, and prognostication of lymphomas [e.g., T and B cell non-Hodgkin lymphoma (NHL), Hodgkin lymphoma] by analyzing the immunophenotype of the atypical lymphoid cells.
    - Multiple myeloma: Flowcytometry can be used to assess the presence and quantity of abnormal plasma cells in the bone marrow, as well as to monitor disease progression and response to therapy.
    - Bone marrow disorders and myelodysplastic syndromes (MDS): Flowcytometry can help in distinguishing MDS from other bone marrow disorders by analyzing cell surface markers and cytometric patterns.

- *Nonhematological disorders*: Solid tumors such as lung cancers, breast cancers, prostatic cancers, gastrointestinal cancers, etc., can be detected by analyzing specific tumor marker expression.[9-11]

Q5. How is flowcytometry different from immunohistochemistry?

Ans: Flowcytometry and immunohistochemistry (IHC) are both techniques used to analyze cells and tissues based on the surface, cytoplasmic, and nuclear expression of various proteins and cellular properties, but they differ significantly in their methods, applications, and the types of information they provide.[12,13] Comparison of the two techniques (also depicted in **Table 1**):

- *Principle and technique*:
  - Flowcytometry:
    - Principle: Analyzes cells or particles as they flow in a liquid stream through a laser beam. It measures light scatter and fluorescence emitted by labeled cells to determine various characteristics.
    - Technique: Cells are suspended in a fluid and passed through a flow cytometer where they are individually analyzed by lasers. Detectors measure FSC (size), SSC (granularity), and fluorescence (specific markers).
  - Immunohistochemistry:
    - Principle: Detects and visualizes specific antigens in tissue sections or cell preparations using antibodies that are conjugated to enzymes or fluorochromes.
    - Technique: Tissue or cell samples are fixed onto slides, treated with specific antibodies, and then visualized using either colorimetric reactions (enzyme-linked) or fluorescence microscopy.
- *Sample preparation*
  - Flowcytometry:
    - Sample type: Requires cells to be in a single-cell suspension, often obtained from blood, bone marrow, or tissue dissociation.
    - Preparation: Cells are stained with fluorescently labeled antibodies or dyes and then analyzed in a fluidic system.
  - Immunohistochemistry:
    - Sample type: Works with tissue sections or cell preparations on slides, typically requiring preservation of tissue architecture.
    - Preparation: Tissues are fixed (often with formalin), embedded in paraffin or frozen, sectioned, and then stained with antibodies.

TABLE 1: Comparison of flowcytometry and immunohistochemistry.

Aspects	Flowcytometry	Immunohistochemistry (IHC)
Sample type	Single-cell suspension	Fixed tissue sections
Data	Quantitative, high-throughput	Qualitative, spatially detailed
Applications	Immune profiling, cell sorting	Tissue architecture, disease diagnosis
Throughput	High (~10,000 cells/second)	Low (manual examination)
Automation	Easily automated	Limited automation
Spatial information	Lacks spatial context	Provides spatial and subcellular context

- *Data output*
  - *Flowcytometry:*
    - Output: Provides quantitative data on individual cells, including cell counts, percentages, and intensity of fluorescence for multiple parameters simultaneously. It generates histograms or scatter plots.
    - Resolution: Can analyze thousands of cells per second and provides detailed information on cell populations.
  - *Immunohistochemistry:*
    - Output: Provides qualitative and semiquantitative data on the localization and expression levels of antigens within tissue sections. It produces visual images that show staining patterns.
    - Resolution: Provides spatial context and detailed morphology of antigen expression within tissue structures.
- *Applications*
  - *Flowcytometry:*
    - Applications: Used for analyzing and sorting individual cells based on multiple parameters. It is commonly used in immunology, hematology, oncology, and cell biology for applications such as cell counting, cell sorting, immunophenotyping, and measuring cell functions.
  - *Immunohistochemistry:*
    - Applications: Used for detecting and visualizing specific antigens within tissue sections. It is commonly used in pathology for diagnosing diseases, understanding tissue architecture, and evaluating protein expression in various cancers and other conditions.
- *Advantages and limitations*:
  - *Flowcytometry:*
    - Advantages: High-throughput analysis, quantitative data, ability to analyze multiple markers simultaneously, and the capability to sort cells
    - Limitations: Requires single-cell suspension, cannot provide spatial information, and requires specialized equipment and reagents.
  - *Immunohistochemistry:*
    - Advantages: Provides spatial context and morphological details, suitable for fixed tissue samples, and can reveal tissue-specific antigen localization.
    - Limitations: Typically less quantitative than flowcytometry, slower throughput, and may require extensive sample preparation and interpretation.

To conclude:
- Flowcytometry is ideal for detailed, quantitative analysis of individual cells in suspension, allowing for the analysis of multiple parameters in a high-throughput manner.[12,13]
- Immunohistochemistry is best suited for examining the localization and expression of specific proteins within the context of tissue architecture, providing valuable spatial information.

Both techniques can be complementary depending on the research or diagnostic needs. For example, flowcytometry might be used to identify specific cell populations, while IHC might be used to investigate the expression of markers in tissue samples.[1,2]

Q6. **What are the indications for flowcytometric testing?**

Ans: Flow cytometric testing is used for a variety of clinical and research purposes due to its ability to analyze multiple parameters of individual cells rapidly and simultaneously. Common indications for flow cytometric testing are as follows:
- *Hematologic malignancies*:
    - *Diagnosis and classification*: Identifying and classifying types of leukemia (e.g., ALL, AML, lymphomas, plasma cell disorders, and mast cell disorders based on cell surface markers and immunophenotyping)
    - *Minimal residual disease (MRD) monitoring*: Detecting residual disease after treatment to monitor for relapse.
    - *Prognostication*: Few markers are known to have prognostic significance.
- *Benign disorders*:
    - Diagnosis of PNH by detecting and quantifying PNH clones on leukocytes and RBCs.
    - *Platelet flowcytometry*: Use of CD41, CD61 and Cd42a, and Cd42b helps in diagnosing disorders such as Bernard–Soulier and Glanzmann syndromes.
    - Platelet aggregometry can also be performed by flowcytometry.
    - *OFT and EMA binding test*: OFT helps in indicating presence of HS. While EMA binding test is one of the recommended tests for diagnosing HS by measuring binding of EMA by RBCs.
    - *Immunodeficiency disorders*:
        - PIDs: Diagnosing congenital immunodeficiencies by analyzing immune cell populations, such as T cells, B cells, and NK cells, to assess immune function.
        - Acquired immunodeficiencies: Monitoring HIV/AIDS progression by evaluating CD4+ and CD8+ T cell counts and function.
    - Autoimmune diseases: Assessing immune cell subsets and activation markers to aid in the diagnosis and monitoring of autoimmune diseases such as SLE and rheumatoid arthritis.
- *Transplantation*:
    - Stem cell enumeration in hematopoietic stem cell transplantation (HSCT) is crucial for optimizing the success of the procedure, particularly by assessing the yield (number of stem cells collected) and ensuring sufficient stem cell numbers for graft engraftment. Proper enumeration of hematopoietic stem cells (HSCs) guides the transplant process by providing critical information, influencing decisions.
    - *Graft-versus-host disease (GVHD)*: Evaluating T-cell activation and other markers to monitor for GVHD following organ or stem cell transplantation.
    - *Engraftment monitoring*: Assessing donor cell engraftment and chimerism in stem cell or bone marrow transplant patients.
- *Infection monitoring*:
    - *Viral infections*: Evaluating immune responses and monitoring infection progression, such as in HIV or viral hepatitis, by analyzing immune cell subsets.
    - *Fungal and bacterial infections*: Identifying and quantifying pathogens and assessing immune responses to infections.
- *Quantitative and functional analysis*:
    - *Cell cycle analysis*: Assessing cell cycle stages and proliferation rates using specific dyes or markers.
    - *Functional assays*: Measuring cellular functions such as intracellular calcium levels, cytokine production, or oxidative burst activity.

- *High-throughput screening for drug discovery*: Evaluating large numbers of cells in drug development and screening assays to assess the effects of compounds on cell populations.
- *Vaccine development and monitoring*: Flowcytometry can measure the activation and differentiation of immune cells (especially T cells and B cells) in response to vaccination. Assessing the immune response to vaccines by analyzing specific immune cell subsets and markers helps in its development.
- *Cancer research and diagnostics*: Flowcytometry aids in identifying and validating biomarkers for various cancers, assisting in both diagnosis and therapeutic development. Isolating specific cell populations by sorting for further research in cancer biology.

Flowcytometry is a versatile tool with a broad range of applications. Its ability to provide detailed, multiparameter analysis of individual cells makes it invaluable in diagnosing diseases, monitoring disease progression, evaluating treatment efficacy, and conducting research across various fields including oncology, immunology, and infectious diseases.[9,11,14]

Q7. What is the role of quality control in flowcytometric immunophenotypic testing?

Ans: Quality control (QC) is crucial in flow cytometric immunophenotypic testing to ensure the accuracy, reliability, and consistency of the results. Effective QC practices help maintain the integrity of the data and are essential for accurate diagnosis and research findings. Here are the key roles of QC in flow cytometric immunophenotypic testing:

- *Instrument calibration and performance monitoring*:
  - *Calibration of the flow cytometer*: QC includes regular calibration of the flow cytometer and daily QC checks example by running C and ST beads (cytometer set-up and tracking beads are used to define the baseline performance of the cytometer) or reference samples to ensure that the detectors and optics are properly aligned, which is essential for the accuracy of fluorescence measurements.
  - *Laser and detector performance*: Regular monitoring of laser intensity and detector sensitivity is necessary to ensure consistent performance. Drift in laser intensity or detector malfunction can lead to inaccurate fluorescence measurements.
  - *Fluorescence calibration*: Using calibration beads that are fluorescently labeled with known intensities helps validate that the flow cytometer is accurately detecting and distinguishing between different fluorochromes.
- *Reagent and antibody quality*:
  - *Antibody titration*: Ensuring the proper titration of antibodies is essential to prevent over-saturation or undersaturation of cell markers, which can distort the results. Antibody titration should be checked as part of QC to verify that each antibody is used within its optimal concentration range.
  - *Antibody lot-to-lot consistency*: QC includes confirming that antibodies from different lots perform consistently and provide the same staining patterns, ensuring that there are no discrepancies between different batches of reagents.
  - *Reagent stability*: QC also monitors the storage conditions and expiration dates of reagents (antibodies, dyes, and buffers) to ensure they remain effective and stable over time.
- *Sample handling and preparation*:
  - *Cell viability*: QC checks cell viability to ensure that the cells used in the immunophenotypic analysis are alive and not affected by poor sample handling, such as cell aggregation or lysis. Viable cells ensure reliable results.

- *Sample preparation standardization*: QC ensures that samples are prepared according to standardized protocols, including appropriate fixation, permeabilization, and staining procedures, which helps eliminate variability that could affect staining patterns and analysis.
- *Compensation and fluorescence spillover*:
  - *Compensation for fluorescence spillover*: QC involves setting up and checking compensation controls to correct for spectral overlap between different fluorochromes. Without proper compensation, fluorescence signals from different channels may overlap, leading to incorrect identification of cell populations.
  - *Bead controls for compensation*: Use of compensation beads with known fluorescence intensities is part of the QC process to verify and correct for spectral overlap.
- *Gating strategy and data analysis*:
  - *Gating consistency*: QC ensures that the gating strategy used for analysis is consistent and accurate. Consistent gating helps ensure that the correct populations of cells are being analyzed, reducing the risk of misidentification or data interpretation errors.
  - *Reproducibility of results*: QC includes checking for the reproducibility of results between different runs and operators. This is achieved by comparing the results from different instruments, different days, or different personnel to ensure that the flowcytometry data is stable and reliable.
  - *Data review*: QC ensures that the data analysis process is standardized, including the setting of thresholds for positive and negative populations and the evaluation of scatter plots and histograms to check for any abnormalities in the data.
- *Control samples and reference data*:
  - *Use of control samples*: Negative control and positive control samples are integral to QC. These controls help verify the performance of the staining panel and antibodies, ensuring that the expected patterns are seen in known populations.
    - Negative controls are used to ensure there is no nonspecific binding of antibodies.
    - Positive controls are used to confirm that the flow cytometer can detect the target antigen effectively.
  - *Reference data*: QC includes comparison with established reference data or normative ranges for immunophenotypic testing to ensure the accuracy of the results and to detect potential anomalies.
- *Operator training and proficiency*:
  - *Standard operating procedures (SOPs)*: QC requires that all operators adhere to established SOPs for flow cytometric analysis. This ensures uniformity and reduces human error.
  - *Operator proficiency testing*: Operators must be trained and proficient in handling the flow cytometer, preparing samples, performing staining, and analyzing data. Regular proficiency tests and performance reviews help maintain high-quality results.
- *Troubleshooting and error detection*: QC processes help in identifying potential errors or problems early. These can include issues like clogging of the flow cytometer, instrument drift, or incorrect reagent concentrations, and prompt corrective action can be taken to avoid the generation of unreliable data.
- *Documentation and traceability*: Record keeping—QC requires thorough documentation of all procedures, reagents, instrument calibrations, and QC checks. This ensures traceability and helps in identifying any inconsistencies or issues that may arise in the future.

- *EQUAS (external quality assurance programs)*: Regular participation in EQUAS [conducted by College of American Pathologists (CAP) or chimera in India] leads to harmonization of different labs and ensures that flow cytometric testing yields consistent results across different laboratories and settings, enhancing the reliability of reports, multicenter studies, and collaborations.

Quality control in flow cytometric immunophenotypic testing plays a vital role in ensuring the accuracy, reliability, and consistency of the results. By maintaining rigorous QC practices, laboratories can deliver high-quality data for clinical diagnosis and research, ultimately leading to more accurate patient outcomes and scientific discoveries.[15,16]

Q8. What reagent and panel optimization is needed for flowcytometry?

Ans: Optimizing reagents and panels in flowcytometry is essential for ensuring accurate, reproducible, and efficient results, especially in complex immunophenotyping, biomarker analysis, and other applications.[17]
- *Reagent optimization*:
  - *Antibody selection and titration:*
    - Antibody selection: Choosing appropriate antibodies is crucial for detecting the markers of interest on cells. These antibodies should:
      - Be specific for the target antigen without cross-reactivity.
      - Be validated for use in flowcytometry applications.
      - Be compatible with the fluorochromes used in the experiment.
      - Be directly conjugated to fluorochromes (fluorochrome-conjugated antibodies) to reduce background staining.
    - Antibody titration: Titrating antibodies is essential to find the optimal concentration to maximize signal without saturating the antigen-binding sites. Over-concentration can cause nonspecific binding, while under-concentration may result in insufficient staining.
  - *Fluorochrome selection:*
    - Fluorochrome compatibility: When designing a multicolor panel, it is essential to select fluorochromes with distinct emission spectra to minimize spectral overlap. Overlap can lead to incorrect compensation, which can distort the results.
    - Brightness of fluorochromes: The choice of fluorochrome should match the abundance of the antigen being detected. Rare antigens require bright fluorochromes, while more abundant antigens can be detected with dimmer fluorochromes.
    - Spectral overlap: Minimize spectral overlap between channels by selecting fluorochromes that are spectrally distinct and can be accurately compensated.
  - *Fixation and permeabilization:*
    - Fixation: Fixing cells ensures that the markers remain stable for analysis. Common fixatives include paraformaldehyde (PFA) or methanol, but fixation must be optimized to prevent loss of antigen expression or altered cell morphology. Fixative choice—for surface markers, PFA is commonly used, whereas methanol or acetone is used for intracellular markers (after permeabilization).
    - Permeabilization: To stain intracellular markers, cells need to be permeabilized. The permeabilization protocol should be optimized depending on the target antigen and cell type. Common agents include saponin, Triton X-100, and methanol. Remember overpermeabilization may disrupt the cell structure, while underpermeabilization may prevent antibody binding.

- *Buffers and blocking agents:*
  - Buffer selection: The choice of buffers is critical for minimizing nonspecific binding and maintaining cell integrity during staining. Common buffers include phosphate-buffered saline (PBS) or FACS buffer (PBS with 2% FBS).
  - Blocking: Blocking agents (e.g., human IgG, BSA, or serum proteins) can help reduce nonspecific antibody binding, which is essential for improving the specificity of staining.
  - Viability dyes: In some applications, the use of viability dyes (e.g., 7-AAD, DAPI, or propidium Iodide) is important to exclude dead cells from analysis.
- Panel optimization:
  - *Marker selection:*
    - Target markers: The first step in panel optimization is to carefully select cell surface or intracellular markers that define the specific populations you wish to analyze. Common markers include CD3, CD4, CD8, CD19, and CD56, but these vary depending on the research or clinical application.
    - Specificity and sensitivity: Choose markers that are highly specific for the population of interest to avoid cross-reactivity or misclassification of cells.
    - Redundancy: Avoid using markers that are highly redundant, as this can complicate the analysis and increase reagent consumption.
  - *Panel complexity and fluorochrome selection:*
    - Designing multicolor panels: The number of colors used in a flowcytometry experiment can range from 2 to 30 or more.[17] When designing multicolor panels, select fluorochromes that are:
      - Distinct in emission spectra
      - Bright enough to detect dim populations
      - Compatible with each other to minimize spectral overlap
    - Spectral flowcytometry: Newer spectral flow cytometers allow the detection of more than 30 parameters simultaneously. In such cases, fluorochrome selection should be based on their emission spectra, with compensation minimized by using spectral compensation algorithms.
    - Fluorescence minus one (FMO) controls: To fine-tune gating strategies and set compensation, FMO controls are essential. They help determine the exact contribution of each fluorochrome to the overall signal.
    - Compensation: Compensation for spectral overlap—compensation ensures that fluorescence from one channel does not spill over into another. This is crucial when using multiple fluorochromes in a panel. Proper compensation can be achieved through:
      - Single-stained control samples
      - Compensation beads with specific fluorochrome labels
    - Bead-based compensation: Compensation beads are often used for more accurate compensation, especially in multicolor flowcytometry.
    - Optimization of panel reproducibility:
      - Control samples: Always include appropriate control samples such as negative controls, positive controls, and isotype controls to ensure that staining is specific and to correct for any potential artifacts.

- Validation: Before finalizing a flowcytometry panel, perform extensive validation by testing different biological samples to confirm the accuracy and consistency of the results.
- Reproducibility: Ensure that the optimized panel can be reliably reproduced across different days, instruments, and operators by running the panel on different samples and comparing the results.

Conclusion

Reagent and panel optimization in flowcytometry is essential for obtaining reliable and reproducible data. Key strategies include selecting and titrating appropriate antibodies, choosing compatible fluorochromes, optimizing fixation and permeabilization protocols, and designing efficient and reproducible multicolor panels. Ensuring that these factors are carefully optimized will lead to more accurate immunophenotyping and biomarker analysis.[18-20]

REFERENCES

1. Shapiro HM. Practical Flow Cytometry. New Jersey, United States: John Wiley & Sons; 2003.
2. Herzenberg LA, Parks D, Sahaf B, Perez O, Roederer M, Herzenberg LA. The history and future of the fluorescence-activated cell sorter and flow cytometry. Clin Chem. 2002;48(10):1819-27.
3. Perfetto SP, Maecker HT. Flow cytometry: A practical approach. Oxford, United Kingdom: Oxford University Press; 2006.
4. Nolan JP, Condello D. Spectral flow cytometry. Curr Protoc Cytom. 2013;63(1):1-10.
5. Basiji DA, Ortyn WE, Liang L, Venkatachalam V, Morrissey P. Cellular image analysis and imaging by flow cytometry. Clin Lab Med. 2007;27(3):653-70.
6. Bandura DR, et al. Mass cytometry: Technique for real-time mass analysis of single cells. Journal of Analytical Atomic Spectrometry. 2009;24(2):239-45.
7. Goddard G, Mariampillai A. Acoustic focusing flow cytometer: design, operation, and applications. Cytometry Part A. 2011;79:107-17.
8. Dittrich PS, Manz A. Lab-on-a-chip: microfluidics in drug discovery. Nat Rev Drug Discov. 2006;5(3):210-8.
9. Arber DA, et al. The 2016 revision to the World Health Organization classification of lymphoid neoplasms. Hematol Oncol. 2016;34(4):230-9.
10. Tretter T, et al. T cells and autoimmunity. J Immunol. 2007;179:1-6.
11. Miedema F, Miedema K. HIV and the immune system. Clin Immunol. 2007;123(2):131-9.
12. Timm D, Zerfas BL. Comparison of flow cytometry and immunohistochemistry. Cytometry Part A. 2017; 91(3):245–250.
13. Shankey TV, Nunes EA. Flow cytometry in the diagnosis and classification of hematologic malignancies. Cancer J. 2007;13(2):101-13.
14. Harris LJ, et al. Flow cytometry for stem cell enumeration and monitoring stem cell therapy. Stem Cells and Cloning: Advances and Applications. 2005;1(1):1-10.
15. Van der Velden VH, et al. Flow cytometric immunophenotyping for the diagnosis and monitoring of hematologic malignancies: Quality control and challenges. Leukemia Res. 2014;38(3):258-70.
16. Mayer C, et al. Quality control in flow cytometry: Understanding errors and their impact on clinical results. J Clin Lab Analysis. 2013;27(5):362-74.
17. McDonald T, et al. Designing and optimizing multi-color flow cytometry panels for immunophenotyping. FrontImmunol. 2017;8:60.
18. Loken MR, et al. Compensation and the interpretation of multi-color flow cytometry data. Meth Cell Biol. 1999;57:359-80.
19. Osborne EM, et al. Flow cytometry analysis of human immune cells: optimization, validation, and troubleshooting. J Clin Lab Analysis. 2004;18(6):267-77.
20. Gonzalez M, et al. Optimization of sample preparation and staining in flow cytometry for cell analysis. Meth Mole Biol. 2017;1478:43-56.

16. Cytogenetics

Vandana Puri, Tanvi Gupta

Q1. What is cytogenetics?

Ans: Cytogenetics is the study of number, structure, and function of chromosomes within cells, in tissue samples, blood, or bone marrow (BM) samples. It plays a central role in the diagnosis, risk stratification, treatment selection, and disease monitoring in hematological malignancies as it gives a glance to whole genome at once.

Q2. What are the different types of cytogenetic techniques?

Ans: Cytogenetics techniques are broadly categorized into conventional and molecular cytogenetics.

Conventional cytogenetics	Molecular cytogenetics
Karyotyping	• FISH • Chromosomal microarray • Optical genome mapping

Karyotyping: Chromosomal analysis has been the gold standard for cytogenetic studies, which involves visualization of metaphases stained to reveal characteristic banding patterns, under a microscope. It permits single-cell and genome-wide analysis of chromosomal alterations, though at a limited resolution.

Fluorescence in situ hybridization (FISH): FISH represents the methodology to detect specific nucleotide sequences by using fluorescently labeled DNA probes that will hybridize with specific chromosome regions, allowing detection of genetic abnormalities.

Chromosomal microarray (CMA): Microarrays detect submicroscopic chromosomal imbalances, including copy number variations (CNVs) and loss of heterozygosity (LOH).

Optical genome mapping (OGM): OGM is an emerging next-generation cytogenomic approach, offering comprehensive, high-resolution detection of structural genome variation in a single assay. The technology is based on imaging ultra-long (>150 kbp) DNA molecules labeled at a specific 6 bp sequence motif (CTTAAG).

TABLE 1: Comparison of different cytogenetic techniques.

	Karyotyping	FISH	CMA	OGM
Analyte	Metaphase	DNA in interphase	DNA	DNA
Genome coverage	Whole	Targeted	Whole	Whole
Distinction b/w cell clones	Yes	Yes	No	No
Turn around time (TAT)	4–7 days (depends on sample type and indication)	4 hours to 4 days	3–7 days	7–10 days
Resolution	5–10 Mb	100 kb	<50 kb	~0.5–5 kb (SVs), ~500 kb (CNVs)
Sensitivity	2–3 out of 20 metaphases	1–10%	10–20%	5–20%
Abnormalities detected	Aneuploidies, large structural changes	Specific sequences, microdeletions, gene amplifications	Submicroscopic imbalances, CNVs, LOH detection	Balanced and unbalanced SVs (insertions, deletions, inversions, translocations), CNVs, aneuploidies

(CNVs: copy number variations, LOH: loss of heterozygosity; SVs: structural variations)

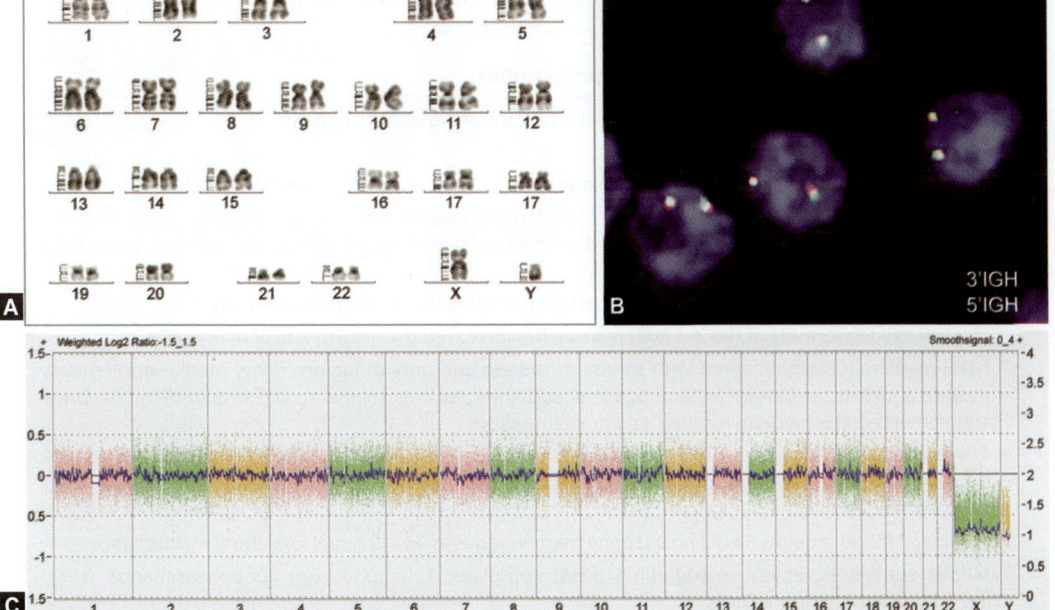

FIGS. 1A TO C: (A) GTG-banded karyogram of a normal male (46,XY) derived from a bone marrow specimen. (B). Interphase FISH analysis showing normal signal pattern (2 Fusion) for *IGH* gene using a break apart probe, (3′ end of IGH gene: red signal and 5′ end of IGH gene: green signal) (C) SNP array in a normal male: Data is shown in whole genome view (WGV) and expressed as the weighted log2 ratio of the copy number on the left Y-axis (blue line), and the chromosome number on the X-axis.

CHAPTER 16: Cytogenetics

Q3. **What are the preferred samples for cytogenetics in hematology?**

Ans: Samples for cytogenetics in hematology include:
- Bone marrow
- Peripheral blood
- Fresh tissue (lymph node, spleen, and extranodal tumorous infiltrate)
- Effusion and cerebrospinal fluid
  The tissue of choice should be where the disease is most expressed **(Table 2)**.

TABLE 2: Samples for cytogenetics.

Source of preferred sample	Condition
Peripheral blood	Lymphoproliferative disorders, such as chronic lymphocytic leukemia (CLL)
Bone marrow	• Myeloproliferative neoplasms (MPN) • Myelodysplastic neoplasms (MDS) • Acute leukemias
Bone marrow enriched 138 positive cells	Myeloma
Lymph nodes or affected primary sites	Lymphomas

Q4. **How are cytogenetic studies especially karyotyping and FISH done?**

Ans: The first step in conventional cytogenetics is the requirement of chromosomes in metaphase **(Box 1)**. For this, the culture of the chromosomes is required. Culture technique depends on the sample taken [peripheral blood (PB), BM, amniotic fluid, etc.].

BOX 1A: Method of conventional cytogenetic studies.

- *Collection of blood*: Blood is collected in a sterile tube containing sodium heparin
- *Separation and culture*:
  - Maintaining a strict aseptic culturing technique is important as microbes may lead to failure
  - Cultures may be incubated in an open or closed system. Open cultures can exchange gases with the atmosphere surrounding the culture. Closed systems are sealed tightly and do not exchange gases with the atmosphere
  - The 5% CO_2 adjusts the culture medium to pH 7.25–7.40 via the buffer in the medium
  - The low oxygen formula of the 2–5% O_2 mixture has increased the growth rate of many cell types
  - Basal medium is supplemented with serum for protein and growth factors. Other media supplements include antibiotics, l-glutamine, and optional additions, such as selenium, and insulin medium. Once supplemented, the medium is called a complete medium
  - Cultures that are valuable or may be needed for future use may be frozen in medium with 5–10% dimethyl sulfoxide (DMSO) or glycerol to prevent ice crystal formation and kept in liquid nitrogen until they are needed
  - Peripheral blood requires 69–72 hours, bone marrow requires 16–18 hours for culture maintenance
  - Mitotic stimulants: Phytohemagglutinin (PHA) stimulates T lymphocytes; lipopolysaccharide (LPS), IL-2 stimulates B lymphoid cells
- *Harvest procedures*:
  - The first step in most harvest procedures is to arrest cells in metaphase which is done using colcemid
  - The second major step in harvesting cells is treatment with a hypotonic saline solution (10–20 minutes) to increase cell volume so that the chromosomes have adequate space to spread out during slide preparation concentration of 0.075 M (0.56%) is commonly used

Continued

CHAPTER 16: Cytogenetics

Continued

- ○ The third constant feature of chromosome harvesting is the fixation of the cells. Fixation is done with a 3:1 ratio of methanol and glacial acetic acid
- **Steps of banding**:
  - ○ The chromosomes are spread out, fixed, banded and stained using GTG banding (G banding by trypsin using Giemsa) allow examination with a microscope
  - ○ The cells are then photographed and arranged into a karyotype (an ordered set of chromosomes)
  - ○ The karyotype will show the chromosomes of an individual arranged in pairs and sorted according to size and centromere position
- **Analysis**:
  - ○ Routine chromosome analysis refers to the analysis of chromosomes that have been banded using trypsin (a serine protease) followed by Giemsa staining
  - ○ This creates a unique banding pattern on the chromosomes
  - ○ Generally, 20 cells are analyzed to rule out chromosome abnormalities

---

BOX 1B: Wet lab procedure of FISH studies.

An overview of the FISH procedure on a PB or a BM sample, for hematologic neoplasms analyses:

1. *Sample collection and harvesting*:
   - Approximately 1–2 mL bone marrow or PB sample is collected into a sodium heparin tube
   - Cells are exposed to a hypotonic solution and then fixed using modified Carnoy's fixative (Methanol: acetic acid 3:1)
   - Plasma-cell enrichment is desirable in MM cases to enhance test sensitivity

2. *Slide preparation*:
   - Spread a thin layer of sample on a slide and allow to air-dry
   - Treat with methanol-acetic acid (3:1) fixative to preserve cell morphology and DNA

3. *Pretreatment*:
   - *Dehydration*: Pass slides through graded ethanol (70%, 85%, 100%) and air-dry
   - *Digestion*: Apply enzyme (e.g., pepsin) to remove proteins and improve probe access

4. *Probe addition and hybridization*:
   - Add fluorescently labeled DNA probes targeting specific genes or loci [e.g., 1p/1q, del(17p), IGH translocations]
   - Denaturation of DNA strands of is done by heating the slides at approximately 75°C for 5 minutes
   - Incubate the slides in a hybridizer (humid chamber) at approximately 37°C, typically overnight.

5. *Post-hybridization washes*:
   - Remove nonspecifically bound probes using a series of washes—stringency adjusted by temperature and salt conditions
   - Counterstain (e.g., DAPI) to visualize nuclei

6. *Microscopy and analysis*:
   - Examine slides under a fluorescence microscope with appropriate filters
   - 200 interphase nuclei are analyzed for signal pattern and compared to established cut-offs to confirm positive or negative status for each probe

7. *Reporting*: Numbers of signals per cell and percentage of abnormal cells are compared against lab-specific thresholds

Q5. Are cytogenetic studies still relevant in the era of molecular diagnostics?

Ans: Cytogenetic information in hematologic conditions is crucial to clinicians for diagnosis, risk stratification, and prognosis; hence, chromosomal analysis is performed in almost all cases of leukemias, myelodysplastic neoplasms (MDS), and lymphomas. Dedicated risk stratification systems are based on cytogenetic anomalies in AML and MDS.

FISH is the cornerstone for detecting prognostically significant genetic aberrations in chronic lymphocytic leukemia (CLL) and multiple myeloma. In MM, CD138+ cell selection greatly enhances FISH detection sensitivity. Enrichment also improves detection of key high-risk abnormalities like t(4;14), del(17p), amp(1q), and IgH translocations, directly influencing treatment. In CLL, interphase FISH on peripheral blood or bone marrow rapidly identifies key aberrations—del(13q), +12, del(11q), and del(17p)—that stratify patients into different risk groups.

While the clinical utility of molecular techniques e.g., NGS is undeniable, chromosome banding and FISH with SNP array integration will likely continue to serve as the gold standard of cytogenetic testing for hematologic malignancies.[1,2]

This is not true of solid tumors, in which the specimens are often fixed before a small portion is obtained for chromosome analysis. With increasing appreciation of the value of chromosome findings in epithelial tumors, fresh frozen tissue must be sent for cytogenetic analysis.

Q6. What are the pitfalls in the cytogenetic evaluation? (already described in Q2.)

Ans: Cytogenetic evaluation is a cornerstone in diagnosing and prognosticating hematological disorders, however, there are inherent limitations that can impact the accuracy of results. To ensure comprehensive assessment and optimal patient care, it is imperative to integrate complementary hematological and molecular techniques, whenever required **(Table 3)**.

TABLE 3: Description of limitations of various cytogenetic techniques.

Limitation or pitfall	Description
Culture failure	Insufficient or hemodiluted BM samples can lead to suboptimal metaphase yield, thereby inconclusive results
Limited resolution	Conventional cytogenetics detects abnormalities ≥5–10 Mb; so, smaller structural variations or cryptic aberrations may be missed
Targeted approach	FISH analysis is abnormality specific, therefore cannot identify aberrations in regions not targeted by the probes used
Interpretation challenges	Chromosomal analysis requires specialized expertise, particularly when dealing with metaphases exhibiting poor morphology and complex rearrangements
Inability to detect balanced rearrangements	Balanced structural abnormalities e.g., translocations and inversions cannot be detected by CMA

TABLE 4: Comparison of cytogenetic evaluation.

Technique	Conventional cytogenetics	Fluorescence in situ hybridization	Microarray
Sample required	Fresh sample	Cells in fixative solution	DNA
Resolution	>10 Mb	>100 Kb	>15 Kb
Genome view	Whole genome	Locus specific	Whole genome
Limitations	*Poor results:* • Low cell growth • Normal metaphases • Poor quality of chromosomes • Presence of cryptic aberrations	Only known mutation can be detected	No detection of balanced translocations
Lab hands-on/analysis	3/1 hour	30/15 minutes	3–5 days/1–2 hours

Q7. What is the role of cytogenetics in myelodysplastic neoplasms?

Ans: Diagnostic evaluation of MDS should always include microscopic examination of adequate BM and PB smears, coupled with chromosome analysis, mutation analysis, and immunophenotypic evaluation by multiparameter flow cytometry.[1]

Acquired cytogenetic aberrations are detected in approximately 45% of patients with MDS and are well established as independent prognostic factors in MDS **(Table 4)**.

According to recent WHO classification of MDS hematolymphoid tumors, MDS entities are grouped into two families: (1) those with defining genetic abnormalities and (2) those that are morphologically defined.

The MDSs with defining genetic abnormalities are now grouped together and comprise MDS-5q, MDS with low blasts and *SF3B1* **mutation (MDS-***SF3B1***), and MDS with biallelic *TP53* inactivation. This last diagnosis supersedes MDS-5q and MDS-***SF3B1***.** The qualifier "low blasts" has been added to MDS-5q and MDS-*SF3B1* **for clarity**.[2]

TABLE 5: Myelodysplastic neoplasms (MDS) with defining genetic abnormalities.

MDS subtype	Cytogenetics
MDS with low blasts and 5q deletion	5q deletion alone, or with one other abnormality other than monosomy 7 or 7q deletion
MDS with low blasts and SF3B1 mutation	Absence of 5q deletion, monosomy 7, or complex karyotype
MDS with biallelic TP53 inactivation	Usually complex

The diagnostic criteria for MDS-5q have not changed and require conventional cytogenetics for diagnosis.

Therefore, studying the karyotype at diagnosis is essential to:
- Confirm clonality.
- Classify patients according to the WHO-defined MDS subgroups.

- Stratify patients according to their prognosis, which will determine the most suitable treatment.
- Cytogenetic risk classification has the strongest prognostic impact in the Revised International Prognostic Scoring System (IPSS-R) for MDS.

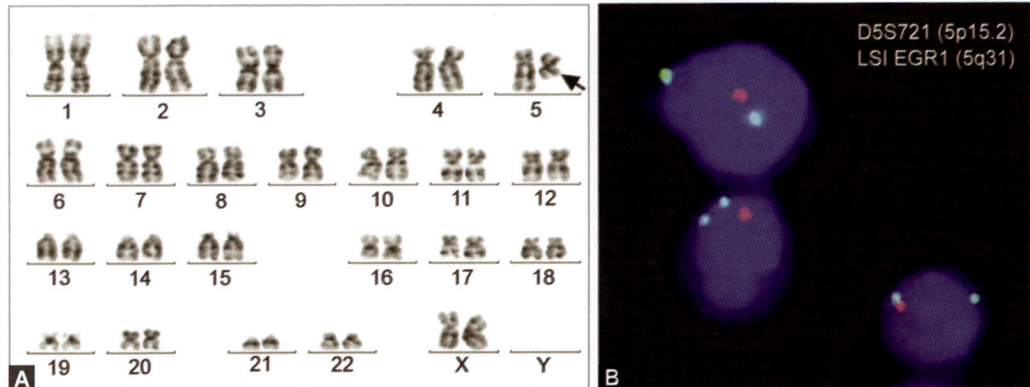

FIGS. 2A AND B: (A) GTG banded karyogram showing deletion 5q (arrow) (B) Interphase FISH analysis showing abnormal signal pattern (1 red 2 green) indicating deletion 5q, (5p15.2: green signal 5q31: red signal).

Q8. What is the role of cytogenetics in acute myeloid leukemia?

Ans: Acute myeloid leukemia (AML) is a genetically diverse hematological disorder. The detection of cytogenetic and molecular alterations is fundamental to diagnosis, risk stratification and treatment of AML. WHO focuses on AML by classifying them on the basis of cytogenetic and molecular genetic subgroups. Conventional cytogenetic studies (karyotyping) are used to detect large (5-10 MB) structural and numerical abnormalities, which are identified in approximately 50-60% of adult patients and approximately 70-80% of pediatric cases of AML.[4] Approx 20-25% of pediatric AML and 40-50% of adult AML have a normal karyotype as do not harbour any clonal cytogenetic abnormalities. In some instances, it can be cryptic abnormality which needs further analysis either by FISH or molecular testing e.g., inv(16(p13q24), t(5;11) (q35;p15). While many of these cytogenetically normal AML cases harbour clonal mutations that are prognostically significant e.g., NPM1, CEBPA, FLT3D, IDH1/2 etc. Conventional cytogenetic analysis is mandatory in the evaluation of AML. If conventional cytogenetics fails, FISH is an alternative to detect specific abnormalities like RUNX1::RUNX1T1, CBFB::MYH11, KMT2A (MLL), and MECOM (EVI1) gene fusions, or myelodysplasia-related chromosome abnormalities, e.g., deletion 5q, 7q, or 17p.[3]

Unbalanced clonal abnormalities: del(5q)/t(5q)/add(5q); 27/del(7q); 18; del(12p)/t(12p)/(add)(12p); i(17q), 217/add(17p) or del(17p); del(20q); and/or idic(X)(q13) are defined as myelodysplasia defining entities. AML with myelodysplasia-related cytogenetic abnormality is a defined entity.[3]

Complex karyotype is defined as ≥3 unrelated chromosome abnormalities in the absence of other class-defining recurring genetic abnormalities; excludes hyperdiploid karyotypes with three or more trisomies (or polysomes) without structural abnormalities. It is considered an adverse prognostic factor.

Monosomal karyotype, defined by the presence of two or more distinct autosomal chromosome monosomies or one single autosomal monosomy in the presence of structural abnormalities, has been identified as a poor prognostic factor independently of complexity.[4]

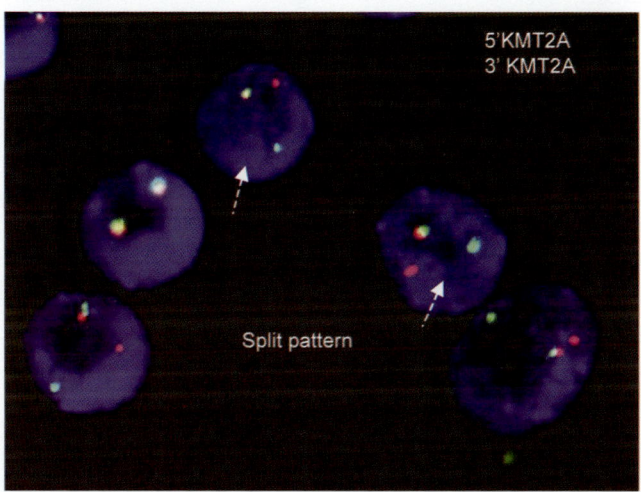

FIG. 3A: Interphase FISH analysis showing abnormal signal pattern (1 red 1 green 1 fusion) for *KMT2A* gene rearrangement using a break apart probe. (5' end of *KMT2A* gene: Red signal and 3' end of *KMT2A* gene: Green signal).

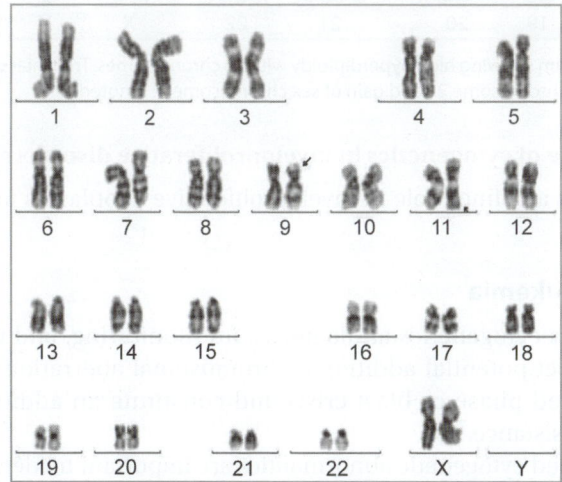

FIG. 3B: GTG banded karyogram showing a balanced translocation between chromosomes 9 and 11 at band levels 9p21 and 11q23, leading to KMT2A gene rearrangement.

Q9. **What is the role of cytogenetics in acute lymphoblastic leukemia?**

Ans: Cytogenetic abnormalities are seen in >75% of B-acute lymphoblastic leukemia (B-ALL) and they usually define specific entities. Cytogenetic abnormalities in B-ALL can be divided into two main groups according to their risk.
1. *Good risk*: t(12;21)(p13;q22) and the high hyperdiploidy karyotype, accounting for 50% of pediatric B-ALL (1–10 years old).
2. *High risk*: t(9;22)(q34;q11.2) (20–30% in adults), low hypodiploidy/near haploidy (6% in any age group), complex intrachromosomal amplification of chromosome 21 (iAMP21) (mainly affecting older children), t(17;19) (q22;p13) (1% in childhood), and *KMT2A* translocations [t(11q23;v)] (80% in the newborns and 13% in adults)].[5]

Recent cytogenetic classifications lack information in up to 50% of patients with ALL due to the low incidence of some aberrations that are beyond the resolution of cytogenetics, such as gene microdeletions, e.g., PAX,IKZF1, and abnormalities such as Ph-like ALL. These alterations carry prognostic impact and should be detected using higher-resolution technologies.[6]

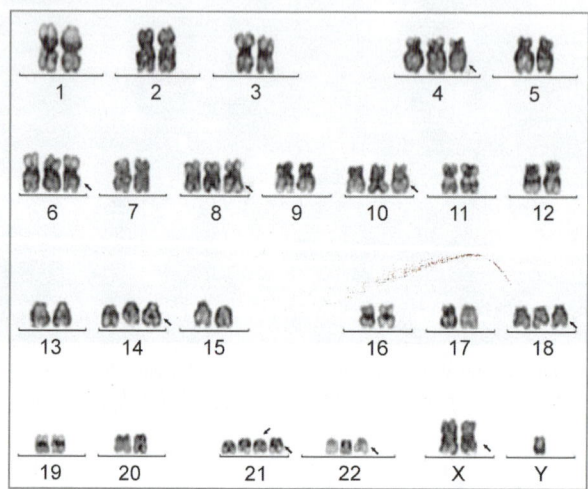

FIG. 4: GTG banded karyogram showing high hyperdiploidy with 56 chromosomes. Trisomies of chromosomes 4, 6, 8, 10, 14, 18 and 22, tetrasomy of chromosome 21 and gain of sex chromosome, X is noted.

Q10. What is the role of cytogenetics in myeloproliferative disorders?

Ans: Cytogenetics has a defined role in myeloproliferative neoplasms for diagnosis and risk stratifications.

Chronic Myeloid Leukemia

The ELN recommends cytogenetics at diagnosis, for monitoring, and whenever treatment failure occurs to detect potential additional chromosomal aberrations (ACAs). ACAs can indicate an accelerated phase or blast crisis and constitute an additional risk factor for treatment failure or resistance.[7]

The WHO has defined cytogenetic abnormalities are important to identify chronic myeloid leukemia (CML) at increased risk of disease progression **(Box 2)**.[2]

According to ELN, the following abnormalities have been proposed as high-risk ACA—trisomy 8 (+8), a second or extra copies of Ph-chromosome (+Ph), i(17q), trisomy (+19), monosomy or deletion of chromosome 7 (−7/7q-), 11q23 or 3q26.2 aberrations, and complex aberrant karyotypes.

Response monitoring in CML: Cytogenetics, by BM cell metaphases, may be useful when performed, but alone is not sufficiently sensitive to monitor response. However, cytogenetics should be done in patients with atypical translocations, rare, or atypical BCR-ABL1 transcripts that cannot be measured by quantitative polymerase chain reaction (qPCR), in patients with treatment failure/resistance to exclude ACA, and with progression to blast phase.[8]

Cytogenetics should be performed every 3 months, until the Ph' chromosome clone is not detected. Karyotyping analysis should then still be performed once a year, since the presence of other chromosomal alterations in negative Ph clones has been described in 5-10% of CML cases. These secondary abnormalities do not have a poor prognosis if dysplasia is not observed, except abnormalities of chromosome 7, which have been described in cases with MDS with risk of transformation to acute leukemia.

> **BOX 2: Features in chronic-phase chronic myeloid leukemia associated with an increased risk of disease progression.**
>
> *At diagnosis*:
> - ≥ 10% blasts in peripheral blood and/or bone marrow
> - ≥ 20% basophils in peripheral blood
> - Additional chromosomal abnormalities in Ph+ cells include the following: 3q26.2 rearrangements, monosomy 7, trisomy 8, 11q23 rearrangements, isochromosome 17q, trisomy 19, trisomy 21, additional Ph chromosome, and/or complex karyotype
>
> *Emerging on treatment*:
> - Resistance to tyrosine kinase inhibitors (TKIs) as defined by the European LeukemiaNet (ELN) in 2020
> - Emergence of additional chromosomal abnormalities
> - BCR::ABL1 kinase domain mutations

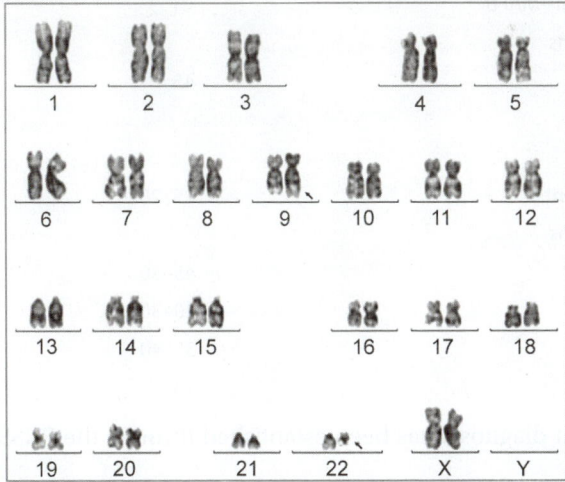

FIG. 5: GTG banded karyogram showing a balanced translocation between the long arms of chromosomes 9 and 22 at band levels q34 and q11.2 respectively, resulting in the formation of Philadelphia chromosome i.e., derivative 22.

Primary Myelofibrosis

Altered karyotype is seen in 30-45% of patients with primary myelofibrosis (PMF). Presence of either del(13)(q12-22) or der(6)t(1;6)(q21-q23;p21.3) is strongly suggestive of PMF. Der(6)t(1;6)(q21-23;p21.3) is a highly specific cytogenetic anomaly that may harbor gene(s) specifically associated with myelofibrosis with myeloid metaplasia.[9]

Cytogenetic abnormalities play an important role in establishing the prognostic impact of patients with PMF, as evidenced in the Genetically Inspired Prognostic Scoring System (GIPSS) for PMF, being based exclusively on genetic (cytogenetic and molecular) markers.

Q 11. What is the role of cytogenetics in multiple myeloma?

Ans: Cytogenetic abnormalities can be detected much more efficiently by the FISH technique (>90% cases) when compared to the conventional cytogenetics in MM (approximately in one-third cases); as plasma cells have low proliferative activity and are limited in number in the bone marrow. FISH plays a pivotal role in the risk stratification of multiple myeloma (MM), especially when combined with CD138-based plasma cell enrichment. Cytogenetic abnormalities are both numerical and structural abnormalities and include trisomies, partial or whole chromosome deletions, gain or amplification and translocations.

TABLE 6: Major cytogenetic abnormalities with their relative frequency in multiple myeloma.

Cytogenetic abnormalities	Frequency in newly diagnosed MM (%)
Primary events	
• IGH translocations	
○ t(11;14)(q13;q32)/IGH-CCND1	20
○ t(4;14)(p16;q32)/IGH-MMSET/FGFR3	10
○ t(14;16)(q32;q23)/IGH-MAF	4
○ t(6;14)(p21;q32)/IGH-CCND3	5
○ t(14;20)(q32;q12)/IGH-MAFB	<1
• Copy number variations	
○ Hyperdiploidy	45
Secondary events	
• Translocation	
○ c-MYC rearrangements	15–20
• Copy number variations	
○ 13q deletion	45–50
○ 1p deletion	20–30
○ 1q gain/amp	35–40
○ 17p deletion	10

Prognosis in MM at diagnosis has been established through the R-ISS and the IMWG risk stratification model.

TABLE 7: mSMART 4.0: Classification of active MM cytogenetic risk stratification.

High risk cytogenetic abnormalities	Standard risk cytogenetic abnormalities
• Del17p and/or TP53 mutation	MM with no HR abnormalities including isolated:
• Bi-allelic del 1p	• Trisomies
• t(4;14),t(14;16), or t(14;20) plus either Gain/Amp 1q or Del 1p	• t(11;14)
• Gain/Amp 1q plus Del 1p	• t(6;14)

CHAPTER 16: Cytogenetics   157

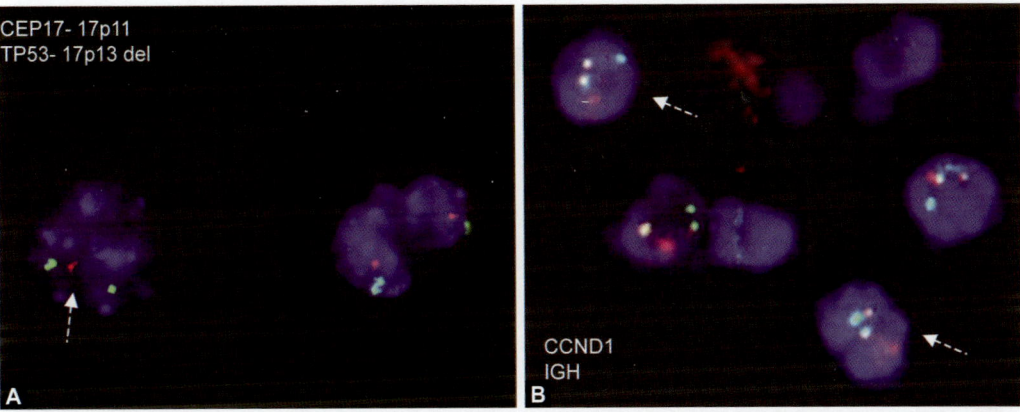

FIGS. 6A AND B: (A) Interphase FISH analysis showing abnormal signal pattern (1 red 2 green) indicating deletion 17p. (B) Interphase FISH analysis showing abnormal signal pattern (2 fusion 1 red 1 green) indicating CCND1-IGH translocation.

REFERENCES

1. Cross NCP, White HE, Colomer D, Ehrencrona H, Foroni L, Gottardi E, et al. Laboratory recommendations for scoring deep molecular responses following treatment for chronic myeloid leukemia. Leukemia. 2015;29(5):999-1003.
2. Li W. The 5th Edition of the World Health Organization Classification of Hematolymphoid Tumors. In: Li W (ed). Leukemia. Brisbane (AU): Exon Publications; 2022.
3. Döhner H, Wei AH, Appelbaum FR, Craddock C, DiNardo CD, Dombret H, et al. Diagnosis and management of AML in adults: 2022 recommendations from an international expert panel on behalf of the ELN. Blood. 2022;140(12):1345-77.
4. Pasquini MC, Zhang MJ, Medeiros BC, Armand P, Hu ZH, Nishihori T, et al. Hematopoietic Cell Transplantation Outcomes in Monosomal Karyotype Myeloid Malignancies. Biol Blood Marrow Transplant J Am Soc Blood Marrow Transplant. 2016;22(2):248-57.
5. Moorman AV, Ensor HM, Richards SM, Chilton L, Schwab C, Kinsey SE, et al. Prognostic effect of chromosomal abnormalities in childhood B-cell precursor acute lymphoblastic leukaemia: results from the UK Medical Research Council ALL97/99 randomised trial. Lancet Oncol. 2010;11(5):429-38.
6. Gökbuget N, Boissel N, Chiaretti S, Dombret H, Doubek M, Fielding A, et al. Diagnosis, prognostic factors, and assessment of ALL in adults: 2024 ELN recommendations from a European expert panel. Blood. 2024;143(19):1891-902.
7. Wang W, Cortes JE, Tang G, Khoury JD, Wang S, Bueso-Ramos CE, et al. Risk stratification of chromosomal abnormalities in chronic myelogenous leukemia in the era of tyrosine kinase inhibitor therapy. Blood. 2016;127(22):2742-50.
8. Hochhaus A, Baccarani M, Silver RT, Schiffer C, Apperley JF, Cervantes F, et al. European Leukemia Net 2020 recommendations for treating chronic myeloid leukemia. Leukemia. 2020;34(4):966-84.
9. Dingli D, Grand FH, Mahaffey V, Spurbeck J, Ross FM, Watmore AE, et al. Der(6)t(1;6)(q21–23;p21.3): A specific cytogenetic abnormality in myelofibrosis with myeloid metaplasia. Br J Haematol. 2005;130(2):229-32.

17 Molecular Diagnostics

Sanjeev Kumar Gupta, Gadha K Leons

Q1. What are the basic techniques for isolation of deoxyribonucleic acid (DNA) or ribonucleic acid (RNA) for molecular diagnostics?

Ans: Isolation of nucleic acids (DNA or RNA) is the starting point for most of the molecular biological assays. Both DNA and RNA extraction methods are critical for downstream applications, such as polymerase chain reaction (PCR), sequencing, and gene expression analysis.[1,2] Although a number of extraction methods are listed in the following text, the two most commonly used methods are the organic extraction and the silica membrane-based kit.

The choice of extraction method depends on the sample type, downstream application, and the required purity and yield of the nucleic acids, e.g., the purity and yield of DNA are better with the silica membrane-based kit than with the organic extraction.

Isolation of nucleic acids involves four main steps:
1. *Cell lysis:* The cells or tissues are lysed to release the cellular contents, e.g., by sodium dodecyl sulfate (SDS) detergent.
2. *Separation:* The nucleic acid (DNA or RNA) is separated from other cellular components such as proteins, lipids, etc., e.g., by proteinase K enzyme.
3. *Precipitation:* Cold ethanol or isopropanol is used to precipitate the nucleic acid.
4. *Washing and resuspension:* The precipitated nucleic acid is washed with ethanol to remove impurities and then resuspended in nuclease-free water or buffer.

Deoxyribonucleic Acid Isolation

The DNA can be separated using various methods based on the biological sample, with two main methods being organic extraction (phenol-chloroform method) and adsorption method (silica-based commercial kits); besides the less common nonorganic method (salting out).[1]
- *Organic extraction* involves a phenol-chloroform mixture which denatures and precipitates proteins, leaving the DNA in the aqueous phase (phenol-chloroform method). This method is labor intensive and time-consuming.
- *Silica-based methods* rely on silica particles or membranes that bind to the DNA (silica matrices or silica column-based DNA extraction method). Commercially available kits such as Thermo Fisher Purelink Genomic DNA extraction kit and QIAGEN DNeasy Blood kit are based on this method.

Different types of DNA isolation methods include:
- Phenol-chloroform method
- Silica column-based DNA extraction method
- Silica matrices (binding of negatively charged DNA with silica covered with positively charged ions)
- Salting-out method (lysis buffer, SDS, and proteinase K)
- Alkaline extraction (NaOH and SDS detergent based)
- Chromatography-based DNA extraction method
- Magnetic beads
- Filter paper-based DNA extraction method
- Cellulose-based paper (Whatman FTA cards)
- Ethidium bromide—cesium chloride (EtBr-CsCl) gradient centrifugation method
- Cetyltrimethylammonium bromide (CTAB) extraction (especially plant and bacterial DNA)
- Chelex-100 extraction

The quality and quantity of the extracted nucleic acid is assessed using spectrophotometry (e.g., nanodrop spectrophotometer) or gel electrophoresis. Spectrophotometry involves estimation of nucleic acid concentration by measuring the amount of light absorbed by the sample at specific wavelengths. The absorption peak for nucleic acids and proteins are approximately 260 and 280 nm respectively. The A260/A280 ratio is approximately 1.8 for double-stranded DNA (dsDNA). A ratio of <1.7 indicates protein contamination.

Ribonucleic Acid Isolation

The instability of RNA and the widespread presence of ribonuclease (RNase) enzymes make RNA extraction more challenging than DNA extraction. One of the most commonly used RNA extraction methods is using the TRIzol (TRI) reagent, a monophasic solution of phenol and guanidinium isothiocyanate for lysis.

Phenol-chloroform mixture separates the homogenate into aqueous and organic phases (phase separation). The RNA remains in the aqueous phase which is precipitated using isopropanol or ethanol.

Other RNA extraction methods include silica spin-column absorption, and isopycnic gradient centrifugation, and methods using specialized RNA extraction columns.[2]

The RNA yield and integrity (RIN or RNA integrity number) is better with the traditional phenol-chloroform method whereas the purity of RNA (A260/A280 ratio ~2) is better with the silica-based column extraction. A260/280 ratio of approximately 2 is considered as pure RNA without protein or phenol contamination.

Q2. **What is the role of PCR techniques in the diagnostic laboratory?**

Ans: PCR techniques play a significant role in diagnostic laboratories due to their high sensitivity, specificity, and versatility. These can help in diagnosis, classification, and in adopting the best treatment strategies. PCR can also detect genetic biomarkers associated with certain cancers or genetic disorders, thereby allowing to predict the potential risk or early diagnosis before the onset of clinical symptoms.[3]

Hematology and hemato-oncology: PCR is commonly used to detect genetic aberrations in both benign hematological disorders like thalassemia as well as malignant hematological disorders such as acute and chronic leukemias. The various genetic aberrations where PCR-based techniques can help include recurrent translocations and fusions, mutations, expression of oncogenes, tumor suppressor genes, tumor-related virus, and drug resistance genes.

Some specific examples of PCR applications in hemato-oncology include:
- Recurrent fusion detection using qualitative reverse transcriptase PCR (RT-PCR), e.g., t(9;22); BCR::ABL1 in chronic myelogenous leukemia (CML), t(8;21); RUNX1::RUNX1T1 in acute myeloid leukemia (AML), inv(16) or t(16;16); CBFB::MYH11, t(12;21); ETV6::RUNX1 in B-cell acute lymphoblastic leukemia (B-ALL), t(4;11); KMT2A::AFF1, t(1;19); TCF3::PBX1, t(15;17); PML::RARA in APML, etc.
- Quantitation of BCR::ABL1 load and other mutations using real time quantitative PCR (RQ-PCR).
- Point mutation detection, e.g., Janus kinase 2 (JAK2) mutation.
- PCR as initial step for fragment analysis (e.g., NPM1 mutation), Sanger sequencing (e.g., of KIT, CEBPA, BRAF, CALR, MPL, imatinib resistance mutation analysis, etc.), next-generation sequencing (NGS), and multiplex ligation dependent probe amplification (MLPA).

Virology: PCR can be used to detect viral nucleic acids to determine subtype, genotype, and strands of the viruses. Qualitative and quantitative detection, with the addition of real time PCR, of viral nucleic acids and in turn viral loads help in diagnosing and monitoring the viral infections, such as human immunodeficiency virus type 1 (HIV-1), hepatitis B virus (HBV), and human cytomegalovirus (IICV), and most recently severe acute respiratory syndrome coronavirus 2 (SARS-CoV-2).

Infectious diseases: PCR is widely used for the detection, screening, or diagnosis of infectious diseases. PCR techniques help in the identification and genetic characterization of various pathogens including viruses, bacteria, fungi, and parasites. PCR is also used to identify and monitor pathogenic microbial loads and is especially useful in identifying pathogens that are difficult to culture. Thus, PCR provides valuable information for epidemiological studies, treatment selection, and monitoring of infectious diseases.

Q3. **How is the validation and quality control of PCR-based assays done?**

Ans: Quality control and validation are crucial steps in any kind of PCR-based assays.[4] Quality control for PCR-based assays are done by adding positive and negative control samples. Positive controls are used to monitor assay precision and accuracy. Negative controls are used to detect contamination and nonspecific amplification.

No-template controls (NTC) are used to detect carryover contamination. Reference genes with stable expression are used as internal controls to normalize the gene expression analysis by quantitative PCR (qPCR). The frequency of quality control (QC) sample analysis depends on the experimental design and expected variability.

Validation of PCR-based assays consider the assay's sensitivity, specificity, limit of detection, precision (intra- and interlaboratory), and recovery (experimental yield/theoretical yield). The validation of a test is especially critical for lab developed tests (LDTs) as compared to the commercial test kits, which still need verification of the performance characteristics of the test. If possible, the validation of the results may be done by performing other orthogonal tests/assays.

Q4. What is single nucleotide polymorphism?

Ans: Single nucleotide polymorphisms (SNPs) are genomic variants present at a single base position of DNA sequence. An SNP occurs when a single nucleotide (adenine, thymine, cytosine, or guanine) in the DNA sequence is altered.[5]

A variation is classified as SNP if > 1% of a population shows a nucleotide variation at a specific position in the DNA sequence. SNPs are present throughout the genome almost once every 1,000 bp on average, resulting in around 4–5 million SNPs in a person's genome.

The variations can be deletion or insertion of a base pair or can be transition or transversion. SNPs can occur within genes, in noncoding regions, or in intergenic regions between genes.

The SNPs within genes can be either synonymous or sometimes known as silent mutation (no change in amino acid sequence, due to the degeneracy of the genetic code) or nonsynonymous (change in amino acid sequence) which may either be missense (results in a different amino acid) or nonsense (results in a premature stop codon).

The SNPs occurring in noncoding or intergenic regions can still have impact on gene function through gene splicing, transcription factor binding, influencing promoter activity (thereby altering gene expression), etc.

The SNPs can often be associated with certain diseases or conditions and thus act as biomarkers to help evaluate individual's genetic predisposition to develop a disease, drug response, or track the inheritance of disease-causing variants within families.[5]

There are various databases that serve as repositories for SNPs such as 1,000 Genome Project and NCBI dbSNP database. Additionally, there are databases that link SNPs association to various studies such as genome-wide association studies (GWAS central), pharmacogenomics (PharmGKB), and other areas of genomic research to help study the genetic basis of complex traits and diseases.

In summary, SNPs are the most common type of single nucleotide variation in the human genome and serve as important tools for genetic and genomic research and clinical applications.

Q5. What are the limitations of molecular assays?

Ans: The major limitation of the molecular assays is the occurrence of false-positive and false-negative result.[6]

False-positive

- Nonspecific amplification from direct or indirect contamination (environmental factors or host gene) can result in false-positive results especially if the amplicons are similar in size or have the same melting temperature in melting curve analysis.
- Carryover contamination of PCR reagents or setup equipment.
- PCR assays cannot differentiate between live, injured, dead cells, or cells existing in a viable but nonculturable (VBNC) state.

False-negative

- The genetic aberrations such as insertions or deletions or mutations can sometimes cause the PCR to give false-negative results.
- Pathogen loads are below the limit of detection.
- Presence of PCR inhibitors.

Other Limitations

Limited Multiplexing Capability

The number of genes/targets that can be detected simultaneously is limited. High-density microarrays can detect the most targets in parallel, but are slower and more expensive than other methods.

Quantification Assays are Technically Demanding

Even though real-time PCR (qPCR) is a quantitative assay, the reference genes (internal controls) or control samples must be included in the assay; and calibration curves and standard curves analyzed for accurate results.[6]

Q6. What is the basic principle of fluorescence in situ hybridization?

Ans: Fluorescence in situ hybridization (FISH) is a technique that uses fluorescently labeled probes to detect and localize the presence or absence of specific DNA or RNA sequences within cells or tissue samples. The basic principle of FISH involves the hybridization of the fluorescently labeled probe to its complementary target sequence.[7]

Probe preparation: DNA or RNA probes complementary to the target sequence are synthesized and labeled with fluorescent dyes, such as fluorescein, rhodamine, or cyanine, directly or indirectly using haptens, like biotin or digoxigenin, that are incorporated into the probe, which are then detected using fluorescently labeled antibodies or avidin/streptavidin conjugates.

Sample preparation: Cells or tissue samples are prepared for FISH by fixing the sample with chemical fixatives such as formaldehyde or methanol-acetic acid. The double-stranded DNA or RNA is then denatured into single strands, by heating or treatment with alkaline solutions, to make the region of interest accessible for the probe.

Hybridization: The probe is added to the denatured sample and allowed to hybridize under specific conditions, such as optimum temperature and buffer composition, to the target sequence. Unbound or nonspecifically bound probes are removed by washing with buffers in particular washing conditions.

Detection: The hybridized probes are then visualized using fluorescence microscope and the results (fluorescent signals) are interpreted to determine the presence and location of the sequence within the cell or tissue.

When indirect labeling is used, additional detection steps using fluorescently labeled antibodies or avidin/streptavidin conjugates are performed to amplify the signal.

The FISH has numerous applications in genetic research, diagnostics, and species identification. It can detect chromosomal abnormalities, identify specific genes, study gene expression patterns, and analyze the spatial distribution of genetic elements within cells and tissues. FISH is a versatile technique that combines the specificity of nucleic acid hybridization with the sensitivity of fluorescence detection, making it an essential tool in modern molecular biology and cytogenetics.[7]

Q7. What are the clinical indications for FISH testing in hematological disorders?

Ans: Fluorescence in situ hybridization is routinely used for detecting structural chromosomal abnormalities such as chromosomal translocations, deletions, insertions, and amplifications in hematological disorders.[8,9]

The FISH technique is considered when there are no metaphases available for conventional cytogenetics or to clarify complex or abnormal conventional cytogenetic findings.

The FISH can be particularly useful in the following diagnostic scenarios:
- Recurrent chromosomal translocation detection in CML (BCR::ABL1), AML (RUNX1::RUNX1T1, CBFB::MYH11), APML (PML::RARA), B-ALL [mixed lineage leukemia (MLL/KMT2A) rearrangements, TCF3::PBX1] as an alternative to RT-PCR and conventional cytogenetics.
- Abnormalities with a high frequency of "false-negative" cytogenetics, e.g., CLL (del13q14, del17p13, del11q22), multiple myeloma [t(4;14)/FGFR3::IGH], chronic eosinophilic leukemia (del4q12/FIP1L1::PDGFRB).
- Interphase FISH, when conventional cytogenetics fails or is not possible, like, on fixed tissue.
- To clarify abnormal or complex conventional karyotypic findings.
- As a surrogate marker for a primary genetic event, e.g., CHIC2 deletion as a marker of del4q12/FIP1L1::PDGFRB.

In summary, FISH testing is used to detect specific chromosomal abnormalities that are important for diagnosis, classification, and management of various hematological malignancies, especially when conventional cytogenetics is limited or unable to identify the genetic changes.

Q8. What are the types of FISH probes routinely used in hematologic malignancies?

Ans: There are mainly three different types of FISH probes that are used to detect DNA sequences:
1. *Locus specific probes (LSPs):* LSPs bind to a specific region/gene of a chromosome, thus enabling the detection of microdeletions and microduplications of a region/gene within a particular chromosome.
2. *Centromeric or alphoid repetitive probes:* These probes bind to the repetitive sequences in the middle of each chromosome, which can be used to determine aneuploidies. These probes can be used to determine the missing genetic material from a particular chromosome when used along with LSPs.
3. *Whole chromosome probes (WCPs):* WCPs are used to map or paint the whole chromosome. These are a collection of small fluorescently labeled probes which bind to a different sequence along a particular chromosome.

The types of FISH probes usually used in hematological malignancies are:
- *Break-apart probes:* Break-apart probes are used to detect gene translocations, particularly in scenarios where a gene has multiple possible partners and so, it is difficult to check for each individual partner separately. Two differently labelled probes (e.g., green and red) are taken that bind to different areas (proximal and distal) of one of the two genes involved in translocation. The separate signals (green and red) indicate a cell with translocation whereas, the fusion signal (e.g., yellow) indicates intact gene and is observed in a normal cell. Examples include ABL1 break-apart probes and KMT2A (previously MLL) break-apart probes used in B-cell acute lymphoblastic leukemia, IGH break-apart probes in B-cell lymphomas and MYC break-apart probes.
- *Dual-color fusion probes:* Fusion probes are used to detect gene fusions in a cell. Differently labeled probes complementary to each of the two genes involved in the fusion is used. A fusion signal indicates the presence of the gene fusion and two separate signals indicate

a normal cell. Examples include BCR::ABL1 fusion probes in B-ALL/CML and IGH::BCL2 dual fusion probe for follicular lymphoma.
- *Dual-color/tricolor probes:* Dual-color probes contain a mixture of a gene-specific probe and a control probe (e.g., centromeric probe). They are used to detect gene amplifications, deletions, and aneusomies.

Examples include ERBB2/CEN17 dual-color probe for HER2 status in breast cancer, BCR/ABL1/ASS1 in B-ALL.

Some of the FISH probes routinely used for the diagnosis and monitoring of hematological malignancies include:[8,9]
- *Acute lymphoblastic leukemia*
    - t(9;22)/BCR::ABL1
    - t(12;21)/ETV6::RUNX1
    - t(1;19)/TCF3::PBX1
    - t(4;11)/KMT2A (previously MLL) rearrangements
    - Hyperdiploidy
    - Ph-like ALL panel [includes ABL1 and ABL2 rearrangements, platelet-derived growth factor receptor B (PDGFRB) rearrangements, JAK2 rearrangements, cytokine receptor-like factor 2 (CRLF2) rearrangements, etc.]
- *Acute myeloid leukemia*
    - t(8;21)/RUNX1::RUNX1T1
    - inv(16)/CBFB::MYH11
    - t(15;17)/PML::RARA
- *Chronic myeloid leukemia*
    - t(9;22)/BCR::ABL1
- *Chronic lymphocytic leukemia*
    - Del(13q14)
    - Del(11q22)
    - Del(17p13)
    - +12
- *Plasma cell myeloma*
    - Del (13q14)
    - Hyperdiploidy
    - t(4;14)/FGFR3::IGH
- *T-cell lymphoma*
    - inv(7)/TCRB rearrangement
    - inv(14)/TCRAD rearrangement
    - t(2;5)/ALK rearrangement
- *B-cell lymphoma*
    - t(14;18)/IGH::BCL2
    - t(8;14)/MYC::IGH
    - BCL6 rearrangements
- *Myelodysplastic syndrome*
    - 5q deletion

These FISH probes allow for the detection of chromosomal abnormalities, gene rearrangements, and copy number changes that are important for diagnosis, classification, and monitoring of various hematological malignancies. FISH provides advantages over conventional cytogenetics in terms of sensitivity as well as speed.

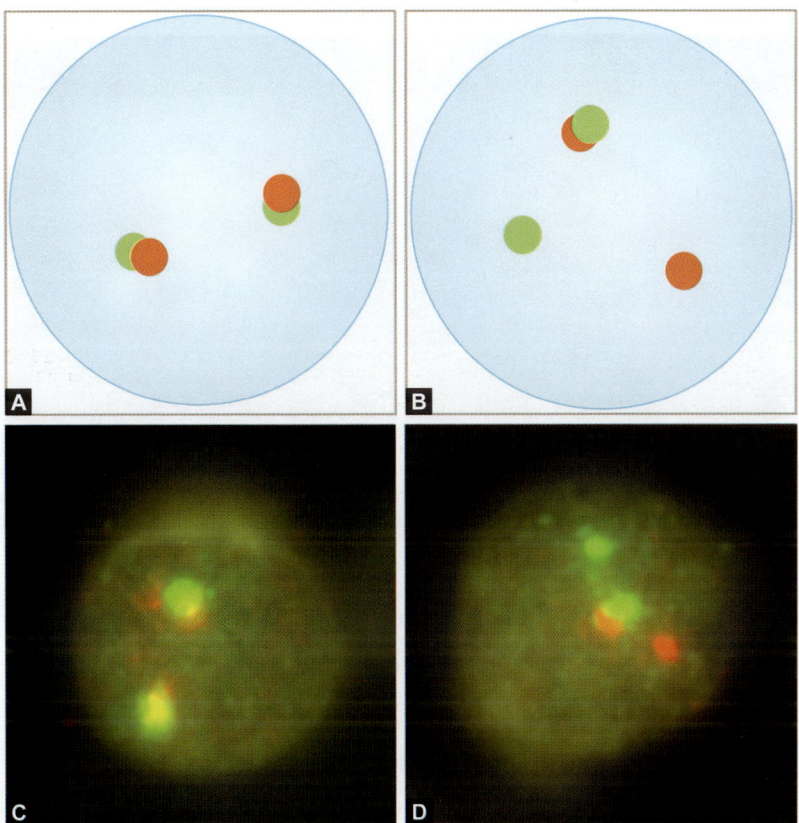

FIGS. 1A TO D: Break-apart (BA) probe scheme in FISH (A) Normal cell showing two green-red (2GR) fusion signals. (B) Aberrant cell showing one green-red (1GR) fusion signal, one separate green (1G) and red signal (1R) each, resulting from a chromosome rearrangement involving the probe locus (C) Normal pattern of 2 fusion (2GR) signals of ABL1 BA probe (D) 1 fusion (1GR) and split of red-green (1G,1R) signal suggesting ABL1 rearrangement.

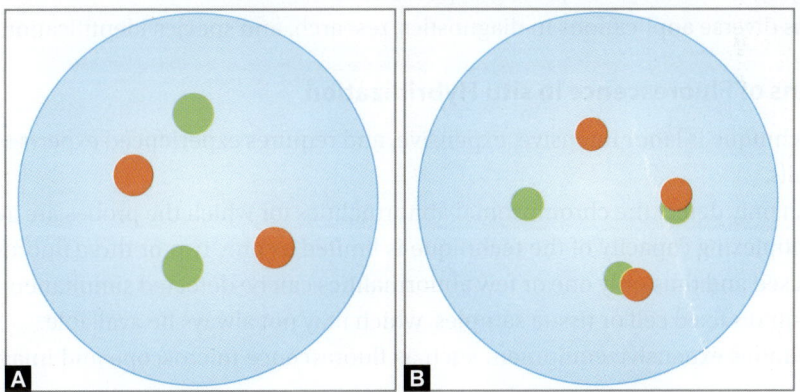

FIGS. 2A TO D: *Continued*

Continued

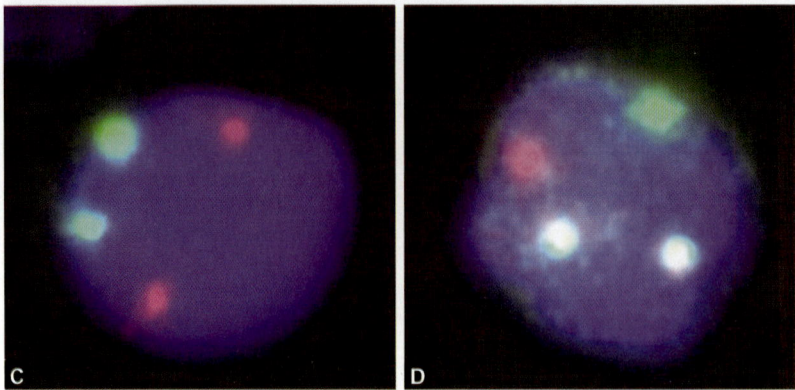

FIGS. 2A TO D: Dual-color dual fusion probe scheme in FISH: (A) Normal cell showing two green (2G) and two red (2R) signals. (B) Aberrant cell showing two green-red (2GR) fusion signals resulting from a reciprocal translocation alongwith 1G and 1R signals. (C) Normal pattern of two green (2G) and two red (2R) signals using ETV6/RUNX1 dual color dual fusion probe (D) 2 fusion (2GR) signals suggesting reciprocal translocation ETV6/RUNX1 alongwith 1G (ETV6) and 1R (RUNX1) signals.

Q9. What are the advantages and limitations of FISH?

Ans: Fluorescence in situ hybridization technique is routinely used in diagnosis of hematologic malignancies.[10]

Advantages of Fluorescence in Situ Hybridization

- FISH has a faster turnaround time compared to conventional cytogenetics and a large number of cells can be analyzed in a short period.
- High sensitivity and specificity of the techniques makes it possible to detect single copy genes and chromosomal abnormalities that can be missed in conventional cytogenetics.
- FISH can be performed on nondividing or terminally differentiated cells, unlike conventional cytogenetics which require metaphase cells.
- FISH has diverse applications in diagnostics, research, and species identification.

Limitations of Fluorescence in situ Hybridization

- FISH technique is labor intensive, expensive, and requires experienced experts to interpret the results.
- FISH can only detect the chromosomal abnormalities for which the probes are available.
- The multiplexing capacity of the technique is limited as only two or three fluorescent dyes can be used and thus only one or few abnormalities can be detected simultaneously.
- FISH requires fixed cell or tissue samples, which may not always be available.
- FISH requires expensive equipment such as fluorescence microscope and image analysis system.
- Interpretation of FISH results require expertise to distinguish true signals from artifacts and for setting a cutoff for the FISH probes.

- Co-localization (signals from two FISH probes overlap because the chromosomes happen to be in the same place on the slide and appear as one) and cross-hybridization (the probe binds to regions with repetitive sequences) can occur.

In summary, while FISH offers advantages in sensitivity, specificity, and speed, it has limitations in terms of multiplexing, cost, and is technically demanding.

Q10. **How is clonality detected by immunoglobulin and T-cell receptor (*TCR*) gene rearrangements?**

Ans: Clonality can be detected by analyzing immunoglobulin (Ig) and *TCR* gene rearrangements using molecular techniques like PCR and is a valuable tool for the diagnosis of B-cell and T-cell lymphoid malignancies.[11]

Clonality assessment of the Ig or *TCR* genes is a useful supplementary tool for the diagnosis of B-cell and T-cell lymphoid malignancies.

During B-cell and T-cell development, the immunoglobulin heavy chain gene and the TCR genes undergo rearrangement, resulting in a unique rearranged sequence in each mature lymphocyte.

The Ig rearrangement process involves the random selection and joining of variable (V), diversity (D), and joining (J) gene segments, and TCR involves the rearrangement of α, β, γ, and δ genes. The junctions between the gene fragments contain random insertions and deletions, making each rearrangement unique to a single lymphocyte.

In lymphoid malignancies like lymphomas, a transformed lymphocyte clonally expands, resulting in a population of identical cells with the same Ig or *TCR* gene rearrangement. Therefore, the unique clonal rearrangement is considered as "DNA fingerprints" for the malignant cells and can be detected using PCR-based assays.

Primers targeting conserved regions of the Ig and *TCR* genes are used to amplify the rearranged Ig and TCR gene segments. The size and sequence of the amplified fragments are used to assess clonality. In a clonal population, the amplicons will be of identical size and sequence, while a polyclonal population (healthy/normal sample) will have multiple amplicons with different sizes and sequences.

Minimal residual disease (MRD) assessment can also be done using these clonal markers.

In summary, the detection of clonal Ig or *TCR* gene rearrangements by PCR-based assays is a valuable tool for diagnosing lymphoid malignancies, determining lineage, and monitoring disease status and response to treatment.[11]

Q11. **What are the pitfalls in immunoglobulin and *TCR* clonality testing?**

Ans:

Technical Pitfalls[12]

- *Bands/peaks observed may vary in size:*
    - Bands/peaks outside the expected size range—could indicate true rearrangements, should confirm with sequencing or could be nonspecific products.
    - Undersized bands/peaks—could be due to internal deletions in *VH/Vkappa/Vlambda* gene [somatic hypermutations (SHM) related] and should be confirmed by sequencing.
    - Oversized bands/peaks—could be due to extended amplification from downstream J gene and should be confirmed by sequencing.

- Multiple clonal signals—could be due to biallelic rearrangements or multiple rearrangements per allele, which needs to be interpreted in the context of the expected number of rearrangements, or biclonality.
- Lack of clonal signal and polyclonal Gaussian curve—could be due to low DNA input, poor DNA quality, or lack of B/T cells in the sample. Lack of clonal signal could also be due to the presence of SHM in the malignant cells.

Biological Pitfalls

- Selective amplification and pseudoclonality—this can be due to low level of template, that is, very few T/B cells, leading to preferential amplification of a specific rearrangement.
- Oligoclonal T-cell repertoire in peripheral blood of elderly individuals, immunodeficient patients, or transplant patients—this is due to incomplete or aberrant immune system.
- Oligo/monoclonality in histologically reactive lesions—this can be an exaggerated immune response with dominant specificity.

These pitfalls can be addressed by a few potential solutions including:
- Confirming DNA quality and quantity.
- Performing multiple PCR replicates using the same or independent DNA samples.
- Integrating the molecular data with immunohistology and flow cytometry findings.
- Considering the clinical context and percentage of suspect cells.

Q12. How detection of MRD is done using immunoglobulin/*TCR* gene rearrangements as PCR targets?

Ans: Minimal/measurable residual disease is an important biomarker of patient's response to therapy and in guiding treatment decisions.[13] The MRD in lymphoid malignancies can be detected by using clonal Ig and *TCR* gene rearrangements as PCR targets which brings the sensitivity of detection of MRD up to 10^{-4} or 10^{-5}.

Allele-specific RQ-PCR is the gold standard technique for the sensitive and accurate assessment of MRD; EuroMRD Consortium have developed extensive guidelines. New generation of PCR techniques such as digital droplet PCR (ddPCR) and amplicon-based NGS are being tried as a potential alternative for RQ-PCR.

The unique rearranged Ig and *TCR* gene sequences in the malignant cells are identified using PCR and sequencing, at diagnosis, and these patient-specific rearrangements are then used for tracking MRD in follow-up samples.[13]

The RQ-PCR assays use allele-specific oligonucleotide (ASO) primers to detect the specific Ig/TCR rearrangements and in turn, MRD.

The MRD assessment helps determine the prognosis and potential risk of relapse in hematological malignancies such as acute lymphoblastic leukemia, chronic lymphocytic leukemia, and lymphomas.

The detection of MRD using Ig and *TCR* gene rearrangements as PCR targets is a powerful sensitive tool, which informs clinical management of hematological malignancies.

REFERENCES

1. Gupta N. DNA extraction and polymerase chain reaction. J Cytol. 2019;36(2):116-7.
2. Nandi Jui B, Sarsenbayeva A, Jernow H, Hetty S, Pereira MJ. Evaluation of RNA Isolation methods in human adipose tissue. Lab Med. 2022;53(5):e129-33.

3. Wang M, Cai J, Chen J, Liu J, Geng X, Yu X, et al. PCR Techniques and Their Clinical Applications. Polymerase Chain Reaction. IntechOpen; 2023.
4. Smith M. Validating real-time polymerase chain reaction (PCR) Assays. Encyclopedia of Virology. 2021;35-44.
5. Brumfield RT, Beerli P, Nickerson DA, Edwards SV. The utility of single nucleotide polymorphisms in inferences of population history. Trends Ecol Evol. 2003;18:249-56.
6. Morshed MG, Lee M-K, Jorgensen D, Isaac Renton JL. Molecular methods used in clinical laboratory: prospects and pitfalls. FEMS Immunol Med Microbiol. 2007;49(2):184-91.
7. Shakoori AR. Fluorescence in situ hybridization (FISH) and its applications. Chromosome Structure and Aberrations. 2017;343-67.
8. Wan TSK, Ma ESK. The role of fish in hematologic cancer. Inter J Hemato Oncol. 2012;1(1):71-86.
9. Hu L, Ru K, Zhang L, Huang Y, Zhu X, Liu H, et al. Fluorescence in situ hybridization (FISH): an increasingly demanded tool for biomarker research and personalized medicine. Biomark Res. 2014;2(1):3.
10. Gozzetti A, Beau MML. Fluorescence in situ hybridization: Uses and limitations. Semin Hematol. 2000;37(4):320-33.
11. Gazzola A, Mannu C, Rossi M, Laginestra MA, Sapienza MR, Fuligni F, et al. The evolution of clonality testing in the diagnosis and monitoring of hematological malignancies. Ther Adv Hematol. 2014;5(2):35-47.
12. Groenen PJ, Langerak AW, van Dongen JJ, van Krieken JH. Pitfalls in TCR gene clonality testing: teaching cases. J Hematop. 2008;1(2):97-109.
13. van der Velden, Dombrink VHJ, Alten J, Cazzaniga G, Clappier E, Drandi D, et al. Analysis of measurable residual disease by *IG/TR* gene rearrangements: quality assurance and updated EuroMRD guidelines. Leukemia. 2024;38(6):1315-22.

18. Next-generation Sequencing

Shrinidhi Nathany

Q1. What do you understand by sequencing of tumor cells?

Ans: Sequencing of tumor cells includes sequencing the genome of the tumor cells.[1] This is achieved after microdissection of the tumor from formalin fixed paraffin embedded tissue (FFPE) and ascertaining the tumor percentage in the background of normal tissue. The cancer genome comprises both somatic and germline deoxyribonucleic acid (DNA), including the tumor infiltrating inflammatory cells. It can be done using different technologies ranging from the first generation Sanger sequencing to the sophisticated next-generation sequencing (NGS) technologies. **Figure 1** depicts how a tumor fraction on a slide is ascertained by microdissection.

Q2. What is next-generation sequencing?

Ans: Next-generation sequencing is second-generation sequencing which is also known as massively parallel sequencing. It has evolved since the first machine by Roche. Roche 454 to fourth generation nanopore sequencers. All machines have different technologies on which the sequencing happens which include sequencing by synthesis, ion-semiconductor sequencing, single molecule real time sequencing, and nanopore sequencing.[2] Although the basic principle of sequencing by synthesis and incorporation of deoxynucleotide triphosphates

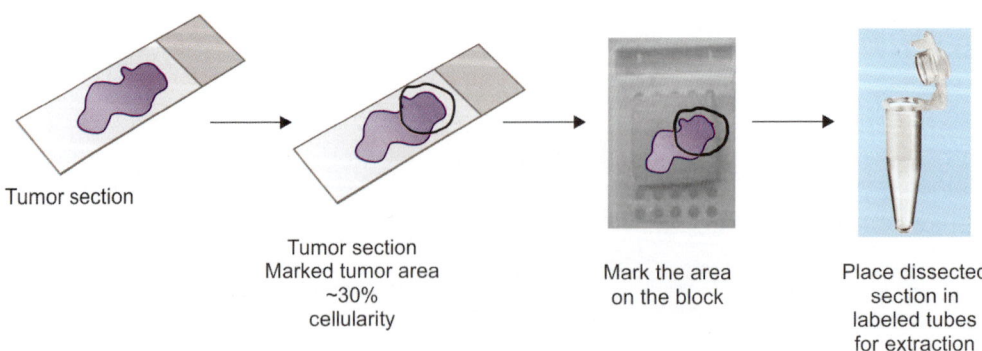

FIG. 1: Tumor microdissection.

(dNTP) is common to Sanger method and the NGS, the major difference lies in the throughput and assays uses.

Q2. **What are the various methods of performing next-generation sequencing?**

Ans: The two broad methods are short-read and long-read sequencing.
1. *Short-read sequencing*: The short-read sequencing method typically includes sequencing by synthesis or synthesis by ligation. Each of these utilizes either a polymerase or ligase enzymes for extension of numerous strands of DNA. The advantage also lies in the premise that these can be controlled synchronously or can be done in real time, depending on the approach which is used.[2,3] Examples of short-read sequencing methods include Illumina's single stranded DNA amplification approach, as well as clonal amplification-based methods from Ion torrent, SOLiD, and Roche.
2. *Long-read sequencing*: This technology enables sequencing longer lengths of base pairs typically 5,000–30,000 bp. The major advantage of this over-short read sequencing is the elimination of amplification bias and a better consensus sequence assembly owing to better overlay of sequences. Currently, two such platforms are available, which include the single molecular real time (SMRT) sequencer from PacBio Biosciences' and the Oxford Nanopore's long-read sequencing platforms.

Q3. **What are the various applications of NGS in hematological diseases?**

Ans: The applications of NGS based testing range across the entire spectrum of hematologic diseases from benign to malignant.[4]
- *Diagnosis:* Most of the diseases enlisted in the World Health Organization (WHO) HEME five classification now mandate molecular testing for correct diagnosis. Examples include acute myeloid leukemia (AML) with recurrent genetic abnormalities, myeloproliferative neoplasia, myelodysplastic syndromes (MDS), as well as the myeloid/lymphoid neoplasms with germline predisposition.
- *Risk stratification*: Recommendations for risk stratification, international prognostic index (IPI) for chronic lymphocytic leukemia (CLL), MDS, and even myeloma mandate molecular testing for optimal risk stratification in order to optimally triage patients for chemotherapy versus transplant.
- *Predisposition*: Genetic testing helps to find the predisposed and then cascade testing can also detect healthy carriers in the family. This is especially important in the context of inherited bone marrow failure syndromes, primary immunodeficiency diseases as well as myeloid/lymphoid neoplasms with germline predisposition. Germline testing is also important in the context of stem cell transplant especially in case of sibling/related donors and autologous transplants. Screening donors for any potential germline variants is good clinical practice.
- *Precision*: In the era of personalized/precision medicine it is important to find potential targets such as FLT3, IDH, KIT, FGFR, platelet-derived growth factor receptor (PDGFR), etc., for which Food and Drug Administration (FDA) approved small molecule inhibitors are available. Genomic inspired treatment of AML is now a part of a trial which has been launched by the National Cancer Institute (NCI) in the United States known as myeloMATCH, which is trying to ascertain the utility of rapid NGS in hematologic malignancies in deciding what induction would be offered to the patient.

HEMATOLOGIC MALIGNANCIES

NGS in Myeloid and Lymphoid Neoplasms

Myeloproliferative Neoplasms (MPNs)

CML: Confirmatory tests include FISH, PCR, and karyotyping to detect BCR-ABL1 rearrangements. Monitoring of kinase domain mutations is crucial for managing TKI resistance.

Philadelphia-negative MPNs: JAK2 V617F, CALR, and MPL mutations define most cases of PV, ET, and PMF. Techniques like allele-specific PCR or fragment analysis aid detection.

MDS/MPN Overlap Syndromes

NGS has helped recognize recurrent mutations in overlap syndromes—TET2, SRSF2, ASXL1 in CMML; SETBP1, ETNK1 in aCML; JAK2/CALR/SF3B1 in MDS/MPN with ring sideroblasts.

Myelodysplastic Syndromes (MDS)

SF3B1 mutations now define a diagnostic category (MDS with ring sideroblasts). TP53 mutations are linked to poor prognosis and resistance to lenalidomide in del(5q) MDS.

Acute Myeloid Leukemia (AML)

Modern AML classification integrates recurrent mutations such as NPM1, FLT3 (TKD/ITD), IDH1/2, CEBPA, and structural rearrangements (RUNX1-RUNX1T1, CBFB-MYH11, PML-RARA). RNA sequencing detects novel and known fusions.

Germline Predisposition Syndromes

Recognition of germline mutations (e.g., RUNX1, ETV6, DDX41) in patients with high variant allele fractions or family histories is essential, particularly when considering sibling donors. Though skin fibroblasts are ideal for testing, buccal swabs are commonly used.

NGS in Lymphoid Neoplasms

B-cell Malignancies

CLL: Somatic hypermutation status of IGHV is prognostic. TP53 mutations necessitate alternative therapies over chemoimmunotherapy.

Hairy cell leukemia: BRAF V600E mutation is pathognomonic and targetable.

Waldenström's macroglobulinemia: MYD88 L265P mutation distinguishes it from mimickers.

T-cell Neoplasms

Monoclonality in T-cell lymphomas is confirmed via TCR rearrangement. ALK rearrangements in anaplastic large cell lymphoma are best assessed by IHC or FISH.

Plasma Cell Disorders

IGH translocations involving genes like CCND1, MMSET, and MAF drive prognosis. Mutations in TP53 and the NF-κB pathway are linked with treatment resistance and progression.

Molecular Subtypes of DLBCL

Recent genomic efforts have redefined DLBCL into distinct genetic subgroups beyond the traditional GCB versus ABC classification. The Schmitz classification divides DLBCL into four major clusters:

1. *MCD (MYD88/CD79B):* Frequently ABC subtype, associated with extranodal disease, especially in the CNS and testes.
2. *BN2 (BCL6 fusions/NOTCH2):* More indolent, linked to marginal zone lymphomas.
3. *N1 (NOTCH1 mutations):* Poor prognosis, enriched in ABC phenotype.
4. *EZB (EZH2/BCL2):* Mostly GCB origin with t(14;18), often harboring EZH2 gain-of-function mutations.

These have now been further refined in the LymphGen algorithm into:
- ST2 *(SGK1/TET2):* Possibly derivable from germinal center exit B cells.
- A53 *(aneuploid-rich subtype):* Associated with TP53 mutation, often chemo-resistant.
- NGS enables molecular subclassification of DLBCL, which has profound implications for targeted therapy and clinical trial enrollment (e.g., EZH2 inhibitors in EZB subtype).

NGS in Precursor Lymphoid Leukemias

BCP-ALL: RT-PCR or RNA-NGS detects fusions like BCR-ABL1, TEL-AML1, and more recently, Ph-like ALL fusions.

T-ALL: While molecular stratification is limited, recurrent chromosomal abnormalities may eventually guide targeted interventions.

Screening

Thalassemia carriers: Prenatal screening of carriers of thalassemia using NGS has been in vogue. Even the use of NGS in antenatal setting on maternal cell free DNA to look for possible chromosomal anomalies leading to failure to thrive, or inherited marrow failure syndromes have been reported.

Inherited Platelet Disorders

In case of unexplained cytopenia at a young age, usually a working diagnosis of immune thrombocytopenia (ITP) is made and treatment is rendered. However, in approximately 12% cases the diagnosis is modified owing to refractoriness to platelet therapy, and variants may be detected in transcription factor genes such as *ETV6* and *RUNX1* which are also known to cause myeloid/lymphoid neoplasms with germline predisposition. Usually, a thorough family history along with a whole-exome sequencing at diagnosis can save some lead time into the disease course of the patient.

Q4. What are targeted resequencing, whole-exome sequencing, and whole-genome sequencing? What are the important considerations in choosing the most appropriate NGS method?

Ans:

Targeted Resequencing

This is a targeted NGS method where regions or hotspots of genes are targeted by various enrichment methods such as hybrid capture, HALOPLEX, amplification, and then sequenced. The entire coding regions or all genes are not sequenced.[11] Panels are designed of variable sizes based on already published literature, and hotspots are determined as per databases available. Specific primers are designed using a tiled approach or a gapped approach and then a panel is made specific to the disease.

Whole-exome Sequencing

This type of sequencing involves sequencing the entire protein coding region of the genome, i.e., the exons. Human genome has 180,000 exons, constituting about 1% of the human genome. Typically, the DNA is extracted and enrichment for exons is done by different techniques like array-based capture or in solution capture and then sequenced using a high throughput sequencer. Depending on whether the sample of interest or disease question is germline or somatic, the depth of coverage is determined.

Whole-genome Sequencing

This involves sequencing the entire genome including both exons and introns.

Q5. What parameters should be monitored when reading an NGS report? What is variant allele frequency?

Ans: While reading an NGS report the following need to be checked and given due consideration.[12]

- *Identifiers:* The patient's demographic details, sample collection and receiving time, the type of sample, the working clinical diagnosis, and other clinical parameters, and cytogenetics if available for better correlation of genomic findings. The dates are important in order to ascertain sample viability.
- *Variants:* The genes, variants, and variant allele frequency along with assertion criteria as per association of molecular pathology guidelines should be read.
- *Quality metrics:* The depth of coverage of the entire panel employed, as well as on target percentage should be read. As per NCI match, a depth of coverage of 500–1,000× for somatic, 30–100× for germline, and 30,000× for liquid biopsy are recommended. For fusion, this is not applicable, and each assay has its own cutoff to definitively call a fusion. The assay sensitivity is also important especially in the context of a test assaying measurable residual disease. These assays require lower limits of detection to ascertain for deeper responses.
- *Gene panel:* The contents, i.e., the genes which have been tested, along with type of alterations which have been tested: e.g., single nucleotide variations, insertions, deletions, copy number alterations, and fusions. Some panels are DNA only and may not interrogate for fusions, so it is important to pay heed in the given clinical context, so as to not miss out on any potential targets.
- *Variant allele frequency:* Percentage of sequence reads observed matching a specific DNA variant divided by the overall coverage at the locus.

Q6. What is the difference between germline and somatic mutations? Which type of mutations are implicated in hematological diseases and how?

Ans:
Somatic mutation: "A somatic mutation describes any alteration at the cellular level in somatic tissues occurring after fertilization. These mutations do not involve the germline and consequently do not get transmitted to progeny.[13] Somatic mutations are a part of aging and occur either spontaneously as a result of errors in DNA repair mechanisms or a direct response to stress. Mutations can cause spectrum of diseases ranging from benign to malignant. On NGS if the tumor is sequenced it can detect somatic and germline mutations, although may

still miss approximately 3% germline variants, since NGS may not be able to detect large indels with optimal sensitivity.

Germline mutation: These occur in the germ cells and are usually passed on from one generation to the other. These usually are inherited and depending on penetrance it may or may not result in phenotypic manifestations. They may be passed in autosomal dominant, recessive, codominant, or X-linked inheritance modes. Depending on the genetic make-up of parents, it will depend if a recessive gene shall manifest phenotypically or not. Apart from developmental malformation syndromes and mental retardation syndromes, 73 genes have been enlisted by the American College of Medical Genetics and Genomics to be implicated in inherited cancer predisposition. Because of this, WHO Heme classification also has a category known as myeloid/lymphoid neoplasms with germline predisposition.

Q7. How is NGS helpful in the management of myelodysplastic syndrome and acute myeloid leukemia?

Ans: Major advances in NGS over the past decade have unraveled close to 50 driver alterations in MDS.[14] In targeted sequencing, on an average at least 1 mutation is detected in all MDS patients. Not one single mutation that is 100% pathognomonic for MDS, and it is a functional genetic cluster which ultimately drives the disease and determines outcomes. Traditionally, MDS diagnosis has been based on cytomorphology, flow cytometric immunophenotyping and cytogenetics, and now NGS. However, NGS cannot be the standalone test, and is considered a complementary tool to the already in-vogue modalities. The inclusion of SF3B1 and tP53 in WHO classification mandate testing, as the cutoff for percentage of blasts and ringed sideroblasts also become different. Similarly, SF3B1 and TP53 are also independent prognostic factors determining outcomes of chemotherapy and transplant in MDS.

Q8. How is NGS helpful in the management of inherited bone marrow failure syndromes?

Ans: Inherited bone marrow failure syndromes are a group of heterogeneous disorders, which result due to mutations in implicating genes.[15] The disorders with their implicated genes are listed in the **Table 1**.

TABLE 1: Next-generation sequencing (NGS) for inherited bone marrow failure syndromes.	
Disease	**Genes**
Fanconi anemia	• AR: FANCA (60%), FANCC (14%), BRCA2 (FANCD1) (3%), FANCD2 (3%), FANCE (3%), FANCF (2%), FANCG (XRCC9) (10%), FANCI (1%), BRIP1 (FANCJ) (2%), FANCL, FANCM, PALB2 (FANCN), RAD51C (FANCO), SLX4 (FANCP), ERCC4 (FANCQ, XPF), BRCA1 (FANCS), UBE2T (FANCT), XRCC2 (FANCU), MAD2L2 (FANCV, REV7), RFWD3 (FANCW) • AD: RAD51 (FANCR) • XLR: FANCB (2%)
Dyskeratosis congenital (DC) and related telomere biology disorders	• XLR: DKC1 (15–20%) • AD: TINF2 (TIN2) (11–20%), TERC (5%), NAF1 • AR: CTC1, NOP10, NHP2, WRAP53 (TCAB1), STN1, POT1 • AD and AR: RTEL1 (5–10%), TERT (5%), ACD (TPP1), PARN

Continued

Continued

Disease	Genes
Diamond–Blackfan anemia	• AD: RPS19 (25%), RPL11 (6–7%), RPS26 (6%), RPS10 (2–3%), RPL35A (3%), RPS24 (2%), RPS17 (1%), RPL5, RPL15, RPL17, RPL19, RPL26, RPL31, RPS7, RPS19, RPS20, RPS28, RPS29 • XLR: GATA1, TSR2
Shwachman–Diamond syndrome	AR: SBDS (95%), DNAJC21, EFL1 AD: SRP54

(AD: autosomal dominant; AR: autosomal recessive; XLA: X-linked recessive)

Considerations in inherited marrow failure syndromes which need elucidation include:
- *Somatic gene rescue:* The cells in which an in vivo somatic genetic event has happened that partially or totally counterpoises the effect of the pathogenic germline mutation, may gain a selective advantage over nonmodified cells. This forms the concept of somatic gene rescue. This affects cells in these patients via two mechanisms. One end of the spectrum is that an acquired variation may improve cell fitness and rescue from a deleterious phenotype. The other end is that it may provide fitness toward malignant transformation. This phenomenon has been seen across the spectrum of these diseases and hence it is important to monitor for potential therapeutic implications.
- *Somatic reversion:* The implicated mutation reverts to wildtype. So in patients with high clinical suspicion of Fanconi anemia with normal chromosomal breakage study this should be suspected. In such cases, alternate specimen like cultured skin fibroblasts may be utilized to test the same or testing of other family members may provide clues to diagnosis.

Attributing to the phenotypic overlap, atypical presentation, and genetic heterogeneity among these syndromes, NGS-based gene panel testing is often preferred, as it has the ability to analyze multiple genes simultaneously and is also cost-effective. However, few intronic regions and large deletions not detected or covered in NGS may be tested by Sanger method using multiplex ligation probe assay, etc.

Q9. What are the drawbacks or limitations of NGS?

Ans: NGS is a robust technology and now with different modifications and advancements, it has achieved a sensitivity of close to approximately 95%. However, there are challenges and limitations for the same.[16]

Limitations include:
- *Cost:* In an economically restrained society like India, where more than one-third inhabit rural lowlands, affording a comprehensive NGS based test is a challenge.
- *Technical challenges:*
    - *Sequence errors*: These may occur due to artifacts that initiate from library preparation, the sequencing process, or data analysis (e.g., read mapping, variant calling) resulting in improper calling of DNA bases or sequence variants.
    - *Short-read sequencing* is intrinsically prone to miss structural variants such as longer insertions and deletions.
    - *Minimal residual disease (MRD) detection* is restricted by the background noise of NGS. Already known mutations are reidentifiable at a variant allele fraction as low as 1%.

Thus, the sensitivity of MRD detection by NGS is limited compared to quantitative real-time PCR (qPCR) which typically offers sensitivities of 10–4 to 10–6, or sometimes even more sensitive digital droplet PCR (ddPCR) which can detect up to 1 mutant copy of DNA as well.
- *Discrepancies in reporting format:* Since currently there are no consensus recommendations for NGS based testing and reporting in India, each lab has its own format, and own methodology. Some information is typically missing from all reports, which on monitoring makes it difficult to interrogate for MRD.
- *Biological challenges:*
  - Defining clinical impact of variants detected is a challenge. Many variants of uncertain clinical significance are detected. Additionally, variants implicated both in myeloid malignancies as well as clonal hematopoiesis of indeterminate potential are also detected. This poses a dilemma since not too much data and no consensus guidelines are available for definitively ascertaining the same. For example, AML, DNMT3A mutations can persist in the post-therapeutic period despite continuous remission without affecting the relapse rate in the absence of coincidental gene mutations. Using in-silico computational tools may not always be clinically meaningful and NGS reporting guidelines do not currently recommend assigning an assertion solely on the basis of computational evidence. Additionally, detection of copy number variants on NGS follows a normalization based on conserved regions and some technologies utilize number of reads generated. This again may not be as definitive as FISH.

REFERENCES

1. Martelotto LG, Baslan T, Kendall J, Geyer FC, Burke KA, Spraggon L, et al. Whole-genome single-cell copy number profiling from formalin-fixed paraffin-embedded samples. Nat Med. 2017;23(3):376-85.
2. Satam H, Joshi K, Mangrolia U, Waghoo S, Zaidi G, Rawool S, et al. Next-generation sequencing technology: current trends and advancements. Biology (Basel). 2023;12(7):997.
3. Qin D. Next-generation sequencing and its clinical application. Cancer Biol Med. 2019;16(1):4-10.
4. Jennings LJ, Arcila ME, Corless C, Kamel-Reid S, Lubin IM, Pfeifer J, T, et al. Guidelines for validation of next-generation sequencing–based oncology panels: a joint consensus recommendation of the Association for Molecular Pathology and College of American Pathologists. J Mol Diagn. 2017;19(3):341-65.
5. Alshemmari SH, Rajan R, Emadi A. Molecular pathogenesis and clinical significance of driver mutations in primary myelofibrosis: A Review. Med Princ Pract. 2016;25(6):501-9.
6. Reiter A, Gotlib J. Myeloid neoplasms with eosinophilia. Blood. 2017;129(6):704-4
7. Kayser S, Levis MJ. Clinical implications of molecular markers in acute myeloid leukemia. Eur J Haematol. 2019;102(1):20-35.
8. Coccaro N, Anelli L, Zagaria A, Specchia G, Albano F. Next-generation sequencing in acute lymphoblastic leukemia. Int J Mol Sci. 2019;20(12):2929.
9. Falini B, Martelli MP, Tiacci E. BRAF V600E mutation in hairy cell leukemia: from bench to bedside. Blood. 2016;128(15):1918-27.
10. Cardona-Benavides IJ, de Ramón C, Gutiérrez NC. Genetic abnormalities in multiple myeloma: prognostic and therapeutic implications. Cells. 2021;10(2):336.
11. Pei XM, Yeung MHY, Wong ANN, Tsang HF, Yu ACS, Yim AKY, et al. Targeted sequencing approach and its clinical applications for the molecular diagnosis of human diseases. Cells. 2023;12(3):493.
12. Schmid S, Jochum W, Padberg B, Demmer I, Mertz KD, Joerger M, et al. How to read a next-generation sequencing report-what oncologists need to know. ESMO. 2022;7(5):100570.

13. Zoller J, Trajanova D, Feurstein S. Germline and somatic drivers in inherited hematologic malignancies. Front Oncol. 2023;13:1205855.
14. Madaci L, Farnault L, Abbou N, Gabert J, Venton G, Costello R, et al. Impact of Next-generation sequencing in diagnosis, prognosis, and therapeutic management of acute myeloid leukemia/myelodysplastic neoplasms. Cancers (Basel). 2023;15(13):3280.
15. Muramatsu H, Okuno Y, Yoshida K, Shiraishi Y, Doisaki S, Narita A, et al. Clinical utility of next-generation sequencing for inherited bone marrow failure syndromes. Genet Med. 2017;19(7):796-802.
16. Alkan C, Sajjadian S, Eichler EE. Limitations of next-generation genome sequence assembly. Nat Methods. 2011;8(1):61-5.

19. Evaluation of Lymph Node

Rajan Duggal

CASE

A 45-year-old male presented with fever, weight loss, and bilateral cervical and axillary lymph node enlargement for 1 month. He was treated for tubercular lymphadenitis with antitubercular medicines for 2 months but there was no response to the treatment.

Q1. **What is the preferred histological diagnostic test for this patient? Why excisional biopsy is preferred over Tru-cut biopsy for the diagnosis of lymphoma?**

Ans: The preferred histological diagnostic test for suspected lymphoma patient is excision biopsy.

Excision biopsy is preferred over Tru-cut biopsy due to following reasons:[1,2]
- Since this patient has cervical and axillary lymph nodes which are more accessible group of lymph nodes. Tru-cut biopsy would have been considered if the lymph nodes were deep seated (like retroperitoneal lymph nodes, etc.).
- Lymph node architecture is best appreciated on excision biopsy sample. The relationship of different compartments of the lymph node such as cortex, paracortex, medulla, vasculature, and the sinuses with each other is best visualized in excision biopsy.
- If the lymphomatous pathology is focal/partial then it can be easily missed in Tru-cut biopsy. For example:
  - If the Reed–Sternberg cells/classical Hodgkin cells are seen only in the interfollicular areas and the Tru-cut biopsy is not able to sample the paracortex, then diagnosis of interfollicular Hodgkin lymphoma can be missed.[3]
  - In situ follicular neoplasia and in situ mantle cell neoplasia can be missed.
  - Sometimes lymphoma shows only partial effacement of the lymph node architecture. Further testing including immunohistochemistry (ICH) is also better appreciated if adequate representative tissue is available.

Q2. **What is the architecture of lymph node in benign and malignant diseases and what is the role of morphology in lymphoma evaluation?**

Ans: Benign pathologies show no effacement of the lymph node architecture. The relationship between cortex, paracortex, sinuses, vascular structures, and medulla is well preserved in benign lesions of the lymph node.[4,5]

Malignant diseases show effacement of the lymph node architecture. The relationship between cortex and paracortex is lost. For example, in follicular lymphoma, the neoplastic follicles are seen in cortex and paracortex with attenuated mantle zone layer. The sinusoidal architecture is lost in neoplastic lesions except in anaplastic large cell lymphoma where sometimes lymphoma cells are proliferating with in the sinuses (intrasinusoidal pattern).[5,6]

Role of morphology in lymphoma evaluation: Morphology plays a significant role in lymphoma diagnosis. The low magnification is helpful in assessing pattern. Examine each lymph node compartment capsule, sinuses **(Table 1)**, vasculature **(Table 2)**, paracortex **(Table 3)**, and cortex **(Table 4)**. **Table 5** shows pattern-based approach to lymphoma diagnosis.

TABLE 1: Abnormal findings in lymph node sinuses.	
Morphological abnormality in the lymph node sinusoidal architecture	**Morphological differential diagnosis**
Sinusoidal dilatation by histiocytes	• Rosai–Dorfman disease • Langerhans cell histiocytosis
Lymphocyte trafficking	• Viral infections • Lymphoma/Leukemia
Atypical clustering of cells in the expanded sinuses	• Metastatic disease • Anaplastic large cell lymphoma

TABLE 2: Abnormal vascular findings in lymph node.	
Morphological abnormality in the lymph node vascular architecture	**Morphological differential diagnosis**
Prominent hilar vessels	Vascular transformation of sinuses secondary to blockage of efferent lymphatics
Increased vascular elements	• Angioimmunoblastic T-cell lymphoma • Bacillary angiomatosis
Plump high-endothelial venules vascular hyalinization	• Angioimmunoblastic T-cell lymphoma (AITL) • Castleman disease (hyaline-vascular variant)
Primary vascular neoplasm	• Hemangioma • Angiomyolipoma • Kaposi sarcoma

TABLE 3: Paracortical expansion.	
Reactive conditions	**Lymphomatous conditions**
• Viral infection • Dermatopathic	• Marginal zone lymphoma • Lymphoplasmacytic lymphoma • Early involvement of CLL/SLL • T-cell lymphoma

TABLE 4: Follicular/Nodular pattern of cortical expansion.

Reactive conditions	Lymphomatous conditions
• Florid follicular hyperplasia • Progressive transformation of germinal centers	• Follicular lymphoma • Pediatric follicular lymphoma • Nodular lymphocyte predominant Hodgkin lymphoma • Nodular sclerosis Hodgkin lymphoma • Mantle cell lymphoma • Marginal zone lymphoma

TABLE 5: Pattern-based approach to lymphoma diagnosis.

Morphological patterns	Differential diagnosis
Small lymphocytes (blue looking lymphomas)	• CLL/SLL • Mantle cell lymphoma • Marginal zone lymphoma (MZL)
Follicles	Follicular lymphoma and reactive lymphoid proliferations
Follicles and some diffuse areas	Follicular lymphoma, MZL, AITL, and reactive processes
Mixed small and large cells, no definite pattern	• T-cell/histiocyte—cell rich large B-cell lymphoma • EBV positive lymphoid proliferation • T-cell lymphoma
Sinusoidal pattern	ALCL, metastatic lesions
Polymorphous with scattered large cells	Hodgkin, EBV positive lymphoproliferative disorder
Clusters/aggregates of large cells	High grade follicular lymphoma, large B-cell lymphoma with IRF4 rearrangement
Diffuse sheets of large cells	Diffuse large B-cell lymphoma
Increased stromal component	AITL, Kaposi sarcoma
Interfollicular pale cells	Marginal zone lymphoma, T-cell lymphomas

Abnormal Capsular Findings

- Thinning of the capsule is seen when there is rapid expansion of the nodal parenchyma by the malignant process.
- Thickening of the lymph node capsule is seen in chronic inflammatory processes, indolent B-cell lymphomas and nodular sclerosis Hodgkin lymphoma
- Extracapsular extension of the pathology is often seen with lymphomatous lesions.

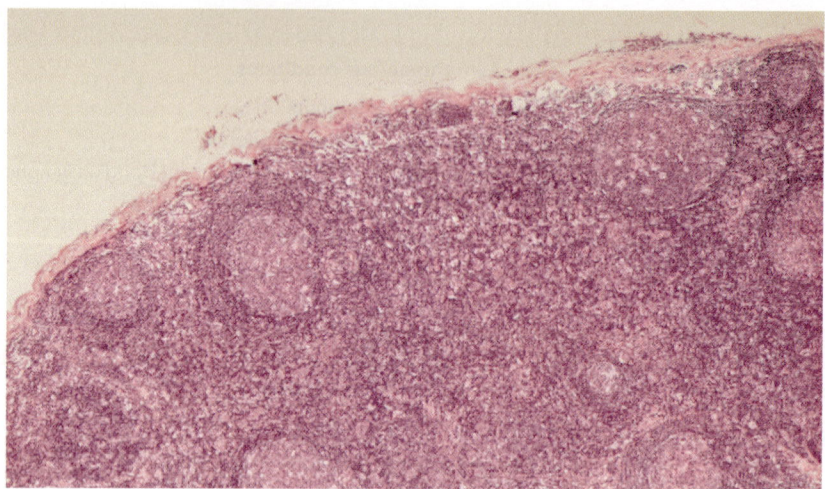

FIG. 1: Section from reactive lymph node show secondary follicles with preserved mantle zones and expanded paracortex. The paracortex is punctuated by endothelial venules (H&E staining, original magnification 10×).

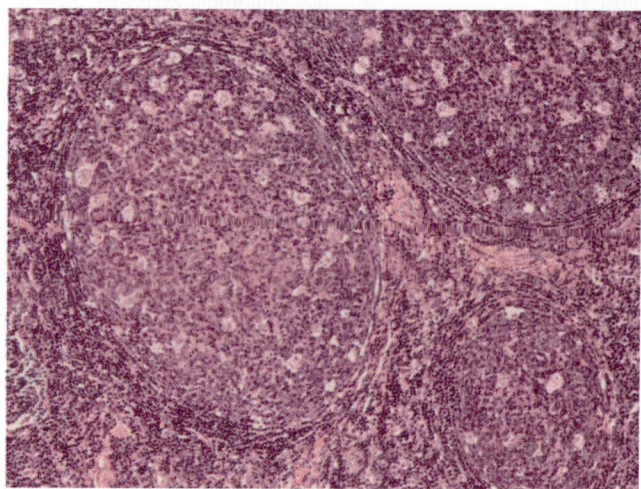

FIG. 2: Lymph node follicle showing presence of tingible body macrophages in the germinal center with preserved mantle zone, thereby indicating reactive secondary follicle (H&E staining, original magnification 20×, enlarged view of previous picture).

Q3. How should the immunohistochemical evaluation of lymph node be done? How IHC markers differentiate various subgroups of lymphomas?

Ans: Immunohistochemistry can have five different staining categories:[7-9]
1. Small B-cell lymphoma
2. Intermediate sized B-cell lymphoma
3. Large cell lymphoma
4. Hodgkin lymphoma
5. T-cell lymphoma

Small B-cell lymphoma IHC panel **(Table 6)**: CD3, CD20, CD5, CD23, CD10, BCL2, BCL6, CD10, Cyclin D1, SOX11, and Ki-67

Intermediate sized B-cell lymphoma IHC panel: LCA, CD3, CD20, CD5, CD23, CD10, BCL2, BCL6, CD10 , Cyclin D1, SOX11, TdT, CD16, CD56, EBV, and Ki-67

Large cell lymphoma IHC panel: CD3, CD20, CD30, BCL6, PAX5, MUM-1, ALK, and Ki-67

Hodgkin lymphoma IHC panel: LCA, CD3, CD20, CD15, CD30, Pax5, Mum-1, and EBV

T-cell lymphoma IHC panel: CD3, CD20, CD2, CD5,CD7, CD43, CD4, CD8, PD-1, BCL6, CD10, EBV, ALK, Granzyme, perforin, and CD21

TABLE 6: Small B-cell lymphoma specific immunohistochemistry (IHC) markers.	
Lymphoma type	**IHC marker expression**
CLL/SLL	CD5, CD23, CD20 (dim), LEF-1, and CD200
Mantle cell lymphoma	CD5, CD20, Cyclin D1, and SOX11
Marginal zone lymphoma	MNDA and IRTA
Hairy cell leukemia	CD103, CD11c, CD25, CD123, and CD200

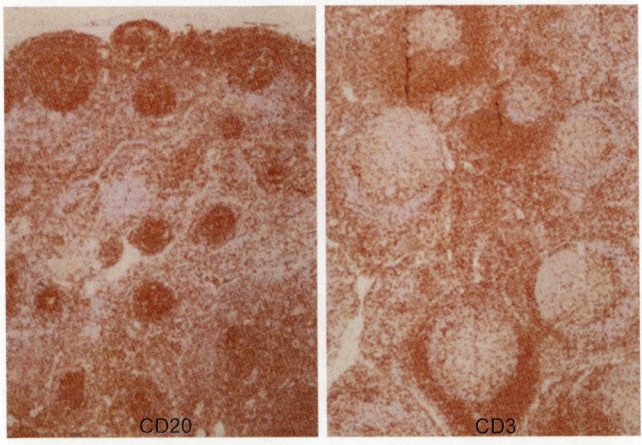

FIG. 3: Photomicrograph highlight normal distribution of B-cells and T-cells. CD20 stains predominantly lymph node follicles (Left image), primordial or secondary; however, CD3 stains the interfollicular compartment (Right) (CD20 and CD3 immunohistochemical stains, original magnification 20×).

Q4. **How reactive B cell rich lymphoid proliferation is differentiated from lymphoma?**

Ans: Most common reactive B cell lymphoid proliferation which can mimic lymphoma are:[10,11]
- Florid reactive lymphoid hyperplasia **(Table 7)**
- Marginal zone expansion **(Table 8)**
- EBV infection **(Table 9)**

TABLE 7: Differentiating florid reactive lymphoid hyperplasia from follicular lymphoma.

Florid reactive lymphoid hyperplasia	Follicular lymphoma
B-cell follicles show retained mantle zone	B-cell follicles show attenuated mantle zone
Reactive follicles show tingible body macrophages	No tingible body macrophages seen
Varying sized lymphoid follicles	Predominantly uniform sized lymphoid follicles with back to back arrangement
Immunohistochemistry: BCL2—negative in center of follicles. The mantle zone is positive	BCL2 positive in center of follicles
CD10—positive in germinal centers	CD10—positive in germinal centers and focally in interfollicular areas
BCL6—positive in germinal centers	BCL6—positive in germinal centers and focally in interfollicular areas
Ki-67 proliferative index—high in the germinal centers and highlight polarization within germinal centers	Ki67 proliferative index—low in the follicular centers and show no Ki-67 polarization. In some cases of high grade follicular lymphoma, Ki-67 proliferative index is high

TABLE 8: Marginal zone expansion versus marginal zone lymphoma.

Marginal zone expansion	Marginal zone lymphoma
The follicles show expanded marginal zone with no effacement of the lymph node architecture	Effacement of the lymph node architecture with expansion of the marginal zone around follicles and in interfollicular areas
Monomorphic appearance of expanded marginal zone cells	The marginal zone lymphoma show heterogenous population composed of intermediate to large cells with monocytoid appearance

TABLE 9: EBV infection versus B-cell lymphoma.

EBV infection	B-cell lymphoma
No effacement of the lymph node architecture	Effacement of the lymph node architecture
Composed of immunoblasts or Reed–Sternberg-like cells which are positive for both CD20 and CD3	All large cells (centroblasts or immunoblasts) show staining for only CD20

Q5. What is the role of flowcytometry in lymphoma diagnosis and how is it done?

Ans: Flowcytometry can provide diagnostic information regarding lymphomatous pathology in a short turnaround time.[12,13]

Flowcytometry is a very useful modality for a rapid diagnosis of mature B-cell non-Hodgkin lymphoma by identifying clonal restriction for kappa or lambda light chains. In addition, it also contributes to the diagnosis and classification of mature T- and NK-cell lymphoid neoplasms. Low-grade indolent lymphomas such as mucosa-associated lymphoid tissue (MALT) lymphoma of the head and neck region might not be at clinical need for a rapid diagnosis, however, in contrast aggressive lymphomas which present with compression of upper airways require an urgent diagnosis. Hence, flowcytometry plays a significant role in rapid diagnosis of aggressive lymphomas.

Excision biopsy tissue is processed using a mechanical disaggregation method. Tissues sampled are placed in a Petri dish and adjoining fatty and necrotic tissue is removed using a surgical scalpel. The useful tissue is fragmented into small tissue fragments with a diameter of 0.2–0.5 cm. To this 1 mL of phosphate-buffered saline (suspension buffer) is added. The sample must be in form of a suspension of single particles for being analyzed by flowcytometry. Analysis of DNA content by flowcytometry is based on the fluorescence intensity of nuclei stained with a fluorochrome specific to the DNA. The ideal cell count for assessment on the flowcytometry is 500,000 cells.

Q6. How is follicular lymphoma diagnosed?

Ans: Follicular lymphoma is diagnosed based on histology of lymph node biopsy. The cut surface of lymph nodes involved by follicular lymphoma may display a vaguely nodular pattern. Follicular lymphoma resembles germinal centers in its cellular composition, with a mixture of centrocytes (CCs) and centroblasts (CBs). The follicles are often crowded, with a back-to-back arrangement. Most neoplastic follicles lack mantle zones, with ill-defined borders. They usually lack polarization of the germinal centers i.e., the physiological demarcation between a centroblast-rich (dark) and a centrocyte-rich (light) zone is absent. Traditionally, follicular lymphoma has been graded as FL1, 2, 3A, and 3B based on the quantification of absolute numbers of centroblasts in 10 consecutive high-power fields.

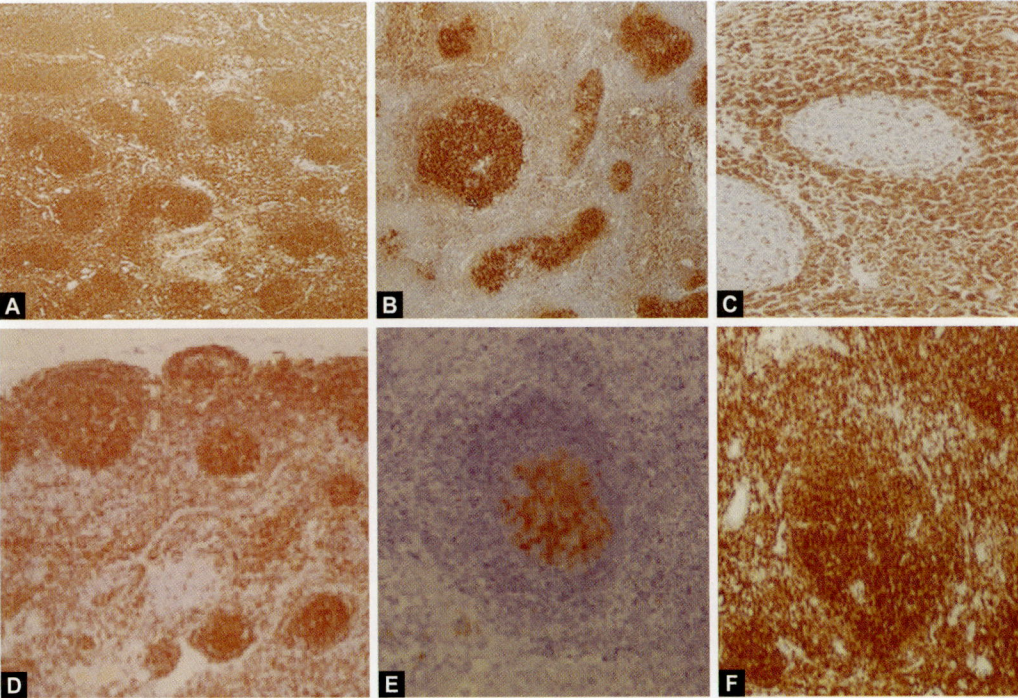

FIGS. 4A TO F: Highlight immunohistochemical pattern of staining in follicular lymphoma. (A) shows CD20 positivity in the follicles and interfollicular areas. (B) shows CD10 staining within follicles and interfollicular areas. (C) shows BCL2 staining the germinal centers thereby indicating neoplastic follicles. (D to F) Highlight immunohistochemical pattern of staining in follicular hyperplasia. (D) shows CD20 positivity predominantly in the follicles and no significant staining in interfollicular areas. (E) shows CD10 staining limited only to germinal centres. (F) shows BCL2 staining the periphery of the germinal centers thereby indicating reactive follicles.

Immunohistochemistry of lymph node is positive for cell surface CD19, CD20, CD10, and monoclonal immunoglobulin, as well as cytoplasmic expression of BCL-2 protein. Normal germinal center cells are BCL-2 negative. The pathological hallmark of follicular lymphoma is translocation t(14;18)(q32;q21) which results in overproduction of the BCL-2 protein, which impairs the apoptosis of germinal center B cells resulting in their overgrowth and thus lymphoma.

Q7. How is diffuse large B-cell lymphoma (DLBCL, NOS) diagnosed?

Ans: Diffuse large B-cell lymphoma, not otherwise specified (DLBCL, NOS), is a lymphoma consisting of medium to large B cells with a diffuse growth pattern. The majority of patients with DLBCL, NOS present with nodal disease. Around 30–40% of cases present with disease confined to extranodal sites at diagnosis.

Most DLBCL, NOS broadly recapitulate the germinal centre differentiation/maturation mechanisms. They are composed of large cells often resembling centroblasts derived from the germinal center and showing mutational signatures of the somatic hypermutation machinery. Tissue architecture of lymph nodes or extranodal sites is partially or totally effaced by medium-to-large sized lymphoid cells (with large cell defined as having nucleus more than twice the size of a small lymphocyte nucleus) that are arranged in a diffuse or vaguely nodular pattern.

Lymphoma cells express CD45 and Pan-B-cell markers (CD19, CD20, CD22, CD79a, and PAX5), but may lack one or more of the B-cell markers and use of more than one B-cell marker may be necessary to confirm B-cell lineage and support the diagnosis. The majority of DLBCL, NOS express BCL2 and the intensity of expression is variable. Similarly, expression of MYC protein is highly variable. BCL2 is considered positive if 50% or more of the tumor cells are positive and MYC is considered positive if at least 40% of the tumor cell nuclei are positive. DLBCL, NOS may express CD5 in 5–10% of cases. CD5+ DLBCL, NOS can be distinguished from the pleomorphic variant of mantle cell lymphoma by the absence of cyclin D1 and SOX11 expression. The activated B-cell-like type (ABC) of DLBCL, NOS has an inferior outcome in response to standard therapies when compared to the germinal centre B-cell group (GCB) in most clinical cohorts.

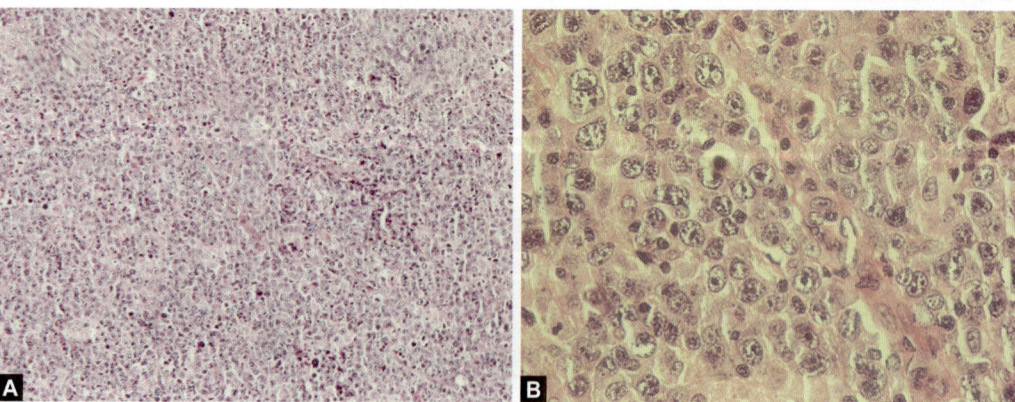

FIGS. 5A AND B: (A) Highlight effacement of the lymph node architecture by an atypical lymphoid infiltrate arranged in diffuse pattern. (B) The lymphoid cells are large in size with moderate cytoplasm, vesicular nucleus and prominent nucleoli suggesting diffuse large cell non-Hodgkin lymphoma.

REFERENCES

1. Osborne BM, Butler JJ. Follicular lymphoma mimicking progressive transformation of germinal centers. Am J Clin Pathol. 1987;88:264-9.
2. Kroft SH. Stratification of Follicular Lymphoma: Time for a Paradigm Shift? Am J Clin Pathol. 2019;151:539-41.
3. Gaffar AB, Seliem RM. Hodgkin lymphoma with an interfollicular growth pattern: A clinicopathologic study of 8 cases. Ann Diagn Pathol. 2018;33:30-4.
4. Jaffe ES, Cook JR. Core biopsy for lymphoma diagnosis? A needling prospect. Blood. 2022;140(24):2525-7.
5. Jegalian AG, Eberle FC, Pack SD, Mirvis M, Raffeld M, Pittaluga S, et al. Follicular lymphoma in situ: clinical implications and comparisons with partial involvement by follicular lymphoma. Blood. 2011;118:2976-84.
6. Syrykh C, Chaouat C, Poullot E, Amara N, Fataccioli V, Parrens M, et al. Lymph node excisions provide more precise lymphoma diagnoses than core biopsies: a French Lymphopath network survey. Blood. 2022;140(24):2573-83.
7. Cho J. Basic immunohistochemistry for lymphoma diagnosis. Blood Res. 2022;57(S1):55-61.
8. Boyd SD, Natkunam Y, Allen JR, Warnke RA. Selective immunophenotyping for diagnosis of B-cell neoplasms: immunohistochemistry and flow cytometry strategies and results. Appl Immunohistochem Mol Morphol. 2013;21(2):116-31.
9. Disanto MG, Ambrosio MR, Rocca BJ, Ibrahim HA, Leoncini L, Naresh KN. Optimal minimal panels of immunohistochemistry for diagnosis of B-Cell lymphoma for application in countries with limited resources and for triaging cases before referral to specialist centers. Am J Clin Pathol. 2016;145:687-95.
10. Chan JKC. An approach to distinction between reactive and malignant lymphoid proliferation. Pathology. 2010;42:S13.
11. Weiss L, O'Malley D. Benign lymphadenopathies. Mod Pathol. 2013;26:S88–S96.
12. Morse EE, Yamase HT, Greenberg BR, Sporn J, Harshaw SA, Kiraly TR, et al. The role of flow cytometry in the diagnosis of lymphoma: a critical analysis. Ann Clin Lab Sci. 1994;24(1):6-11.
13. Stetler-Stevenson M. Flow cytometry in lymphoma diagnosis and prognosis: useful? Best Pract Res Clin Haematol. 2003;16(4):583-97.

20 Lymphoproliferative Disorders

Devasis Panda, Mousumi Kar

Q1. What are B-cell chronic lymphoproliferative disorders (CLPDs)?

Ans: B-cell CLPDs are a group of mature B-cell neoplasms characterized by persistent lymphocytosis and/or lymphoid tissue infiltration.[1] They typically present in older adults and show variable clinical behavior, ranging from indolent to aggressive.

Q2. What are the common B-CLPD entities?

Ans: The common B-CLPDs include:[3]
- Chronic lymphocytic leukemia/small lymphocytic lymphoma (CLL/SLL)
- Mantle cell lymphoma (MCL)
- *Marginal zone lymphoma* (*MZL*): Splenic, nodal, extranodal
- Hairy cell leukemia (HCL)
- Lymphoplasmacytic lymphoma (LPL)
- Follicular lymphoma (leukemic phase)
- Burkitt's lymphoma

Q3. What are the morphological features on peripheral smear and bone marrow?

Ans: Chronic lymphoproliferative disorders predominantly present with lymphocytosis. Lymphocytes are predominantly mature in morphology, however, few signature morphological features can help in subtyping of CLPDs **(Table 1)**.[3]

TABLE 1: Subtyping of chronic lymphoproliferative disorders and their morphological features.		
Entity	**Peripheral smear**	**Bone marrow findings**
Chronic lymphocytic leukemia/ small lymphocytic lymphoma (CLL/SLL)	Small mature lymphocytes with scant cytoplasm, clumped "soccer-ball" such as chromatin and smudge cells	Interstitial or nodular infiltration by small lymphocytes; pseudo follicles (proliferation centers) may be seen in biopsy
Mantle cell lymphoma	Medium-sized lymphoid cells with irregular or cleaved nuclear contours, inconspicuous nucleoli. Often showing blastoid morphology	Nodular or diffuse infiltrate; can resemble other small B-cell lymphomas; cells may involve paratrabecular as well as interstitial areas

Continued

Continued

Entity	Peripheral smear	Bone marrow findings
Marginal zone lymphoma (MZL)	Small to medium-sized lymphocytes with irregular nuclear contours; monocytoid B-cell appearance in some cases. Sometimes cytyoplasmic polar villi noted	Nodular and/or interstitial infiltrate; may involve sinusoids (especially in splenic MZL); variable plasmacytic differentiation
Hairy cell leukemia	Cells with oval kidney/bean shaped nuclei and abundant pale cytoplasm with fine cytoplasmic projections ("hairy" cells)	"Dry tap" due to marrow fibrosis; biopsy shows diffuse or interstitial infiltration with clear area around cells fried-egg appearance; reticulin fibrosis often prominent giving rise to chicken wire like morphology
Lymphoplasmacytic lymphoma	Mixed population of small lymphocytes, plasmacytoid lymphocytes, and plasma cells	Diffuse or interstitial infiltration; plasma cell component with Dutcher bodies and Russell bodies; mast cells may be increased. Serum lakes may be seen
Follicular lymphoma (leukemic phase)	Small to medium-sized lymphocytes with cleaved ("buttock-shaped") nuclei; centrocyte-like cells in blood	Nodular pattern; centrocytes and centroblasts; BCL2-positive germinal centers; paratrabecular aggregates in marrow
Burkitt lymphoma (leukemic phase)	Medium-sized cells with basophilic cytoplasm and multiple cytoplasmic vacuoles	"Starry-sky" appearance due to tingible-body macrophages; high mitotic index; monotonous intermediate-sized cells
Diffuse large B-cell lymphoma (DLBCL)	Large lymphoid cells with vesicular nuclei, prominent nucleoli, and moderate-to-abundant cytoplasm. Often having blastoid bizarre morphology	Diffuse sheets of large, atypical cells; centroblastic, immunoblastic, or anaplastic morphology; high-grade features

Q4. How does flow cytometry help in diagnosis?

Ans: Flow cytometry confirms B-cell lineage, assesses clonality via kappa/lambda light chain restriction, and identifies disease-specific immunophenotypes.

Q5. What are the characteristics of flow cytometric profiles?

Ans: The characteristics of flow cytometric profile are as shown in **Flowchart 1**.

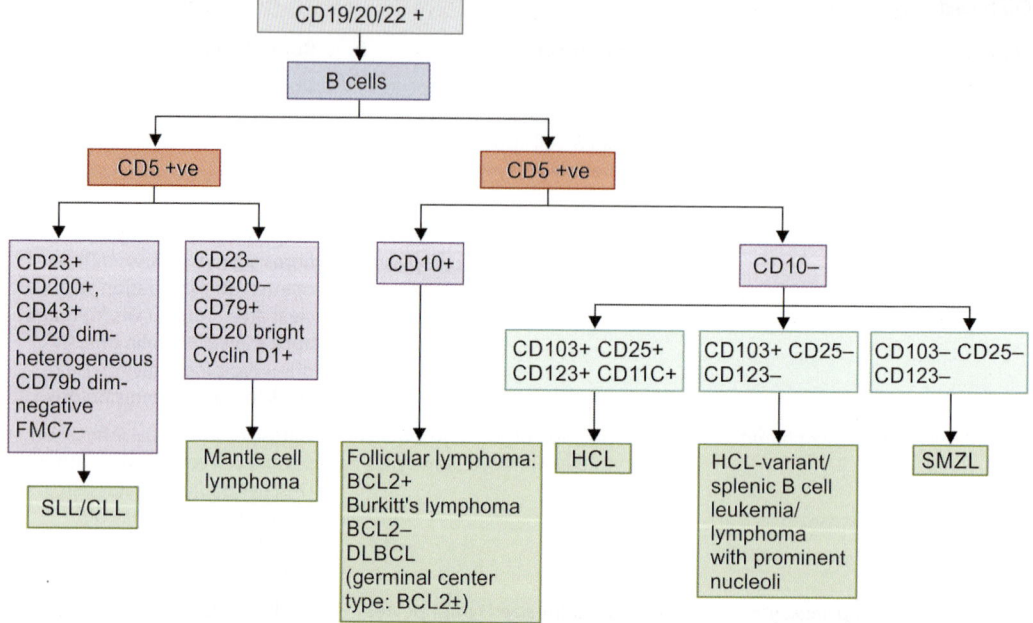

FLOWCHART 1: Characteristics of flow cytometric profile.

(CLL: chronic lymphocytic leukemia; DLBCL: diffuse large B-cell lymphoma; HCL: hairy cell leukemia; SMZL: splenic marginal zone lymphoma; SLL: small lymphocytic lymphoma)

Q6. How does the cell of origin influence the classification and features of B-cell CLPDs?

Ans: The classification of B-cell CLPDs is closely linked to the stage of B-cell differentiation from which the neoplasm arises **(Table 2)**.[4,5] This understanding helps explain their morphological, immunophenotypic, and clinical behavior.

TABLE 2: Classification and features of B-cell CLPDs on the basis of cell of origin.

Cell of origin	Representative CLPDs	Features
Naïve B-cell	MCL	CD5+, Cyclin D1+; t(11;14); more aggressive course
Marginal zone B-cell	MZL	CD5−, CD10−, CD23−; extranodal or splenic involvement
Postgerminal center memory B-cell	HCL, LPL	Aberrant expression (e.g., CD103+ in HCL); indolent clinical course
Germinal center B-cell (centrocyte/centroblast)	Follicular lymphoma, Burkitt lymphoma	CD10+, BCL6+; t(14;18) in FL, t(8;14) in Burkitt; leukemic presentation possible
Plasmacytic differentiation	LPL	CD38+, surface or cytoplasmic IgM+, MYD88 mutation common
Postgerminal/memory B-cell (activated)	CLL/SLL	CD5+, CD23+, CD200+; weak sIg; derived from antigen-experienced B cells

Note: DLBCL may arise from either germinal center B-cells or activated B-cells. Cell-of-origin (COO) classification using immunohistochemistry (e.g., Hans algorithm) or gene expression profiling has prognostic and therapeutic relevance.

(CLL: chronic lymphocytic leukemia; CLPDs: chronic lymphoproliferative disorders; DLBCL: diffuse large B-cell lymphoma; HCL: hairy cell leukemia; LPL: lymphoplasmacytic lymphoma; MCL: mantle cell lymphoma; MZL: marginal zone lymphoma; SLL: small lymphocytic lymphoma; sIg: surface immunoglobulin)

Q7. What are the recent molecular and genetic updates in B-cell CLPDs?

Ans: Molecular diagnostics have enhanced our understanding of B-cell CLPDs and now play a vital role in classification, prognosis, and targeted therapy. Key updates are given in **Table 3**.

TABLE 3: Key updates in B-cell CLPDs.		
Entity	**Key molecular abnormalities**	**Clinical relevance**
CLL/SLL	• *IGHV* mutation status (mutated = better prognosis) • TP53 mutation/del(17p) • NOTCH1, SF3B1, BIRC3 mutations	Risk stratification; TP53 alterations predict poor response to chemoimmunotherapy (prefer BTK inhibitors)
MCL	• t(11;14)(q13;q32) → CCND1–IGH • SOX11 expression • TP53 mutations	SOX11+ classic MCL has worse prognosis; TP53 mutation = aggressive course
MZL (esp. splenic)	• NOTCH2 mutations, • KLF2, TNFAIP3, and • MYD88 (less common)	Aid in subclassification; NOTCH2 associated with splenic MZL
HCL	BRAF V600E mutation (in >95% classic HCL)	Diagnostic marker; BRAF inhibitors used in refractory cases
LPL	• MYD88 L265P mutation (>90% of cases) • CXCR4 mutations (in 30–40%)	MYD88 confirms diagnosis; CXCR4 mutation affects ibrutinib response
FL (leukemic phase)	• t(14;18)(q32;q21) → IGH-BCL2 • CREBBP, EZH2, KMT2D mutations	Diagnostic and prognostic; EZH2 inhibitors under evaluation
Burkitt lymphoma	• MYC rearrangement (usually t(8;14)) • TP53, ID3, TCF3 mutations	MYC translocation is defining; complex karyotype may suggest "double/triple hit" lymphoma
DLBCL (leukemic phase)	• Cell-of-origin stratification (GCB vs. ABC) • MYC, BCL2, BCL6 rearrangements • EZH2 (GCB), MYD88/CD79B (ABC)	COO guides therapy (e.g., ibrutinib in ABC-type); double/triple hit = poor prognosis

(BTK: Bruton's tyrosine kinase; COO: cell of origin; CLL: chronic lymphocytic leukemia; CLPDs: chronic lymphoproliferative disorders; DLBCL: diffuse large B-cell lymphoma; FL: follicular lymphoma; HCL: hairy cell leukemia; LPL: lymphoplasmacytic lymphoma; MCL: mantle cell lymphoma; MZL: marginal zone lymphoma; SLL: small lymphocytic lymphoma)

Q8. How do you differentiate between classic HCL, HCL-variant (now renamed), and splenic marginal zone lymphoma (SMZL)?

Ans: HCL, its variant form, and SMZL can have overlapping features such as *splenomegaly and cytopenias*, but they differ significantly in morphology, immunophenotype, and molecular profile. Accurate distinction is essential for therapy selection and prognosis.

- *Updated nomenclature:*
  - *HCL-Variant* has been *renamed as "Splenic B-cell Lymphoma/Leukemia with Prominent Nucleoli (SBLPN)"* in the 2022 World Health Organization (WHO) classification.
  - International Consensus Classification (ICC) (2022) still refers to it as *"HCL-variant (HCL-v),"* but recognizes it as a distinct entity.
- *Comparison is given in* **Table 4**.[2,6]

TABLE 4: Comparison of classic HCL, HCL-variant/SBLPN, and splenic marginal zone lymphoma (SMZL).

Feature	Classic HCL	HCL-variant/SBLPN	SMZL
Morphology	Small-to-medium cells with *fine cytoplasmic projections* ("hairy" cells); round nuclei	Medium-large cells with *prominent nucleoli*, fewer projections	Small cells with *villous cytoplasm*, round nuclei
Peripheral blood	Pancytopenia, monocytopenia, *dry tap* on BM	Leukocytosis, no monocytopenia	Cytopenia or leukocytosis with circulating villous cells
Immunophenotype	CD19+, CD20+, *CD11c+, CD25+, CD103+, CD123+, Annexin A1+*	CD11c+, CD25–, CD103+/–, CD123–, Annexin A1–	CD11c+, CD25–, CD103–, CD123–, sometimes IgM+, DBA.44–
BRAF mutation	BRAF V600E positive (~90%)	BRAF negative	BRAF negative
TRAP stain	Strongly positive	Weak or negative	Negative
Bone marrow	Diffuse or interstitial infiltration; fried-egg appearance	Interstitial/nodular; no "fried-egg"	Intrasinusoidal pattern
Clinical course	Indolent; good response to cladribine	More aggressive; poor response to cladribine	Indolent, but transformation possible
First-line therapy	Cladribine ± rituximab	Rituximab + chemo (e.g., bendamustine)	Splenectomy or rituximab-based therapy

(HCL: hairy cell leukemia SBLPN: splenic B-cell lymphoma/leukemia with prominent nucleoli)

- *Takeaway for students:*
  - Use *Annexin A1 and BRAF V600E* as key markers to confirm classic HCL.
  - HCL-variant/SBLPN lacks *Annexin A1* and *BRAF* mutation and behaves more aggressively.
  - SMZL can resemble HCL morphologically but lacks the classic immunophenotypic and molecular features.

CHAPTER 21: Lymphoproliferative Disorders

- *Case discussion (Figs. 1 to 3)*:
  - A 54-year-old female, presented with low grade fever, weight loss for last 3 months. Complete blood count (CBC) shows pancytopenia. Splenomegaly—2 cm below costal margin.
  - PS shows lymphocyte preponderance. On high power few lymphocytes show cytoplasmic projections.

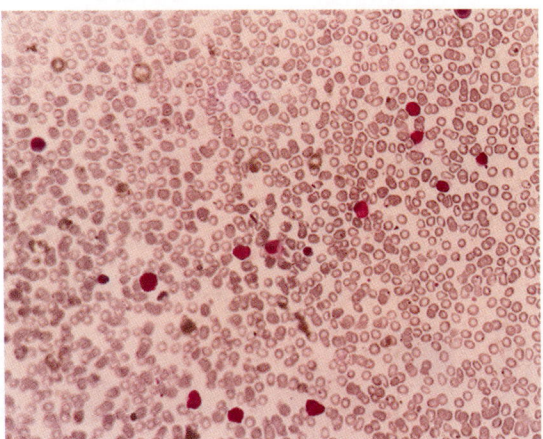

FIG. 1: Low magnification microscopic picture (×20) of peripheral blood showing preponderance of lymphocytes.

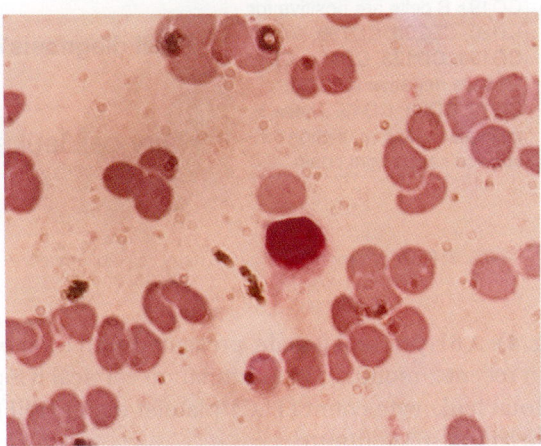

FIG. 2: High power view (×100) of peripheral blood showing mature lymphocytes with cytoplasmic hairy projections.

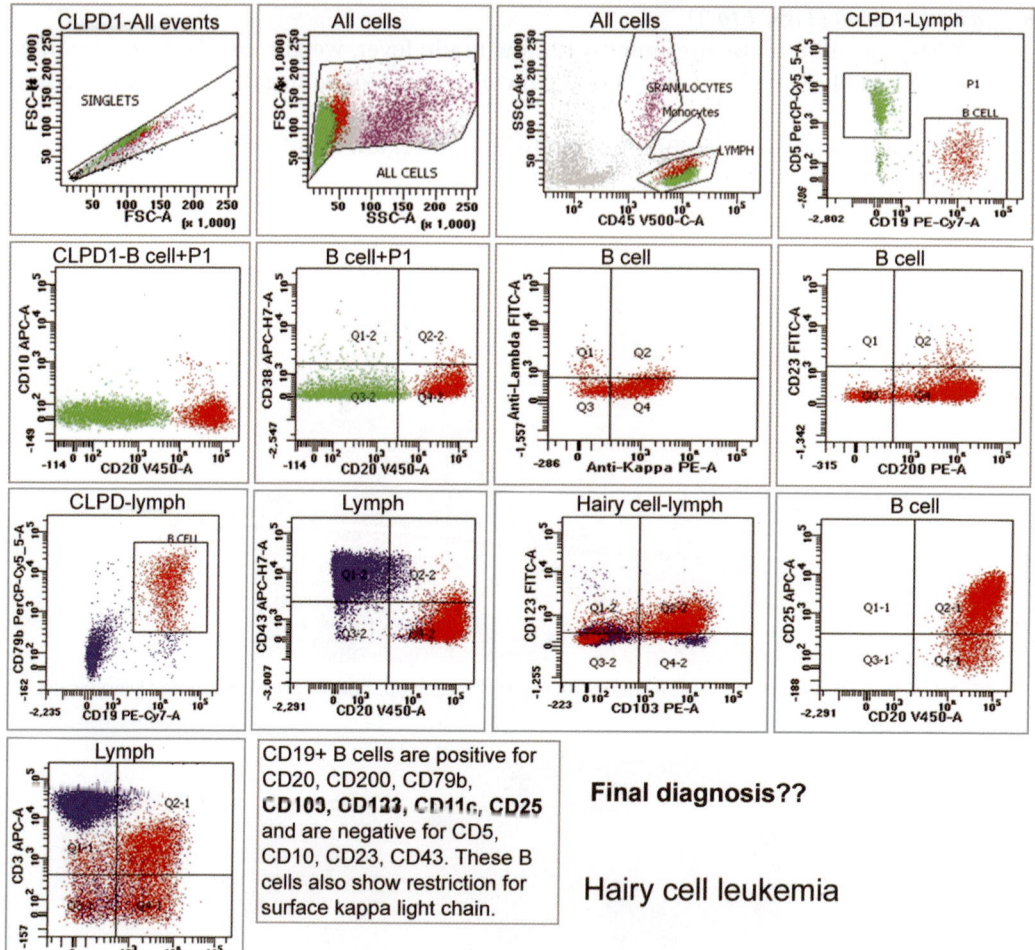

FIG. 3: Flow cytometry analysis of hairy cell leukemia.

- *Case discussion* **(Fig. 4)**: A 61-year-old female, presented with fever on and off in 4 months, weight loss of 5 kg in recent 2 months. On examination cervical lymphadenopathy+. CBC: Hemoglobin (Hb)/total leukocyte count (TLC)/platelet count (PLT)—11.9/74.05/176,000 absolute lymphocyte count—63,000/mm^3.

CHAPTER 21: Lymphoproliferative Disorders

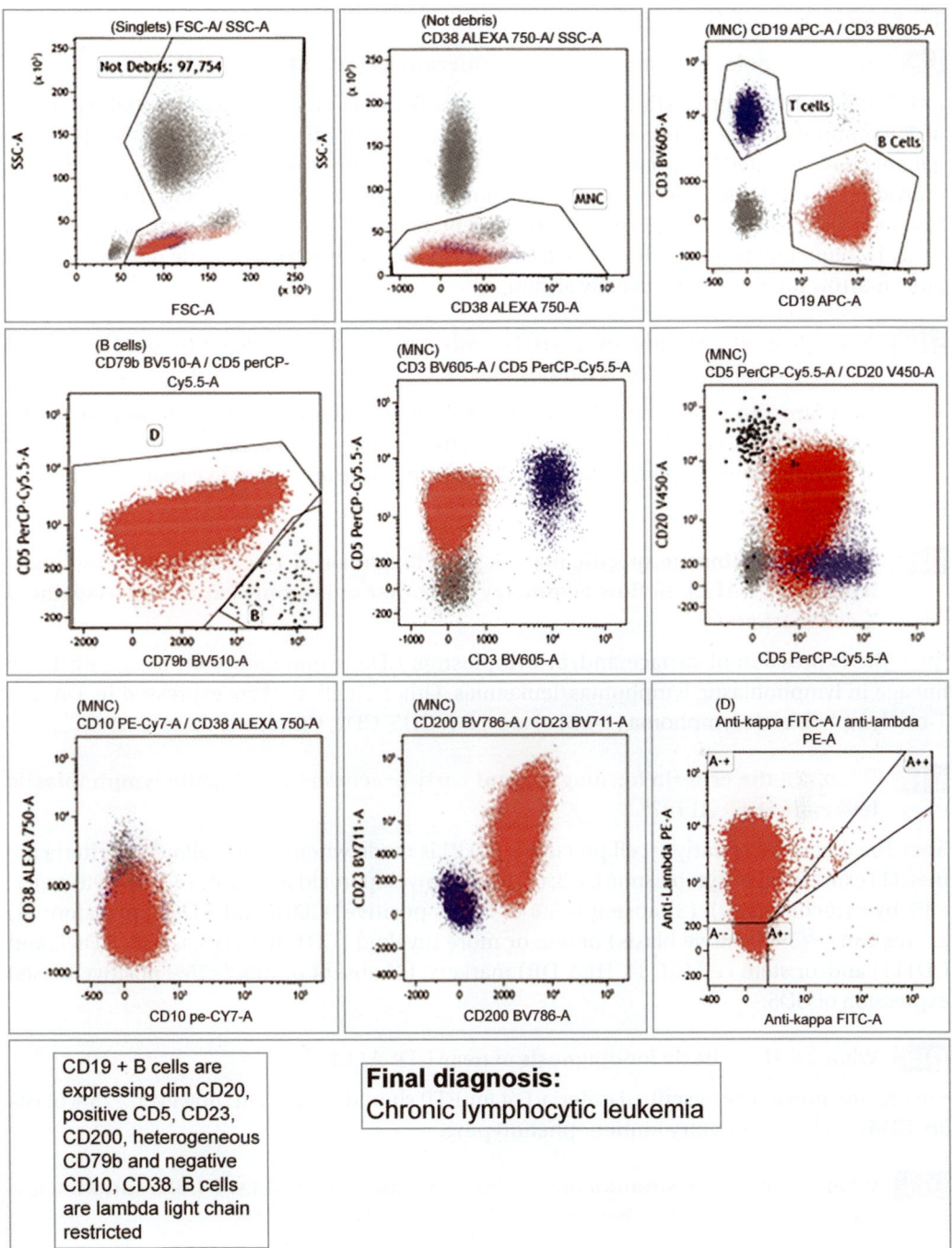

FIG. 4: Flow cytometry analysis of chronic lymphocytic leukemia.

T-LYMPHOID NEOPLASMS

Q9. What is indolent T-lymphoblastic proliferations (IT-LBP)?

Ans: Indolent T-lymphoblastic proliferation is extrathymic in origin and a nonclonal expansion of T-lymphoblasts occurring alone or in association with other disorders. Majority of the patients have isolated lymphadenopathy or an isolated tumor mass in an otherwise healthy individual. It has an immature immunophenotype expressing CD3, TdT, and majority of the cases are CD4/CD8 double positive. CD10, CD99, and CD1a are variably expressed whereas CD34 is frequently negative. The cells, however, do not show atypia or tissue destruction and bone marrow involvement is usually absent.

Q10. Name the non-neoplastic entities added to the recent WHO hematolymphoid malignancies under T-cell lymphomas.

Ans: There are three non-neoplastic entities which have been recently added to the classification of T/NK cell lymphomas in WHO 5th edition, i.e., Kikuchi–Fujimoto disease, IT-LBP, and autoimmune lymphoproliferative syndrome. These are tumor like lesions with T-cell predominance.

Q11. Which is the lineage specific marker for a diagnosis of T-cell acute lymphoblastic leukemia (T-ALL) on flow cytometry and other commonly expressed associated T-cell markers?[7]

Ans: The expression of surface and/or cytoplasmic CD3 is mandatory for assigning T-cell lineage in lymphoblastic lymphomas/leukemias. Other T-cell markers expressed in T-ALLs/T-cell lymphoblastic lymphoma (T-LBLs) are CD7, CD5, CD2, CD1a, etc.

Q12. What are the criteria for diagnosis of early precursor T-cell acute lymphoblastic leukemia (ETP-ALL)?[8]

Ans: The diagnosis of early T-cell precursor (ETP) is made when all the following criteria are met. (1) expression of cytoplasmic CD3; (2) absent myeloperoxidase (<10% by flow cytometry, <3% by cytochemistry); (3) absent (<5% of blasts positive) CD1a and CD8 expression; (4) expression (≥25% positive blasts) of one or more myeloid (CD11b, CD13, CD33, CD65, and CD117) and/or stem cell (CD34, HLA-DR) markers; (5) absent or dim (<75% positive blasts) expression of CD5.

Q13. What are the criteria for diagnosis of near ETP-ALL?

Ans: All the previously described criteria 1–4 for ETP should be present; however, ≥75% blasts are CD5+ on flow cytometry immunophenotyping.

Q14. What are the most common molecular aberrancies in T-ALLs/T-LBLs and what are the subgroups of T-ALL based on molecular markers?

Ans: The most common molecular anomalies in T-ALLs/T-LBLs are mutations affecting the NOTCH1 pathway, translocations of transcription factors to chromosomal regions of TCR loci, and mutations in epigenetic regulators (EZH2, SUZ12, and EED) and chromatin modifiers (PHF6, KDM6A, and USP7).

T-ALL can be divided into four distinct, nonoverlapping genetic subgroups based on specific translocations that lead to aberrant expression of (1) TAL or LMO genes, (2) TLX1, (3) TLX3, and (4) HOXA genes.

Q15. What are T-cell CLPDs?

Ans: These are rare mature T-cell neoplasms characterized by lymphocytosis, often with cytopenias or immune dysregulation. They may be indolent [e.g., T-cell large granular lymphocytic leukemia (T-LGL)] or aggressive [e.g., T-cell prolymphocytic leukemia (T-PLL)].

Q16. What are the major T-CLPDs?

Ans:
- T-cell prolymphocytic leukemia
- T-cell large granular lymphocytic leukemia
- Adult T-cell leukemia/lymphoma (ATLL)
- Sézary syndrome (SS)

Q17. What is the morphological spectrum of T-CLPD?[7]

Ans: The morphological spectrum of T-CLPD is given in **Table 5**.

TABLE 5: Morphological spectrum of T-CLPD.

Entity	Typical morphological feature
T-PLL	Medium-large cells with prominent nucleoli
T-LGL	Large lymphocytes with azurophilic granules
NK-LGL	Granular cytoplasm
ATLL	Flower-shaped (cloverleaf) nuclei
Sézary syndrome	Cerebriform (brain-like) nuclei
Primary cutaneous CD4+ LPD	Small/medium cells with minimal atypia
Indolent GI T-cell LPD	Small lymphocytes in gastrointestinal (GI) biopsy, bland appearance

(ATLL: adult T-cell leukemia/lymphoma; CLPD: chronic lymphoproliferative disorders; NK-LGL: natural killer cell large granular lymphocyte leukemia; LPD: lymphoproliferative disease; T-LGL: T-cell large granular lymphocytic leukemia; T-PLL: T-cell prolymphocytic leukemia)

Q18. How is clonality assessed in T-CLPD?

Ans:
- Polymerase chain reaction (PCR)-based T-cell receptor (*TCR*) gene rearrangement analysis.
- Flow cytometric TCR Vβ repertoire (if available).

Q19. How do you approach a suspected CLPD in the lab?

Ans:
- Peripheral smear review
- CBC with absolute lymphocyte count
- Flow cytometry with lineage markers (CD3, CD19) and extended panels
- Bone marrow aspirate/biopsy
- Cytogenetic/molecular studies if indicated

Q20. What is the flow cytometric approach to diagnosing T-cell CLPDs?[8]

Ans: Flow cytometry is a critical tool in the diagnosis of T-cell CLPDs. It helps in confirming T-cell lineage, assessing aberrant antigen expression, and detecting clonal expansion based on T-cell markers.

Stepwise Flow Cytometric Approach

- *Confirm T-cell lineage:*
  - Use pan-T-cell markers: CD3, CD2, CD5, CD7
  - Identify aberrant loss or dim expression (e.g., loss of CD7 or CD5)
- *Assess CD4/CD8 expression:*
  - Most clonal T-cells are either CD4+ or CD8+
  - Coexpression or double-negativity (CD4–/CD8–) suggests neoplasia
- *Identify LGL expansions:*
  - Use CD57, CD16, CD8 for T-LGL
  - CD56+, CD3– for NK-cell LGL
- *Evaluate TCR expression:*
  - TCR αβ versus TCR γδ can help subtype certain disorders
  - TCR Vβ repertoire analysis (if available) can demonstrate clonality
- *Use of activation and helper markers:*
  - CD25: Seen in ATLL
  - CD26, CD7: Often lost in Sézary syndrome
  - CD10, BCL6, PD1, CXCL13, ICOS: May help identify T-follicular helper phenotype
- *Assess aberrant marker expression:*
  - Neoplastic T-cells may show aberrant coexpression (e.g., CD56) or loss of pan-T antigens like CD5, CD3, CD7, CD2, etc.

Examples of immunophenotypes in common T-CLPDs are given in **Table 6**.

TABLE 6: Immunophenotypes in common T-CLPDs.		
Entity	**Key markers**	**Notes**
T-PLL	CD3+, CD2+, CD5+, CD7+, CD4+/CD8±	Strong CD52 expression; aggressive
T-LGL	CD3+, CD8+, CD57+, CD16+, CD5 dim	STAT3 mutation common
NK-LGL	CD3–, CD56+, CD16+, CD57+	TCR–; may overlap with T-LGL clinically
ATLL	CD3+, CD4+, CD25+, CD7–	HTLV-1 related
Sézary syndrome	CD3+, CD4+, CD26–, CD7–	Cerebriform nuclei; clonality by TCR

(ATLL: adult T-cell leukemia/lymphoma; CLPD: chronic lymphoproliferative disorders; NK-LGL: natural killer cell large granular lymphocyte leukemia; T-LGL: T-cell large granular lymphocytic leukemia; T-PLL: T-cell prolymphocytic leukemia)

Points to Remember

- Always correlate flow cytometry with morphology, clinical features, and *TCR* gene rearrangement studies.
- T-cell neoplasms often show subtle antigen aberrancies, unlike B-cell CLPDs which often have clear clonality via light chains.
- Multicolor panels (≥8–10 colors) are preferred to identify subtle subpopulations.
- WHO/ICC classification should be referenced for final diagnosis.

Q21. What are the essential and desirable diagnostic criteria of T-cell prolymphocytic leukemia?

Ans: *Essential criteria:* (1) Lymphocytosis >5 × 10^9/L with T-PLL immunophenotype in peripheral blood or bone marrow; (2) T-cell monoclonality TCL1A or MTCP1 rearrangement, alternatively TCL1A protein expression.

Desirable: Detection of a juxtaposition of the *TCL1A* or *MTCP1* gene next to a TCR locus mostly the TRA/TRD locus.

Q22. What are the common clinical and laboratory features of T-cell large granular lymphocytic leukemia (T-LGLL)?

Ans: Majority of patients of T-LGLL present have complaints of recurrent infections owing to cytopenias. Up to 80% of cases present with neutropenia complicated by aphthous ulcers of oral mucosa and ulceration or recurrent bacterial infections of the skin, oropharynx, or perirectum. They are frequently associated with autoimmune disorders with rheumatoid arthritis occurring in approximately 20%. Pure red blood cell aplasia leading to transfusion dependent anemia is seen in a minority of cases.

Q23. What are the immunophenotyping and molecular aberrancies in T-LGLL?

Ans: Most T-LGLL show a mature effector memory phenotype (CD3+/CD8+/CD57+/CD45RA+/CD62L–) in majority with few of cases express CD4 either alone or in association with CD8dim (CD4+ T-LGLL). The lymphoid cells usually express other T-cell markers such as CD2, CD3, TCRβ, CD7, and the cytotoxic granule proteins T-cell intracellular antigen 1 (TIA-1), perforin, granzyme B, and granzyme M. They rarely express CD56 and are often negative for CD5.

T-LGLLs show monoclonal *TCR* gene rearrangement. STAT3 and STAT5B mutations are the most commonly recognized gain-of-function genetic lesions in T-LGLL.

Q24. What are the criteria for the diagnosis of NK-LGLL?

Ans: *Essential criteria:* (1) An increase in circulating NK-cells, typically greater than 2 × 10^9/L, persisting greater than 6 months; (2) Flow cytometric evidence of peripheral blood or bone marrow aspirate involvement by a uniform population of surface CD3–, CD16+ NK-cell population; (3) A killer cell immunoglobulin-like receptors (KIRs) restricted pattern of expression, demonstrated by flow cytometry analysis (either a dominant expression of a relevant KIR or lack of them), is accepted as a surrogate marker of clonal expansion; (4) Bone marrow involved by intrasinusoidal cytotoxic CD8+ NK-cells and/or the presence of STAT3 and/or TET2 mutations with NK-cell lineage confirmed by flow cytometry.

*If both 2 and 3 are present, a diagnosis of NK-LGLL can be made in the absence of documented persistence of an absolute peripheral blood NK-cell count of greater than 2 × 10^9/L.

Q25. Which viral marker is associated with adult T-cell leukemia and the major risk factors for infection?

Ans: Adult T-cell leukemia is closely linked to human T-lymphotropic virus (HTLV)-1 infection and the atypical tumor cells are regulatory T-cell origin. The major risk factors and determinants for developing ATLL among people with HTLV-1 infection are: Male sex, older age, higher HTLV-1 proviral load (≥40 copies per 1,000 peripheral blood mononuclear cells), longer duration of infection (>20 years), and younger age at acquisition (infancy or childhood).

Q26. What is the cell of origin of Sézary syndrome and mycosis fungoides and what are the typical immunophenotypic abnormalities?

Ans: The cell of origin of SS cells circulating central memory T cells (CD27+ CD45RA– CD45RO+) or skin-homing CD4+ T cells expressing CLA, CCR4, and CCR7 whereas in MF, the tumor cells are skin-resident memory cells. The neoplastic T cells in SS typically show CD3+, CD4+, and CD8– phenotype with frequent aberrant loss of pan T-cell antigens such as CD2, CD5, CD7, and/or CD26 in the neoplastic cells. Loss of CD7 and CD26 are particularly common in SS.

Q27. What are the features of primary cutaneous T-cell lymphoid lymphomas?

Ans: Features of primary cutaneous T-cell lymphoid lymphomas are given in **Table 7**.

TABLE 7: Cutaneous T-cell lymphomas: epidemiologic, clinicopathological, and prognostic features.

Type and subtypes	Frequency (%)	Clinical features	Histologic features (predominant growth pattern and cytomorphology)	Course	5-year-disease specific survival (%)
Mycosis fungoides (MF)	39	Patches-plaques-tumors	• Epidermotropic infiltrate in all stages; in tumor stage nodular infiltrate with variable epidermotropism • Small lymphoid cell (LC) in early disease (patch). Admixture of medium-sized and large LC in advanced stages (thick plaques, tumors)	indolent	88
MF subtypes:					
Folliculotropic MF	5			Variable	75
Pagetoid reticulosis	1			Indolent	100
Granulomatous slack skin	1			Indolent	100
Sézary syndrome	2	Erythroderma	• Epidermotropic infiltrate • Blood involvement	Aggressive	36
Primary cutaneous CD30+ lymphoproliferative disorders:					
Lymphomatoid papulosis	12	Papules and small nodules	Epidermotropic or dermal infiltrates. Atypical CD30 LC of variable size	Indolent	99

Continued

CHAPTER 21: Lymphoproliferative Disorders

Continued

Type and subtypes	Frequency (%)	Clinical features	Histologic features (predominant growth pattern and cytomorphology)	Course	5-year-disease specific survival (%)
Cutaneous anaplastic large cell lymphoma	8	Tumor(s)	Nodular infiltrate of large CD30. Lymphoid cells with severe nuclear atypia		95
Subcutaneous panniculitis-like T-cell lymphoma	1	Deep seated plaques or nodules	• Subcutaneous infiltrates • Medium-sized LC	Indolent	80
Primary cutaneous γ/δ T-cell lymphoma	<1	Plaques and nodules	• Epidermotropic or dermal nodular infiltrates • Medium-sized to large LC	Aggressive	11
Cutaneous CD8+ aggressive epidermotropic T-cell lymphoma	<1	Erosive or ulcerated plaques and nodules	• Epidermotropic infiltrate • Medium-sized to large LC	Aggressive	31
Primary cutaneous CD4-+ small/medium T-cell lymphoproliferative disorder	6	Solitary nodule	• Dermal nodular infiltrate • Small LC and intermingled medium-sized LC	Indolent	100
Primary cutaneous acral CDS-positive T-cell lymphoma	<1	Solitary nodule	• Dermal nodular infiltrate • Small to medium-sized LC	Indolent	100
Primary cutaneous peripheral T-cell lymphoma, not otherwise specified (NOS)	<1	• Nodule(s). Rarely papules and plaques • No patches	• Nodular infiltrate • Medium-sized to large LC	Aggressive	15
Adult T-cell lymphoma/ leukemia	1	Erythema, papules, plaques-tumors, erythroderma	Epidermotropic or dermal nodular infiltrates medium-sized to large cells	Indolent/ aggressive	Variable
Systemic chronic active Epstein-Barr virus (EBV)-positive disease	<1	Papulo-vesicular eruption	Dermal, often angiodestructive infiltrates small to medium-sized LC	Indolent	Variable

Q28. What are the common intestinal T-cell lymphomas and their diagnostic criteria?

Ans: Intestinal T-cell lymphomas encompass three distinct entities.
1. Enteropathy-associated T-cell lymphoma (EATL)
2. Monomorphic epitheliotropic intestinal T-cell lymphoma (MEITL)
3. Intestinal T-cell Lymphoma, not otherwise specified (NOS)

Enteropathy-associated T-cell Lymphoma

The EATL is an aggressive primary intestinal T-cell lymphoma of intraepithelial lymphocytes (IELs), which exhibits variable cellular pleomorphism and usually occurs in individuals with celiac disease (CD).

Essential Diagnostic Criteria
- An infiltrate of pleomorphic medium-sized to large lymphoid cells.
- Variable inflammatory background often including many eosinophils and histiocytes.
- Uninvolved intestinal mucosa shows features of CD (villous atrophy, crypt hyperplasia, and intraepithelial lymphocytosis).
- T-cell lineage, often with a CD4– CD8– phenotype, with expression of cytotoxic markers.

Desirable Diagnostic Criteria
- CD30 positivity (usually in cases of large cell or anaplastic morphology).
- In problematic cases, presence of JAK1 JH1-kinase and/or STAT3 SH2 domain hotspot mutations could assist in differentiating EATL from MEITL, which usually displays JAK3 and STAT5 mutations and SETD2 inactivation due to mutation or deletion.

Monomorphic Epitheliotropic Intestinal T-cell Lymphoma

The MEITL is an aggressive primary intestinal T-cell lymphoma of intraepithelial T lymphocytes, characterized by monomorphic cytomorphology and epitheliotropism, typically lacking association with CD.

Essential Diagnostic Criteria
- Dense infiltration by relatively monotonous medium-sized or occasionally large lymphoma cells.
- Typically lacking necrosis.
- Epitheliotropism is common.
- No histological evidence of CD in uninvolved mucosa.
- T-lineage, commonly CD3+, CD5–, CD4–, CD8+, CD56+, TIA1+.
- Epstein–Barr virus (EBV) negative.

Q29. What are the features of angioimmunoblastic T-cell lymphoma?

Ans: Angioimmunoblastic T-cell lymphoma (AITL) is an aggressive subtype of peripheral T-cell lymphoma (PTCL), accounting for approximately 15–20% of PTCL cases. The cell of origin is follicular helper T (TFH) cells and characterized by systemic symptoms, immune dysregulation, and polymorphous infiltration of lymphoid tissues.

Immunophenotype: Expression of two or more TFH markers (CD10, BCL6, PD1, CXCL13, CXCR5, ICOS, and SAP) is mandatory for diagnosis apart from presence of other T-cell lineage markers.

Molecular Genetics

Key genetic abnormalities include: TET2 (~80% of cases), DNMT3A (~30–40%), RHOA G17V mutation (~60–70%), and IDH2 (R172 mutation).

Q30. **What are the characteristic features of anaplastic large cell lymphomas (ALCLs)?**

Ans: Anaplastic large cell lymphoma is a rare variant of mature T-cell non-Hodgkin lymphoma (NHL) that arises from T-cells or null cells. It is characterized by large anaplastic cells that express CD30, a hallmark of this disease.

Classification

The recent WHO 2022 classifies ALCL into four distinct clinical and pathological entities **(Table 8)**:
1. Anaplastic lymphoma kinase (ALK)-positive ALCL
2. ALK-negative ALCL
3. Primary cutaneous ALCL
4. Breast implant–associated ALCL

TABLE 8: Characteristic features of anaplastic large cell lymphomas.

Feature	ALK-positive ALCL	ALK-negative ALCL	Primary cutaneous ALCL (pcALCL)	Breast implant–associated ALCL (BIA-ALCL)
Incidence	~3% of NHL; common in children/young adults	Older adults; less common	Rare; affects older adults	Very rare; associated with textured implants
ALK status	Positive (*ALK* gene rearrangements)	Negative	Negative	Negative
Genetics	t(2;5)(p23;q35) → NPM-ALK fusion	DUSP22 (favorable), TP63 (poor prognosis)	No ALK/DUSP22; other T-cell markers	No known specific mutation
CD30 expression	Strongly positive	Strongly positive	Strongly positive	Strongly positive
Common sites	Lymph nodes, skin, bone, soft tissue	Lymph nodes, extranodal sites	Skin (localized nodules/plaques)	Periprosthetic capsule (breast), seroma/mass
Symptoms	B symptoms, systemic involvement	Similar to ALK+ ALCL, often more aggressive	Skin lesions, may ulcerate or regress	Breast swelling, fluid, or mass
Prognosis	Favorable (>70–80% 5-year OS)	Intermediate (~40–60% 5-year OS)	Excellent (>90% 5-year OS)	Excellent if localized; worsens if systemic

(ALK: anaplastic lymphoma kinase; ALCL: anaplastic large cell lymphomas; NHL: non-Hodgkin lymphoma; OS: overall survival)

Q31. **What are the characteristics of peripheral T-cell lymphoma, NOS?**

Ans: Peripheral T-cell Lymphoma, NOS is a diagnosis of exclusion. Most patients present with advanced disease with lymph node involvement, but other sites, including bone marrow, liver, spleen, and extranodal tissues (most commonly skin and gastrointestinal tract), can be involved.

Essential Diagnostic Criteria

- Presence of an abnormal T-cell infiltrate, which is morphologically or immunophenotypically aberrant, and/or monoclonal by ancillary studies.
- The tumor cells are negative or express only one TFH marker (to differentiate from nodal TFH cell lymphomas) and only show Epstein–Barr virus-encoded small RNAs (EBER) in scattered B-cells (to differentiate from EBV-positive nodal T and NK-cell lymphoma).
- Exclusion of other nodal or extranodal mature T and NK cell lymphomas (i.e., ALK+ anaplastic large cell lymphoma, ALK-anaplastic large cell lymphoma, adult T-cell leukemia/lymphoma, extranodal NK/T-cell lymphoma).

Desirable

- Clonal *TCR* gene rearrangements.
- Establish the biological designation of PTCL-TBX21 and PTCL-GATA3.

Q32. **What are the salient features of hepatosplenic gamma delta T-cell lymphoma?**

Ans: Salient features of hepatosplenic gamma delta T-cell lymphoma are given in **Table 9**.

TABLE 9: Salient features of hepatosplenic gamma delta T-cell lymphoma.

Feature	Description
Subcategories	γδ T-cell (majority); αβ vary rare
Common sites	Liver, spleen, bone marrow; may have a leukemic presentation
Symptoms	B symptoms, hepatosplenomegaly, cytopenias
Key markers	CD3+, CD4–, CD8–, CD56+, TCRγδ+, CD5–
Molecular aberrancies	i(7q), ↓8, STAT5B mutations
Prognosis	Poor; median overall survival ~12 months
Best outcomes	Achieved with allogeneic HSCT

REFERENCES

1. Alaggio R, Amador C, Anagnostopoulos I, Attygalle AD, Araujo IBO, Berti E, et al. The 5th edition of the World Health Organization Classification of Haematolymphoid Tumours: Lymphoid Neoplasms. Leukemia. 2022;36(7):1720-48.
2. WHO Classification of Tumours Editorial Board. Haematolymphoid Tumours, 5th edition; Volume 11. Lyon, France: International Agency for Research on Cancer; 2024.
3. WHO Classification of Haematolymphoid Tumours: Lymphoid Neoplasms. 5th ed. Lyon: International Agency for Research on Cancer; 2022.
4. Swerdlow SH, Campo E, Harris NL, Jaffe ES, Pileri SA, Stein H, et al. The 2022 International Consensus Classification of Mature Lymphoid Neoplasms: A report from the Clinical Advisory Committee. Blood. 2022;140(11):1229-50.
5. Jaffe ES, Arber DA, Campo E, Harris NL, Quintanilla-Martinez L. Hematopathology. 3rd ed. Philadelphia: Elsevier; 2021.
6. Matutes E, Oscier D, Montalban C, Owusu-Ankomah K, Garcia Marco J, Houlihan A, et al. Diagnostic value of immunophenotyping and cytogenetics in B-cell chronic lymphoproliferative disorders. Leukemia. 2016;30(4):841-52.
7. Vose J, Armitage J, Weisenburger D; International T-cell Lymphoma Project. International peripheral T-cell and natural killer/T-cell lymphoma study: Pathology findings and clinical outcomes. J Clin Oncol. 2008;26(25):4124-30.
8. Faris NR, Stetler-Stevenson M. Flow cytometric diagnosis of T-cell neoplasms. Clin Lab Med. 2017;37(4):745-62.

21. Myelodysplastic Neoplasm

Aastha Gupta

Q1. When do you suspect myelodysplastic syndrome?

Ans: Myelodysplastic syndrome (MDS) is now termed as myelodysplastic neoplasm (MDS) as per the new WHO proposed in 2022.[1] This has been mainly done to attribute the neoplastic nature of this disease. MDS is suspected when a patient presents with unexplained cytopenia with the presence of acquired and sustained anemia (hemoglobin < 12 g/dL), neutropenia (absolute neutrophil count of <1.8 × 10^9/L) and/or thrombocytopenia (platelet count of <150 × 10^9/L).[2] These cytopenias are not explained by any other condition and the patient may be transfusion dependent. Although there is no specific duration defined, usually the cytopenia is chronic in duration (≥4 months duration).[2] These patients usually complain of fatigue, lethargy, recurrent infection, or bleeding due to underlying cytopenia.

Q2. What is the confirmatory test for MDS?

Ans: Diagnosis of MDS requires a combination of bone marrow aspiration and biopsy, flowcytometry, karyotyping, fluorescence in situ hybridization (FISH), and molecular studies by next-generation sequencing (NGS). Amongst these, the confirmatory tests are: (i) bone marrow morphology if there is presence of ≥10% dysplasia in two or more lineages or increased blasts on bone marrow and/or peripheral smear (≥2% on peripheral smear, >5% on bone marrow); (ii) MDS defining genetic abnormalities by karyotyping/FISH/NGS. These MDS cytogenetic abnormalities comprise of both balanced and unbalanced chromosomal abnormalities. In WHO, genetic types have been updated to include MDS-5q, MDS-SF3B1, and MDSbiTP53.[1] Apart from these, other genetic abnormalities are taken as presumptive evidence of MDS in the setting of persistent cytopenia and absence of morphological features.

Q3. What are the bone marrow findings of MDS?

Ans: Cellular or a hypocellular marrow showing dysplasia in one or more lineages where significant dyspoiesis is present in ≥10% of the cells. For megakaryocytes, micromegakaryocytes are the most specific indicator of MDS. At least 30 or more megakaryocytes should be counted in bone marrow smears/sections. However, it has been suggested but not yet incorporated to increase the threshold for other types of dysmegakaryopoiesis.[3] Other features of dysmegakaryopoiesis include separated lobes and hypolobated megakaryocytes. The erythroid dyspoiesis includes nuclear alterations (nuclear budding, internuclear bridging, karyorrhexis, multinuclearity, and megaloblastoid changes) and cytoplasmic alterations [ring sideroblasts (RS), vacuolization, and aberrant

PAS positivity)]. Dysgranulopoiesis is characterized by hypogranularity, pseudo-Pelger–Huët anomaly, hypersegmentation, and pseudo-Chediak–Higashi granules.[4,5]

Q4. What is ring sideroblast? Why is it considered pathognomonic of MDS? What is the significance of SF3B1 mutation?

Ans: Ring sideroblasts are erythroid precursors with mitochondrial iron granules forming a perinuclear ring.[6] Five or more granules covering one-third or more of the perinuclear area is the defining criteria specially to differentiate from sideroblasts. RS when >15% has been considered as pathognomonic feature of MDS; however, recently the importance of percentage has been diluted by the availability of NGS to detect SF3B1 mutation.

SF3B1 mutation has been recognized as a genetic defining criterion in MDS. MDS with low blast and SF3B1 mutation are identified as low risk. More often than not this has been associated with the presence of RS (≥5%). In a study, a direct correlation of RS% has been demonstrated with SF3B1 mutation.[7] However, as per International Consensus Classification (ICC), irrespective of the number of RS, SF3B1 unmutated cases have been classified as MDS, not otherwise specified (NOS).

Q5. What is the latest classification of MDS and how is it different from previous classification?

Ans: The new classifications of MDS have been primarily based on defining genetic abnormalities, blast percentage, cellularity, and fibrosis.[1,2] The presence of single lineage/multilineage dysplasia has been retained. However, the genetic abnormalities have taken precedence over the morphological criteria. MDS with del 5q and MDS with SF3B1 both have an added feature of low blast (<5% on BM and <2% on PB). MDS with biTP53 has taken take priority with any number of blasts in BM/PB highlighting the grave prognostic implication of biallelic mutated TP53.

Q6. What are the cytogenetic-based risk classifications of MDS?

Ans: Cytogenetic findings were added to the already existing IPSS risk stratification of MDS considering their impact on the overall survival and risk of acute myeloid leukemia (AML) transformation.[4,8] Very good, good, intermediate, poor, and very poor categories were identified and were incorporated into the IPSS-R risk stratification. Complex karyotype with >3 abnormalities is considered as very poor prognostic subgroup, whereas deletion 7, inversion 3, and complex karyotype with up to 3 cytogenetic abnormalities are considered as poor risk subgroup.

Q7. What is the significance of flowcytometry, fluorescence in situ hybridization, and genomic sequencing techniques in the diagnosis of MDS?

Ans: Flowcytometry is the method of choice to understand the immunophenotypic abnormalities in patients of MDS. There have been several publications addressing the same;[9-11] however, due to lack in consensus over sample type to be considered, processing and staining protocols, data analysis, interpretation, and reporting, it has not yet been recommended as the mandatory test in work-up of MDS. European LeukemiaNet International MDS (ELN iMDS) flow working group has been established to bring uniformity on flowcytometry for MDS and published their initial recommendations.[11-13]

Fluorescence in situ hybridization is faster cell interphase-based method to detect chromosomal abnormalities in MDS. The advantage is that it is not dependent on cell metaphases to grow, has less failure rates and faster turn-around time (TAT). However, disadvantage is that only limited number of abnormalities can be identified depending on probes available. Currently, commonly del 5q, del 7q, monosomy 7, trisomy 8, and del 20q can be studied by FISH. It is an additional test but not a replacement for karyotyping.

Genome sequencing by NGS has not only improved the depth and coverage of sequencing, but there has been a significant improvement in TAT and cost due to more demand. The identification of molecular mutations has improved our understanding of clonal hematopoiesis of indeterminate potential (CHIP), clonal cytopenia of undetermined significance (CCUS) and MDS.[14,15] Apart from diagnosis, genome sequencing has established its role in prognostication as well with IPSS-M risk stratification.[16]

Q8. What is the role of epigenetics in the pathophysiology and treatment of MDS?

Ans: MDS is a heterogenous clonal disorder characterized by ineffective hematopoiesis and cytopenia. With the advent of NGS, several driver mutations have been identified in MDS. Two major signal pathways are affected—(i) epigenetic pathways and (ii) RNA splicing pathways.

Epigenetic pathways affect DNA methylation (DNMT3A, TET2, and IDH1/IDH2) and histone/chromatin modification (ASXL1, MLL2, and EZH2) leading to DNA hypermethylation and abnormal histone modification.[17] These changes lead to gene silencing, disruption of normal functioning, and mediation of altered physiology.[18] In view of these findings, hypomethylating agents and inhibitors of histone deacetylases have been used in treatment of MDS.[19] Several studies have shown the efficacy of epigenetic therapy in treating high-risk MDS patients with both clinical improvement and better survival.[19-21]

Q9. What is the difference between clonal hematopoiesis of indeterminate potential, clonal cytopenia of undetermined significance, and clonal hematopoiesis of oncogenic potential?

Ans: Clonal hematopoiesis of indeterminate potential is a pre-MDS condition with no peripheral blood cytopenia, no or mild dysplasia (<10%), <5% blasts, and absence of MDS criteria with presence of one or more MDS-related mutations with variant allele frequency (VAF) ≥ 2%.[22] CHIP is also called as age-related clonal hematopoiesis (ARCH) in view of increasing frequency of these CHIP mutations in elderly healthy individuals. Apart from MDS, CHIP has an increased propensity to progress to myeloproliferative neoplasm (MPN), lymphoid tumors, and even cardiovascular events.[12,22]

Clonal cytopenia of undetermined significance is another pre-MDS condition with presence of one or more cytopenia (same criteria of cytopenia as for MDS) and one or more MDS-related mutations with VAF ≥ 2%. However, with no MDS defining criteria, no or mild dysplasia which is <10% and blasts <5%.[12,22]

Conal hematopoiesis of oncogenic potential (CHOP) mutations are disease-related or even disease-specific lesions that trigger differentiation and/or proliferation of neoplastic cells. Over time, the acquisition of additional oncogenic events converts preleukemic neoplasms into secondary AML. Whereas isolated CHIP-type mutations can be detected in healthy individuals who stay healthy for their lifetime, CHOP mutations are usually associated with manifestation of an overt neoplasm.

Q10. Why MDS with p53 mutation is considered as a high risk?

Ans: TP53, also known as guardian gene, is a tumor suppressor gene which is a master regulator of genomic stability by balancing DNA repair and DNA stress.[23] TP53 mutations have been identified in approximately 5–10% cases of de-novo MDS/AML and approximately 30–40% cases of therapy-related MDS/AML.[24] These patients are associated with a dismal prognosis. TP53-mutated MDS are more frequently associated with complex karyotype which has been a well-established very poor prognostic indicator in IPSS-R.[25] TP53-mutated clones are resistant to chemotherapy with very poor response, if any. MDS with biallelic TP53 mutations are uniformly a poor prognostic group where there is loss of function in both the alleles of TP53.[24-26] At present, there are no targeted therapy for such cases and many prospective trials are under investigation.

Q11. How is hypoplastic MDS differentiated from aplastic anemia?

Ans: Hypoplastic MDS is similar to aplastic anemia in view of hypocellularity and inflammation and also shares features with MDS due to dysplasia, genetic lesions, and cytopenia.[27] It may present with either of the phenotypes and should be treated accordingly. Though, it is differentiated from aplastic anemia by presence of significant dysplasia (>10%) and chromosomal/molecular abnormalities similar to MDS. Many times, there is a gray zone where there is only mild dysplasia with identification of CHIP mutations and it is difficult to differentiate such cases from aplastic anemia. Usually, hypoplastic MDS patients are older in age. If BM display excess of blasts and/or definite genetic lesions are identified in a hypocellular marrow with cytopenia, it becomes easier to diagnose hypoplastic MDS.[28,29]

REFERENCES

1. Khoury JD, Solary E, Abla O, Akkari Y, Alaggio R, Apperley JF, et al. The 5th edition of the World Health Organization Classification of Haematolymphoid Tumours: Myeloid and Histiocytic/Dendritic Neoplasms. Leukemia. 2022;36:1703-19.
2. Arber DA, Orazi A, Hasserjian RP, Borowitz MJ, Calvo KR, Kvasnicka HM, et al. International Consensus Classification of Myeloid Neoplasms and Acute Leukemias: Integrating morphologic, clinical, and genomic data. Blood. 2022;140(11):1200-28.
3. Matsuda A, Germing U, Jinnai I, Iwanaga M, Misumi M, Kuendgen A, et al. Improvement of criteria for refractory cytopenia with multilineage dysplasia according to the WHO classification based on prognostic significance of morphological features in patients with refractory anemia according to the FAB classification. Leukemia. 2007;21(4):678-86.
4. Swerdlow SH, Campo E, Harris NL, Jaffe ES, Pileri SA, Stein H, et al. (2017). WHO Classification of Tumours of Haematopoietic and Lymphoid Tissues. Revised 4th edition. [online] Available from https://publications.iarc.fr/Book-And-Report-Series/Who-Classification-Of-Tumours/WHO-Classification-Of-Tumours-Of-Haematopoietic-And-Lymphoid-Tissues-2017 [Last accessed April, 2024].
5. Della Porta M, Travaglino E, Boveri E, Ponzoni M, Malcovati L, Papaemmanuil E, et al. Minimal morphological criteria for defining bone marrow dysplasia: A basis for clinical implementation of WHO classification of myelodysplastic syndromes. Leukemia. 2015;29:66-75.
6. Cazzola M, Invernizzi R. Ring sideroblasts and sideroblastic anemias. Haematologica. 2011;96(6):789-92.
7. Patnaik MM, Hanson CA, Sulai NH, Hodnefield JM, Knudson RA, Ketterling RP, et al. Prognostic irrelevance of ring sideroblast percentage in World Health Organization–defined myelodysplastic syndromes without excess blasts. Blood. 2012;119(24):5674-7.
8. Greenberg PL, Tuechler H, Schanz J, Sanz G, Garcia-Manero G, Solé F, et al. Revised International Prognostic Scoring System for Myelodysplastic Syndromes. Blood. 2012;120(12):2454-65.

9. Della Porta MG, Picone C. Diagnostic Utility of Flow Cytometry in Myelodysplastic Syndromes. Mediterr J Hematol Infect Dis. 2017;9(1):e2017017.
10. Bento LC, Correia RP, Pitangueiras Mangueira CL, De Souza Barroso R, Rocha FA, Bacal NS, et al. The Use of Flow Cytometry in Myelodysplastic Syndromes: A Review. Front Oncol. 2017;7:270.
11. Valent P, Orazi A, Büsche G, Schmitt-Gräff A, George TI, Sotlar K, et al. Standards and impact of hematopathology in myelodysplastic syndromes (MDS). Oncotarget. 2010;1(7):483-96.
12. Valent P, Orazi A, Steensma DP, Ebert BL, Haase D, Malcovati L, et al. Proposed minimal diagnostic criteria for myelodysplastic syndromes (MDS) and potential pre-MDS conditions. Oncotarget. 2017;8(43):73483-500.
13. Alhan C, Westers TM, Cremers EM, Cali C, Ossenkoppele GJ, van de Loosdrecht AA. Application of flow cytometry for myelodysplastic syndromes: Pitfalls and technical considerations. Cytometry B Clin Cytom. 2016;90(4):358-67.
14. Spaulding TP, Stockton SS, Savona MR. The evolving role of next generation sequencing in myelodysplastic syndromes. Br J Haematol. 2020;188:224-39.
15. Tria FPT, Ang DC, Fan G. Myelodysplastic syndrome: diagnosis and screening. Diagnostics (Basel). 2022;12:1581.
16. Bernard E, Tuechler H, Greenberg PL, Hasserjian RP, Arango Ossa JE, Nannya Y, et al. Molecular international prognostic scoring system for myelodysplastic syndromes. NEJM Evid. 2022;1:EVIDoa2200008.
17. Bond DR, Lee HJ, Enjeti AK. Unravelling the Epigenome of Myelodysplastic Syndrome: Diagnosis, Prognosis, and Response to Therapy. Cancers. 2020;12:3128.
18. Jones PA, Laird PW. Cancer epigenetics comes of age. Nat Genet. 1999;21(2):163-7.
19. Heuser M, Yun H, Thol F. Epigenetics in myelodysplastic syndromes. Semin Cancer Biol. 2018;51:170-9.
20. Fenaux P, Mufti GJ, Hellstrom-Lindberg E, Santini V, Finelli C, Giagounidis A, et al. Efficacy of azacitidine compared with that of conventional care regimens in the treatment of higher-risk myelodysplastic syndromes: a randomised, open-label, phase III study. Lancet Oncol. 2009;10(3):223-32.
21. Kantarjian H, Issa JP, Rosenfeld CS, Bennett JM, Albitar M, DiPersio J, et al. Decitabine improves patient outcomes in myelodysplastic syndromes: results of a phase III randomized study. Cancer. 2006;106(8): 1794-803.
22. Valent P. ICUS, IDUS, CHIP and CCUS: Diagnostic Criteria, Separation from MDS and Clinical Implications. Pathobiology. 2019;86(1):30-8.
23. Bown CJ, Lain S, Verma CS, Fersht AR, Lane DP. Awakening guardian angels: Drugging the p53 pathway. Nat Rev Cancer. 2009:9:862-73.
24. Santini V, Stahl M, Sallman DA. TP53 Mutations in Acute Leukemias and Myelodysplastic Syndromes: Insights and Treatment Updates. Am Soc Clin Oncol Educ Book. 2024;44:e432650.
25. Rücker FG, Schlenk RF, Bullinger L, Kayser S, Teleanu V, Kett H, et al. TP53 alterations in acute myeloid leukemia with complex karyotype correlate with specific copy number alterations, monosomal karyotype, and dismal outcome. Blood. 2012;119:2114-21.
26. Daver NG, Maiti A, Kadia TM, Vyas P, Majeti R, Wei AH, et al. TP53-Mutated Myelodysplastic Syndrome and Acute Myeloid Leukemia: Biology, Current Therapy, and Future Directions. Cancer Discov. 2022;12(11): 2516-29.
27. Fattizzo B, Serpenti F, Barcellini W, Caprioli C. Hypoplastic Myelodysplastic Syndromes: Just an Overlap Syndrome? Cancers (Basel). 2021;13(1):132.
28. Calado RT. Immunologic Aspects of Hypoplastic Myelodysplastic Syndrome. Semin Oncol. 2011;38:667-72.
29. Bennett JM, Orazi A. Diagnostic criteria to distinguish hypocellular acute myeloid leukemia from hypocellular myelodysplastic syndromes and aplastic anemia: Recommendations for a standardized approach. Haematologica. 2009;94:264-8.

22. Myeloproliferative Neoplasm

Anamika Bakliwal

Q1. What are the microscopic features of chronic myeloid leukemia?

Ans: Microscopic features of chronic myeloid leukemia (CML) include:
- *In chronic phase (CP):*
  - The peripheral blood shows leukocytosis due to neutrophils in various stages of maturation, with peaks in the proportions of myelocytes and segmented neutrophils.[1]
  - Blasts typically account for <2% of the white blood cells.
  - Absolute basophilia and eosinophilia are common and sometimes in very rare instances absolute monocytosis may also be present sometimes.
  - Platelet counts are normal or increased.
  - Atypical presentations include marked thrombocytosis without leukocytosis that mimics essential thrombocythemia (ET) or other types of myeloproliferative neoplasm (MPN).
  - The bone marrow is hypercellular, with marked granulocytic proliferation and a maturation pattern similar to that in the blood, including expansion at the myelocyte stage. Dysplasia is absent.
  - The proportion of erythroid precursors is usually significantly decreased.
  - The megakaryocytes are smaller than normal and have hyposegmented nuclei, they are referred to as "dwarf" megakaryocytes.
  - Eosinophils and basophils are usually increased in number and pseudo-Gaucher cells are common.
  - Moderate to marked reticulin fibrosis is seen.
- *In blast phase (BP):*
  - The blast lineage is myeloid, and may include neutrophilic, monocytic, megakaryocytic, basophilic, eosinophilic, or erythroid blasts.
  - In approximately 20–30% of BP cases, the blasts are lymphoblasts.
  - The blasts are often immature and/or heterogeneous, and expression of antigens of more than one lineage is common.
  - In myeloid BP, the blasts express one or more antigens associated with granulocytic, monocytic, megakaryocytic, and/or erythroid differentiation and most lymphoblastic BP blasts are of precursor–B-cell origin but a minority of lymphoblastic BP blasts are of T-cell origin and express T-cell–related antigens.[2]

- Extramedullary blast proliferations are most common in the skin, lymph nodes, bone, and central nervous system (CNS), but can occur anywhere; they may be of myeloid, lymphoid, or mixed-lineage phenotype.
- In bone marrow biopsy specimens, sheets of blasts that occupy focal but substantial areas of the bone marrow.

High-risk chronic CML phase includes:[3,4]
- High ELTS score
- ≥20% basophils in the peripheral blood
- Additional chromosomal abnormalities in Philadelphia (Ph) chromosome–positive (Ph+) cells, including 3q26.2 rearrangements, monosomy 7, isochromosome 17q, and complex karyotype.
- Clusters of small megakaryocytes (including true micromegakaryocytes similar to those seen in myelodysplastic syndromes), associated with significant reticulin and/or collagen fibrosis, which is best assessed in biopsy sections.
- Failure to achieve a complete hematological response to the first line tyrosine kinase inhibitor (TKI).
- Any hematological, cytogenetic, or molecular indications of resistance to two sequential TKIs (excluding explicable causes such as the presence of a kinase domain mutation resistant to the previous choice of TKI).
- Development of new additional chromosomal abnormalities
- Occurrence of compound mutations in the *BCR-ABL1* fusion gene during TKI therapy

Q2. Is dysplasia a common morphologic feature of chronic myeloid leukemia?

Ans: In CML-CP phase, bone marrow shows absence of dysplasia. The 2022 International Consensus Classification replaces the term atypical CML with MDS/MPN with neutrophilia.[4] It is always characterized by leukocytosis with dysplastic features in neutrophils and their precursors. Dysplasia includes abnormal chromatin clumping, hypersegmented or Pelger-Huët forms, and cytoplasmatic hypogranularity.

Q3. What are the variants of BCR-ABL in CML? How the site of the breakpoint in chromosome 22 may influence the phenotype of the disease?

Ans: The two most common isoforms of BCR-ABL are known as e13a2 and e14a2, i.e., BCR exon 13 or BCR exon 14, respectively, spliced to ABL1 exon 2. Collectively, e13a2 and e14a2 account for 98% of CML cases.[5] The majority of these express e14a2. About 10% of cases express both isoforms. The e13a2 isoform was more frequent in males and less common in the elderly. It is known that e13a2 BCR-ABL1 have inferior cytogenetic and molecular responses at various time points after starting imatinib therapy compared to those expressing e14a2, but the underlying reason for this remains unclear. The remaining 2% of CML patients express atypical BCR-ABL1 transcripts that arise from BCR breakpoints outside the M-BCR or downstream of ABL1 exon 2. The most common are e1a2, e19a2, e13a3, and e14a3. Several less common recurrent fusions have also been described (e.g., e6a2). P190 CML was originally associated with a phenotype intermediate between CML and chronic myelomonocytic leukemia (CMML), and recent data have indicated a relatively poor response to imatinib, possibly associated with frequent mutations in epigenetic modifier genes.

The BCR-ABL1 transcript type in any given patient is stable over time since it is determined by the position of the t(9;22) genomic breakpoints.

Rearrangements that give rise to e13a2 and e14a2 BCR-ABL1 have the capability to generate e1a2 mRNA by alternative splicing. Indeed, very low levels of e1a2 transcripts can be detected in most cases of CML prior to treatment but are generally believed to be of no clinical significance.[5] These cases should not be considered as p190 CML since the level of e1a2 expression is typically 100–1,000× lower than that of the predominant isoform, and clonal evolution of p210 to p190 is at best exceedingly rare.

Q4. How quantification of BCR-ABL is done for disease monitoring?

Ans: Monitoring methods include fluorescent in situ hybridization (FISH), and qualitative and quantitative polymerase chain reaction (qPCR).[6] NGS has also been used in the management of CML.

Analysis of mutations of the BCR-ABL kinase domain uses different techniques:
- The direct sequencing of DNA following nested RT-PCR (detect mutations in 10–25% of tumor cells).
- The denaturing-high performance liquid chromatography (D-HPLC) analysis (sensitivity of 5% to 10%).
- The fluorescent-based allele-specific oligonucleotide PCR (ASO-PCR) assays (detect mutations in 0.1–1% of tumor cells).
- RNA-based NGS assay has been used for identification of BCR-ABL1 transcript types, mutation detection, and for simplified molecular testing workflow.

Q5. How is tyrosine kinase mutation detected? What is its relevance?

Ans: Direct sequencing is the method recommended for tyrosine kinase mutation analysis. Direct sequencing may be combined with D-HPLC analysis as it helps in reduction of the number of samples that need to be sequenced. Direct sequencing allows detection of mutations present in ≥ 20% of Ph+ cells.

The D-HPLC has a slightly higher sensitivity, but it alone does not allow characterization of the precise sequence variation underlying an abnormal elution profile. It is performed at diagnosis in accelerated and blastic phase, during CP-in case of imatinib failure, in case of an increase in BCR-ABL transcript levels leading to MMR loss and in case of any other suboptimal response.
- T315I mutation is highly resistant to imatinib, dasatinib, and nilotinib.
- In case of V299L, T315A, or F317L/V/I/C mutations, nilotinib is probably more effective than dasatinib.
- In case of Y253H, E255K/V, or F359V/C/I mutations, dasatinib is probably more effective than nilotinib.
- In case of any other mutation, dasatinib and nilotinib are likely to be similarly effective.

Q6. What is chronic neutrophilic leukemia and how is it morphologically different from chronic myeloid leukemia?

Ans: Chronic neutrophilic leukemia (CNL) is a MPN without BCR-ABL1 mutation, characterized by sustained peripheral blood neutrophilia, bone marrow hypercellularity due to neutrophilic granulocyte proliferation, and hepatosplenomegaly.[7]

The peripheral blood shows neutrophilia. The neutrophils are usually segmented, but there may also be an increase in band forms and neutrophil precursors (promyelocytes, myelocytes, and metamyelocytes). Myeloblasts are almost never observed in the blood. The neutrophils often show toxic granulation and Döhle bodies, but they may also appear normal. It should be noted that toxic granulation and Döhle bodies appear to be more consistently present in plasma cell-associated leukemoid reactions than in CNL. Neutrophil dysplasia is not present. Red blood cell and platelet morphology are usually normal. Megakaryocytes may be cytologically normal or there may be increased smaller forms. Significant dysplasia is not present in any of the cell lineages; therefore, if it is found, another diagnosis, such as atypical CML, should be considered.[7] The diagnosis requires exclusion of reactive neutrophilia and other myeloproliferative and myelodysplastic/myeloproliferative neoplasms and peripheral blood white blood cell count ≥ 25 × 10^9/L. There may be presence of CSF3R p.T618I or another activating CSF3R mutation.

Cytogenetic studies are normal in nearly 90% of cases. In the remaining cases, reported clonal karyotypic abnormalities include gains of chromosomes 8, 9, and 21; del(7q); del(20q) (the most frequently observed abnormality); del(11q); del(12p); and nullisomy 17.

Q7. What are the morphological characteristics of megakaryocyte in polycythemia vera, essential thrombocythemia and myelofibrosis?

Ans:

Polycythemia Vera

Polycythemia vera (PV) is a clonal MPN characterized by erythrocytosis frequently accompanied by leukocytosis, and/or thrombocytosis, and a risk of associated increased hemorrhagic and thrombotic (venous and arterial) risk. JAK2 p.V617F and *JAK2* exon12 mutations have been strongly associated with PV. The morphological features of PV reflect the effective proliferation in the erythroid, granulocytic, and megakaryocytic lineages; i.e., panmyelosis. Bone marrow shows a prominent erythroid proliferation with either normal or reduced myeloid:erythroid ratio. Megakaryocytes are increased in numbers and are frequently larger and have hypersegmented nuclei.[4,8]

Essential Thrombocythemia

Essential thrombocythemia is a chronic MPN characterized by a sustained increase of blood platelet count and increased numbers of large, mature megakaryocytes in the bone marrow and with the risk of thrombosis and/or hemorrhage. The myeloid:erythroid ratio is usually in the normal range. The most striking abnormality is a marked proliferation of megakaryocytes, with a predominance of large to giant forms displaying abundant, mature cytoplasm, and deeply lobed and hypersegmented (staghorn-like) nuclei. Clustering of megakaryocytes is not a prominent feature. Atypical megakaryocytes with hyperchromatic nuclei are not prominent. CD61 or CD42b immunostains can be used to highlight the increased numbers of megakaryocytes.

Primary Myelofibrosis

Primary myelofibrosis (PMF) is a clonal MPN characterized by a proliferation of abnormal megakaryocytes and granulocytes in the bone marrow, which in fibrotic stages is associated with a polyclonal increase in fibroblasts that drive a secondary marrow fibrosis (reticulin fibrosis and/or collagen fibrosis), osteosclerosis, and extramedullary hematopoiesis. The morphologic features of PMF can vary depending on the stage of disease presentation, prefibrotic or fibrotic stages, which are dependent on the fibrosis grades. Since disease progression is associated with progressive accumulation of reticulin and collagen fibrosis and development of osteosclerosis, serial grading of bone marrow fibrosis using reproducible and standard criteria is necessary. Prompt reduction in BM fibrosis postallogeneic stem cell transplant is a favorable marker of overall survival. It is estimated that 30–50% of PMF cases are first detected in the prefibrotic/early stage, with no significant increase in reticulin and/or collagen fibers (i.e., fibrosis grades 0 and 1). Megakaryocyte atypia or "dysplasia" is a component of PMF. Megakaryocyte numbers and their morphological features are best highlighted using an immunostain for either CD42b or CD61 antigens.[4,8]

REFERENCES

1. Arber DA, Orazi A, Hasserjian R, Thiele J, Borowitz MJ, Le Beau MM, et al. The 2016 revision to the World Health Organization classification of myeloid neoplasms and acute leukemia. Blood. 2016;127(20):2391-405.
2. Jabbour E, Kantarjian H. Chronic myeloid leukemia: 2020 update on diagnosis, therapy and monitoring. Am J Hematol. 2020;95(6):691-709.
3. Shahrin NH, Wadham C, Branford S. Defining Higher-Risk Chronic Myeloid Leukemia: Risk Scores, Genomic Landscape, and Prognostication. Curr Hematol Malig Rep. 2022;17(6):171-80.
4. Khoury JD, Solary E, Abla O, Akkari Y, Alaggio R, Apperley JF, et al. The 5th edition of the World Health Organization Classification of Haematolymphoid Tumours: Myeloid and Histiocytic/Dendritic Neoplasms. Leukemia. 2022;36(7):1720-48.
5. Baccarani M, Castagnetti F, Gugliotta G, Rosti G, Soverini S, Albeer A, et al. The proportion of different BCR-ABL1 transcript types in chronic myeloid leukemia. An international overview. Leukemia. 2019;33:1173-83.
6. White HE, Salmon M, Albano F, Andersen CSA, Balabanov S, Balatzenko G, et al. Standardization of molecular monitoring of CML: results and recommendations from the European treatment and outcome study. Leukemia. 2022;36:1834-42.
7. Szuber N, Elliott M, Tefferi A. Chronic neutrophilic leukemia: 2022 update on diagnosis, genomic landscape, prognosis, and management. Am J Hematol. 2022;97(4):491-505.
8. Ng ZY, Fuller KA, Mazza-Parton A, Erber WN. Morphology of myeloproliferative neoplasms. Int J Lab Hematol. 2023;45:59-70.

23. Myeloid Malignancies

Sarjana Tiwari, Nivedita Dhingra

Q1. How is acute myeloid leukemia classified? Is morphological classification of acute myeloid leukemia still relevant?

Ans: Acute myeloid leukemia (AMA) has been classified based on morphological and molecular features.[1] Two types of classification:

1. *Acute myeloid leukemia with defining genetic abnormalities*:
   - Acute promyelocytic leukemia with PML::RARA fusion
   - Acute myeloid leukemia with RUNX1::RUNX1T1 fusion
   - Acute myeloid leukemia with CBFB::MYH11 fusion
   - Acute myeloid leukemia with DEK::NUP214 fusion
   - Acute myeloid leukemia with RBM::MRTFA fusion
   - Acute myeloid leukemia with BCR::ABL1 fusion
   - Acute myeloid leukemia with KMTA21 rearrangement
   - Acute myeloid leukemia with MECOM rearrangement
   - Acute myeloid leukemia with NUP98 rearrangement
   - Acute myeloid leukemia with NPM1 mutation
   - Acute myeloid leukemia with CEBPA mutation
   - Acute myeloid leukemia, myelodysplasia-related
   - Acute myeloid leukemia with other defined genetic alterations

2. *Acute myeloid leukemia defined by differentiation*:
   - Acute myeloid leukemia with minimal differentiation
   - Acute myeloid leukemia without maturation
   - Acute myeloid leukemia with maturation
   - Acute basophilic leukemia
   - Acute myelomonocytic leukemia
   - Acute monocytic leukemia
   - Acute erythroid leukemia
   - Acute megakaryoblastic leukemia

With the advent and uniform use of NPM1, CEBPA, and FLT3-ITD for disease classification and prognostic relevance, the importance of FAB classification has been debatable in present scenario.[1] Data from few large retrospective studies studying its prognostic role on current treatment protocols including bone marrow transplant have been contradictory.

> **Q2.** What is core binding factor acute myeloid leukemia?

Ans: The core binding factor (CBF) is a transcription factor complex comprising a DNA-binding CBFα subunit (RUNX1, RUNX2, or RUNX3) and a non-DNA-binding heterodimerization partner CBFβ subunit (encoded by *CBFB*).[2] RUNX1 is a master transcriptional regulator of adult hematopoiesis expressed by all hematopoietic lineages. RUNX1 and CBFβ form a DNA-binding heterodimer that regulates hematopoietic differentiation. RUNX1T1 is a transcriptional corepressor whose expression is limited to the megakaryocytic and erythrocytic lineages, but not hematopoietic stem and progenitor cells. The *RUNX1::RUNX1T1* fusion resulting from t(8;21)(q22;q22.1) plays a critical role in leukemogenesis by blocking myeloid differentiation but requires other cooperating pathogenic alterations for leukemic development and progression. The CBF is a transcription factor complex comprising a DNA-binding CBFα subunit (RUNX1, RUNX2, or RUNX3) and a non-DNA-binding heterodimerization partner CBFβ subunit (encoded by *CBFB*). *MYH11*, which codes for smooth muscle myosin heavy chain, combines with *CBFB*. The resulting fusion protein interferes with the function of RUNX1/CBFb transcription factor complex, causing dysregulation of myeloid cell growth and differentiation.

> **Q3.** How is acute myeloid leukemia with minimal differentiation diagnosed? How is it different from acute myeloid leukemia with maturation?

Ans: Acute myeloid leukemia with minimal differentiation is an acute leukemia with immunophenotypic but not morphological or cytochemical evidence of myeloid differentiation that lacks defining genetic abnormalities.[3] In AML with minimal differentiation, the blasts express at least two myeloid-associated markers, most often CD13, CD33, and CD117. Most cases also express CD34, CD38, CD123, and HLA-DR. CD7 and TdT are expressed in about 30% of cases. Myeloperoxidase is negative. Markers of specific lineages, including granulocytic (e.g., CD15 and CD65), monocytic (e.g., CD11c, CD14, CD36, and CD64), and B-cell (e.g., CD19), are often absent. AML with maturation is an AML with morphological features of granulocytic maturation that lacks defining genetic abnormalities. Blasts usually show expression of myeloperoxidase and two or more myeloid-associated antigens, such as CD13, CD33, and CD117. Blasts are often positive for CD34 and HLA-DR. They usually express markers associated with granulocytic maturation, including CD11b, CD15, and CD65.

> **Q4.** What is acute erythroid leukemia? What is the significance of TP53 mutation in acute erythroid leukemia?

Ans: Acute erythroid leukemia is a neoplastic proliferation of erythroid cells with features of maturation arrest (increased proerythroblasts) and a high prevalence of biallelic *TP53* alterations.[4]

Essential Diagnostic Criteria

Erythroid predominance, ≥80% of bone marrow elements, of which ≥30% are proerythroblasts.

Desirable Diagnostic Criteria

Evidence of *TP53* mutation—the differential diagnosis of acute erythroid leukemia including both reactive and neoplastic conditions associated with proerythroblast proliferation. Reactive erythroid hyperplasia with a prominent proerythroblast component can be seen in nutritional deficiency and hemolytic anemia. *TP53* mutation analysis is helpful, because reactive proerythroblast proliferation shows no *TP53* mutation and a normal karyotype.

Q5. What are the characteristic features of acute megakaryoblastic leukemia?

Ans: Characteristic features of acute megakaryoblastic leukemia include:[5]
- ≥20% blasts with megakaryocytic differentiation in bone marrow and/or peripheral blood
- Blasts are characteristically positive for megakaryocytic markers by flowcytometry—CD41, CD61, or CD42b.
- Patients with this subtype fall into three clinical groups—children with Down syndrome (DS), children without DS, and adults.
- The majority (>75%) of cases arising in children without DS harbor chromosomal translocations that encode fusion oncogenes that drive . Examples, *CBFA2T3* (*ETO*)::*GLIS2*, *RBM15*::*MRTFA*, *NUP98*::*KDM5A*, and *KMT2A* rearrangements.
- AMKL representing myeloid leukemia of DS has an excellent prognosis.

Q6. What is transient abnormal myelopoiesis?

Ans: Children with constitutional trisomy 21 (DS has a higher propensity to develop myeloid leukemia of DS). This disorder is preceded by a transient preleukemic syndrome termed transient abnormal myelopoiesis (TAM).[6] TAM is characterized by increased circulating blast cells that harbor acquired N-terminal truncating mutations in the key hematopoietic transcription factor gene *GATA1*.[7] In the majority of cases of TAM and silent TAM, the GATA1 mutant clone goes into complete and permanent remission without the need for chemotherapy. However, 10–20% of neonates with TAM and silent TAM subsequently develop myeloid leukemia in the first 5 years of life when persistent GATA1 mutant cells acquire additional oncogenic mutations.

Q7. How is mixed-phenotype acute leukemia diagnosed?

Ans: The diagnosis requires the presence of >20% blasts expressing antigens of two or more lineages or two population of blasts each of a different lineage.[1,8]
- B lineage—CD19 strong along with one of the following strongly expressed—CD10, CD22, CD79, or CD19 (weak) with two or more of the following strongly expressed—CD10, CD22, and CD79
- T lineage—CD3 (cytoplasmic or surface)
- *Myeloid lineage*: MPO or two or markers of monocytic differentiation NSE, CD11c, CD14, CD64, and lysozyme.

Q8. What is the significance of KMT2A rearrangement in hematological malignancies?

Ans: *KMT2A* gene rearrangements result from deletions, duplications, inversions, and translocations at the 11q23 locus. These rearrangements disrupts a 100 kb region in exons 5–11. The resulting derivative chromosome 11 harbors the *KMT2A* promoter and coding regions 5′ to the breakpoint.[9] This rearrangement results in a chimeric protein with a *KMT2A*-encoded N-terminus and a C-terminus encoded by the partner gene.

KMT2A-rearranged leukemias have a distinct gene expression profile resembling early hematopoietic progenitor cells and characterized by the overexpression of *HOX* genes. For AML with *KMT2A* rearrangement, the prognostic impact depends on the fusion partner. Patients with *KMT2A::MLLT3* fusion have an intermediate risk of relapse, whereas other *KMT2A* rearrangements are associated with a poor prognosis. In children, the prognostic impact of fusion partners is debated and might depend on the treatment given. The *KMT2A* fusion partners *ABI1*, *AFDN*, *AFF1*, *MLLT1*, and *MLLT10* have been associated with a high risk of relapse, and *ELL*, *MLLT3*, *MLLT11*, and *SEPTIN6* with a standard risk.

Q9. How is Langerhans cell histiocytosis diagnosed?

Ans: Langerhans cell histiocytosis diagnosis is done by histopathological examination along with immunohistochemistry.[10]

Essential and Desirable Diagnostic Criteria

- *Essential:* Biopsy showing large, round to oval histiocytes with grooved to convoluted nuclei and a Langerhans cell phenotype (CD1a+ and CD207+)
- *Desirable:* Mutation analysis in the MAPK pathway, with sensitive testing for low-frequency allele detection

Q10. What is the role of measurable residual disease monitoring in acute myeloid leukemia?

Ans: Measurable residual disease (MRD) plays a crucial role in prognostication of the disease and helps in decision making between consolidative hematopoietic stem cell transplant or chemotherapy.[11] It is also an important tool to assess response and efficacy of newer drugs and therapeutic. In the post-transplant setting, MRD detection can predict impending relapse and allow for early interventions such as donor lymphocyte infusions (DLI). The techniques used for MRD detection are multiparameter flow cytometry, molecular MRD by qPCR for NPM1; CBFB::MYH11, RUNX1::RUNX1T1, KMT2A::MLLT3, DEK::NUP214, and BCR::ABL1 gene fusions; and WT1 expression. NGS MRD is increasingly being incorporated into clinical practice; however, genes associated with premalignant clonal hematopoiesis (ASXL1, DNMT3A, and TET2) should be excluded from MRD assessment.

Q11. What is chronic myelomonocytic leukemia? How is it diagnosed?

Ans: Chronic myelomonocytic leukemia (CMML) is a myeloid neoplasm with myelodysplastic and myeloproliferative feature.[1,12]

Diagnosis

- *Essential criteria*:
  - Persistent absolute ($\geq 0.5 \times 10^9$/L) and relative ($\geq 10\%$) peripheral blood monocytosis
  - Blasts constitute <20% of the cells in the peripheral blood and bone marrow.
  - Not meeting diagnostic criteria of chronic myeloid leukemia or other myeloproliferative neoplasms (MPN)
  - Not meeting diagnostic criteria of myeloid/lymphoid neoplasms with eosinophilia and tyrosine kinase gene fusions (e.g., *PDGFRA*, *PDGFRB*, *FGFR1*, or *JAK2*)

- *Desirable criteria*:
  - Dysplasia involving ≥1 myeloid lineages
  - Acquired clonal cytogenetic or molecular abnormality
  - Abnormal partitioning of peripheral blood monocyte subsets

Requirements for Diagnosis
- Essential criteria must be present in all cases.
- If monocytosis is ≥1×10^9/L, one or more desirable criteria must be met.
- If monocytosis is <1×10^9/L, desirable criteria 1 and 2 must be met.

Q12. What are the diagnostic criteria for juvenile myelomonocytic leukemia?

Ans: Clinical, hematological, and laboratory criteria (all five criteria are required):[1]
1. Peripheral blood monocyte count ≥ 1×10^9/L
2. Blast and promonocyte percentage of <20% in peripheral blood and bone marrow
3. Clinical evidence of organ infiltration, most commonly splenomegaly
4. No Philadelphia (Ph) chromosome or *BCR::ABL1* fusion
5. No *KMT2A* (*MLL1*) gene rearrangement

Genetic criteria (one criterion is required): Mutation in a component or a regulator of the canonical RAS pathway:
- Clonal somatic mutation in *PTPN11*, *KRAS*, or *NRAS*, or
- Clonal somatic or germline *NF1* mutation and loss of heterozygosity or compound heterozygosity of *NF1*, or
- Clonal somatic or germline *CBL* mutation and loss of heterozygosity of *CBL*
- Noncanonical clonal RAS pathway pathogenic variant or fusions causing activation of genes upstream of the RAS pathway, such as *ALK*, *PDGFRB*, and *ROS1*

Other criteria: Cases that do not meet any of the genetic criteria listed above (or for which genetic testing is not available) must meet at least two of the following criteria in addition to the aforementioned clinical, hematological, and laboratory criteria:
- Increased hemoglobin F for age
- Myeloid (promyelocytes, myelocytes, and metamyelocytes) and erythroid precursors on peripheral blood smear
- Thrombocytopenia with hypercellular marrow often showing a decreased number of megakaryocytes; dysplastic features may or may not be evident.
- Hypersensitivity of myeloid progenitors to granulocyte-macrophage colony-stimulating factor (GM-CSF) as tested in clonogenic assays in methylcellulose or by measuring STAT5 phosphorylation in the absence of or with a low dose of exogenous GM-CSF.

Q13. What is myeloproliferative neoplasm, not otherwise specified?

Ans: Myeloproliferative neoplasm not otherwise specified (NOS) is a diagnosis of exclusion for cases that have definite clinical, laboratory, morphological, and molecular features of an MPN but fail to meet the diagnostic criteria for any of the specific types in this disease category.[1]

Diagnostic criteria: Requires the presence of all three of the following:
1. Presence of features of any one of the following features:
    i. Clinical and hematological features of an MPN (e.g., splenomegaly, leukocytosis, and thrombocytosis) in the absence of significant monocytosis and significant eosinophilia
    ii. Bone marrow hypercellularity with megakaryocytic hyperplasia and varying degrees of granulocytic and erythroid hyperplasia, without dysplastic features
    iii. Clinical and morphological features can be discrepant.
2. Not meeting criteria for any other MPN, myelodysplastic syndrome (MDS), MDS/MPN, or myeloid/lymphoid neoplasms with eosinophilia and tyrosine kinase gene fusions
3. Presence of driver mutations such as *JAK2*, *CALR*, or MPL mutations, or another clonal marker

Requires the absence of both of the following:
- Insufficient clinical data or inadequate bone marrow specimen for accurate evaluation and classification
- Recent history of cytotoxic or growth factor therapy, particularly when dysplastic features are seen.

REFERENCES

1. Khoury JD, Solary E, Abla O, Akkari Y, Alaggio R, Apperley JF, et al. The 5th edition of the World Health Organization Classification of Haematolymphoid Tumours: Myeloid and Histiocytic/Dendritic Neoplasms. Leukemia. 2022;36:1703-19.
2. Borthakur G, Kantarjian H. Core binding factor acute myelogenous leukemia-2021 treatment algorithm. Blood Cancer J. 2021;11:114.
3. Walter RB, Othus M, Burnett AK, Löwenberg B, Kantarjian HM, Ossenkoppele GJ, et al. Significance of FAB subclassification of "Acute myeloid leukemia, NOS" in the 2008 WHO classification: analysis of 5848 newly diagnosed patients. Blood. 2013;121(13):2424-31.
4. Alexander C. A History and Current Understanding of Acute Erythroid Leukemia. Clin Lymphoma Myeloma Leuk. 2023;23(8):583-8.
5. McNulty M, Crispino JD. Acute Megakaryocytic Leukemia. Cold Spring Harb Perspect Med. 2020;10(2):a034884.
6. Bhatnagar N, Nizery L, Tunstall O, Vyas P, Roberts I. Transient Abnormal Myelopoiesis and AML in Down Syndrome: an Update. Curr Hematol Malig Rep. 2016;11:333-41.
7. Groet J, McElwaine S, Spinelli M, Rinaldi A, Burtscher I, et al. Acquired mutations in GATA1 in neonates with Down's syndrome with transient myeloid disorder. Lancet. 2003:361;1617-20.
8. George BS, Yohannan B, Gonzalez A, Rios A. Mixed-Phenotype Acute Leukemia: Clinical Diagnosis and Therapeutic Strategies. Biomedicines. 2022;10(8):1974.
9. Bataller A, Guijarro F, Caye-Eude A, Strullu M, Sterin A, Molina O, et al. KMT2A-CBL rearrangements in acute leukemias: clinical characteristics and genetic breakpoints. Blood Adv. 2021;5(24):5617-20.
10. Goyal G, Tazi A, Go RS, Rech KL, Picarsic JL, Vassallo R, et al. International expert consensus recommendations for the diagnosis and treatment of Langerhans cell histiocytosis in adults. Blood. 2022;139:2601-21.
11. Aitken MJL, Ravandi F, Patel KP, Short NJ. Prognostic and therapeutic implications of measurable residual disease in acute myeloid leukemia. J Hematol Oncol. 2021;14:137.
12. Itzykson R, Fenaux P, Bowen D, Cross NCP, Cortes J, De Witte T, et al. Diagnosis and Treatment of Chronic Myelomonocytic Leukemias in Adults: Recommendations From the European Hematology Association and the European LeukemiaNet. Hemasphere. 2018;2(6):e150.

24. Acute Promyelocytic Leukemia

Rahul Arora

A 36-year-old female presented with complaints of bleeding from gums and fever for 2 weeks duration. Clinical evaluation revealed pallor and ecchymotic patches. Her hemogram showed anemia and thrombocytopenia. White cell count was normal with 80% promyelocytes.

Q1. What are the clinical, morphological, and genetic features of acute promyelocytic leukemia?

Ans: Acute promyelocytic leukemia (APL) is a distinct subtype of acute myeloid leukemia that has specific cytogenetic and clinical findings.[1]

Clinical

A younger median age at presentation, lower median white blood cell count, bleeding related early deaths, characteristics predominance of morphologically abnormal promyelocytes in the peripheral blood and bone marrow, unique karyotypic and molecular genetic characteristics, sensitivity to treatment with all-trans retinoic acid (ATRA) and arsenic trioxide (ATO) are the features which differentiate this subtype of leukemia from other subtypes of acute myeloid leukemia (AML). This disease is the most malignant form of acute leukemia with a severe bleeding tendency and a fatal course of only weeks in affected individuals. It is one of the common hematological emergencies that needs to be diagnosed and managed at the earliest.

The APL is characterized by a balanced reciprocal translocation between chromosomes 15 and 17 [t(15;17) (q21;q21)], which results in a gene fusion involving promyelocytic leukemia (PML) and retinoic acid receptor alpha (RARα)].[2]

Multiple variant translocations involving the *RARα* gene on chromosome 17 have been described. These cases can have morphologic features that overlap with APL. However, because of variation in biology as well as differences in response to pharmacologic doses of ATRA, these cases have been reclassified in the current World Health Organization system as "APL with a variant *RARA* translocation."

- t(11;17)(q23;q21)–*ZBTB16::RARA* (previously known as *PLZF::RARA*), often CD13+, CD56+
- t(5;17)(q35;q21)–*NPM1::RARA*, often CD13-negative, CD56-negative
- t(11;17)(q13;q21–*NuMA::RARA*
- t(17;17)(q21;q21)–*STAT5b::RARA*

Q2. How is acute promyelocytic leukemia diagnosed?

Ans: Acute promyelocytic leukemia is typically diagnosed through a combination of clinical presentation, laboratory tests, and genetic analysis.[2] Here are given the common diagnostic steps.

Clinical Presentation
- *Symptoms:* Fever, fatigue, bleeding, bruising, and weight loss.
- *Physical examination:* Pallor, petechiae, and signs of bleeding.

Laboratory Tests
- *Complete blood count (CBC):* Low/normal or a high white blood cell and low to normal platelet counts.
- *Blood smear:* Abnormal promyelocytes.
- *Coagulation studies:* Prolonged prothrombin time (PT) and partial thromboplastin time (PTT).

Cytochemical and Immunophenotypic Analysis
- *Cytochemistry:* Periodic acid-Schiff (PAS) and myeloperoxidase (MPO) stains.
- *Flow cytometry:* CD13, CD33, CD9, and CD117 markers.

Genetic Analysis
- *Fluorescence in situ hybridization (FISH):* Detects PML::RARA fusion.
- *Reverse transcriptase polymerase chain reaction (RT-PCR):* Confirms PML::RARA transcript.
- *Conventional cytogenetics:* t(15;17) translocation.

Additional Tests
- Bone marrow biopsy and aspirate.
- Imaging studies [e.g., computed tomography (CT) scans] to evaluate organ damage.

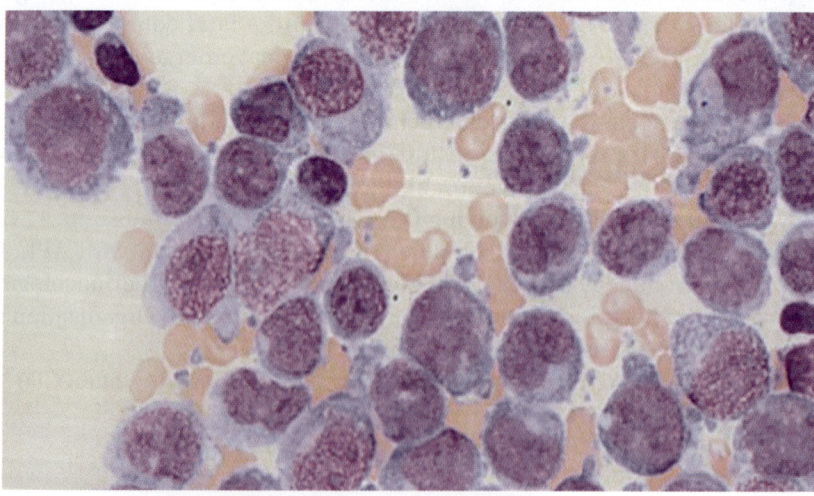

FIG. 1: Acute promyelocytic leukemia.
Courtesy: Dr Jyoti Sawhney.

Diagnostic Criteria

The APL diagnosis requires:
- Presence of abnormal promyelocytes in blood or bone marrow.
- Confirmation of PML::RARA fusion by FISH, RT-PCR, or cytogenetics.
Early diagnosis is crucial for effective treatment and management of APL.

Q3. **Which are the three PML::RARA transcript isoforms?**

Ans: The three main PML::RARA transcript isoforms are:[3]
- *bcr1 (long isoform):* This isoform results from a breakpoint in intron 6 of the *RARA* gene and is associated with approximately 50–60% of APL cases.
- *bcr2 (short isoform):* This isoform results from a breakpoint in exon 6 of the *RARA* gene and is associated with around 20–30% of APL cases.
- *bcr3 (variant isoform):* This isoform results from a breakpoint in exon 3 of the *RARA* gene and is associated with approximately 10–20% of APL cases.

These isoforms vary in their breakpoint locations within the *RARA* gene and affect the resulting PML::RARA fusion protein structure and function.

Q4. **What are the variants of acute promyelocytic leukemia?**

Ans: The cytogenetic hallmark of APL is a translocation involving RARA, the RARα locus on chromosome 17.[2,3] The vast majority of cases of APL contain t(15;17)(q24.1;q21.1).

A number of variant translocations have been described in APL, with t(11;17)(q23;q21.1), t(5;17)(q35;q21.1), and t(11;17)(q13;q21.1) being the most common. Distinguishing between these translocations is important because patients with the variant translocation t(11;17) are almost invariably resistant to ATRA.

Q5. **How is molecular monitoring of acute promyelocytic leukemia done after starting treatment?**

Ans: Molecular analysis of bone marrow collected after the completion of consolidation is crucial to determine relapse risk.[4] The achievement of molecular remission at the end of consolidation corresponds to the new European Leukemia Network (ELN) AML response category "CR without minimal residual disease (CRMRD–)," which is thus a major treatment objective in APL. Real-time quantitative polymerase chain reaction (RQ-PCR) is currently the standard method for molecular monitoring in APL. As compared with qualitative reverse transcription polymerase chain reaction (RT-PCR) tests.

After the completion of consolidation, the response to treatment is again evaluated with a bone marrow aspirate and biopsy. This sample should be tested for the *PML-RARA* fusion transcript using RT-PCR. The goal of APL treatment is the achievement of a molecular CR (CRm), as defined by the absence of the *PML-RARA* fusion transcript using RT-PCR methods with a sensitivity threshold of at least 10^{-3} or 10^{-4}.

With regard to giving precise recommendations for long-term follow-up intervals of patients who have achieved an MRD–status, there are no data. However, it seems reasonable to perform blood counts once a month during the first 12 months after diagnosis, and at 3-4-month intervals during the first 2-3 years.

Q6. **Why is disseminated intravascular coagulation more common in acute promyelocytic leukemia?**

Ans: Disseminated intravascular coagulation (DIC) is more common in APL due to several factors:[5]
- *Release of procoagulant substances:* APL cells contain high levels of tissue factor and cancer procoagulant, which activate the coagulation cascade.
- *Expression of annexin II:* APL cells express annexin II, which binds plasminogen and tissue plasminogen activator, promoting fibrinolysis and coagulation.
- *Impaired fibrinolysis:* APL cells produce inhibitors of plasminogen activator, reducing fibrinolysis and contributing to thrombosis.
- *Cytokine release:* APL cells release proinflammatory cytokines [e.g., tumor necrosis factor alpha (TNF-α), interleukin-1 beta (IL-1β)], which promote coagulation.
- *Abnormal promyelocyte morphology:* APL cells have abnormal morphology, leading to cell lysis and release of procoagulant substances.
- *High cell turnover:* APL is characterized by high cell proliferation and turnover, releasing procoagulant substances.
- *Genetic mutations:* PML-RARA fusion protein disrupts normal cellular function, contributing to coagulopathy.
- *All-trans retinoic acid therapy:* ATRA, used to treat APL, can temporarily worsen coagulopathy.

The DIC in APL is often precipitated by:
- Infection
- Bleeding
- Surgery
- Chemotherapy

Clinical manifestations of DIC in APL are:
- Bleeding (petechiae, ecchymoses)
- Thrombosis (deep vein thrombosis, pulmonary embolism)
- Organ dysfunction (renal, hepatic)
- Laboratory findings (prolonged PT/PTT, low fibrinogen, and elevated D-dimer)
Early recognition and management of DIC are crucial in APL patients.

Treatment Strategies
- Supportive care (transfusions, plasma exchange)
- Anticoagulation (low-molecular-weight heparin) in selected cases
- Fibrinolysis inhibitors (tranexamic acid)
- ATRA and ATO therapy adjustments
- Aggressive infection control and supportive care

Q7. **What is differentiation syndrome and how can it be prevented?**

Ans: Differentiation syndrome (DS), also known as retinoic acid syndrome, is a potentially life-threatening complication in APL patients treated with ATRA and/or ATO.[6]

Pathophysiology
The ATRA and ATO induce differentiation of abnormal promyelocytes into mature cells, leading to rapid cell maturation and release of proinflammatory cytokines, increased vascular permeability, and capillary leak syndrome.

Clinical Features
- Fever
- Weight gain
- Peripheral edema
- Dyspnea
- Hypotension
- Pulmonary infiltrates
- Renal dysfunction
- Cardiac dysfunction

Risk Factors
- High white blood cell count (WBC > 5,000/μL)
- High peripheral blast count
- Poor performance status
- Renal or hepatic impairment
- Prior cardiovascular disease

Prevention and Management
Prevention (Before Features of Differentiation)
- Monitor patients closely during initial treatment.
- Baseline chest X-ray and pulmonary function tests.
- Prophylactic corticosteroids (e.g., dexamethasone 10 mg twice daily) during induction.

Management (After Features of Differentiation)
- Immediate corticosteroids (dexamethasone 10–20 mg twice daily)
- Fluid management (diuresis, fluid restriction)
- Supportive care (oxygen therapy, mechanical ventilation)
- Temporary interruption of ATRA/ATO
- Chemotherapy (e.g., hydroxyurea) to control WBC

Mortality Rate
- *Untreated DS:* 20–50%
- *Treated DS:* < 5%

Early recognition and prompt management are crucial to prevent complications and improve outcomes in APL patients.

Q8. What is the treatment of low risk acute promyelocytic leukemia?

Ans: All-trans retinoic acid and ATO without chemotherapy as the new standard of care for patients with non-high-risk APL (WBC < 10,000/μL).[7,8]

In APL, most deaths occur within the 1st month of diagnosis, approximately one-third of the patients die within 30 days of diagnosis, and 35% of the deaths occur before an ATRA dose. Immediate administration of ATRA at the first suspicion of APL diagnosis is of extreme importance.

In addition to prompt ATRA administration, coagulopathy should be adequately corrected by keeping internationalized normalized ratio (INR) for PT at <1.5–2.0, fibrinogen greater than 100 mg/dL platelets >30,000/µL through blood product transfusions. Invasive procedures, such as central line placements, lumbar punctures, and leukapheresis, should be avoided.

For most low- or intermediate-risk patients (WBC < 10,000/µL) with newly diagnosed APL, recommendation is to use ATRA plus ATO rather than ATRA plus anthracycline-based chemotherapy. This preference places a high value on the lesser toxicity (e.g., myelosuppression, cardiac toxicity), fewer deaths during induction therapy, fewer relapses, and reduced risk of secondary leukemia with this combination. Where ATO is not available for initial use, a standard ATRA plus anthracycline regimen is the recommended alternative for remission induction. Patients who receive induction with ATRA plus chemotherapy benefit when ATO is used for postremission therapy. Most trials of ATO plus ATRA have used intravenous ATO. Although its mechanism of action is not fully understood, (ATO, As_2O_3) has dose-dependent dual effects on APL cells by preferentially inducing apoptosis (at high concentrations) and differentiation (at low concentrations). Initial results suggest that the combination of an oral formulation of tetra-arsenic tetra-sulfide (As4S4) plus ATRA results in similar clinical outcomes. In consolidation too ATRA and ATO can be used based on different trial results.

Q9. Can we treat high risk acute promyelocytic leukemia without chemotherapy?

Ans: High-risk APL is typically treated with a combination of therapies, and while chemotherapy has traditionally been part of the treatment regimen, there are newer approaches that minimize or eliminate chemotherapy.[7,8]

The optimal regimen for patients with high-risk APL remains a debated issue. These patients have a higher possibility of induction mortality due to increased risk of fluid overload, differentiation syndrome, respiratory failure, DIC, and severe bleeding. Hence, controlling leukocytosis and treating DIC early on is critical.

Traditional Treatment

Chemotherapy, usually anthracyclines (e.g., idarubicin or daunorubicin), has been the cornerstone of APL treatment, often combined with ATRA.

Nonchemotherapy Approaches

ATRA + ATO: This combination has become a standard first-line treatment for low-to-intermediate risk APL and is being explored for high-risk patients.[9] ATRA and ATO work together to induce differentiation and apoptosis (cell death) in leukemic cells.

Although ATRA with ATO and an anthracycline is the preferred induction regimen for patients with high-risk APL at most centers, gemtuzumab ozogamicin (GO) remains an alternative to anthracycline, especially for patients ineligible for anthracycline therapy due to cardiac and other comorbidities.

Anthracycline-sparing induction has been explored in high-risk disease in an attempt to mitigate cardiac and hematological toxicity and reduce requirements for supportive care.

Addition of GO, an anti-CD33 antibody conjugated to the cytotoxic agent calicheamicin, to ATRA with ATO in high-risk APL produced a complete response (CR) rate of 98% and a 5-year event-free survival (EFS) rate of 86%.

In addition, aggressive use of hydroxyurea may also be sufficient to allow for a chemotherapy-free approach even in high-risk patients.

Q10. **What are the supportive measures recommended during the treatment of acute promyelocytic leukemia?**

Ans: The supportive measures recommended to treat coagulopathy have not changed during the last decade. Platelet counts and routine coagulation parameters, including PT, activated PTT, and thrombin time, as well as levels of fibrinogen and fibrinogen-fibrin degradation products should be monitored at least daily and more frequently if required. Transfusions of fibrinogen and/or cryoprecipitate, platelets, and fresh-frozen plasma should be given immediately upon suspicion of the diagnosis, and then daily or more than once a day if needed, to maintain the fibrinogen concentration above 100–150 mg/dL, the platelet count above 30×10^9/L to 50×10^9/L, and the international normalized ratio (INR) below 1.5. Supportive treatment should be continued during induction therapy until disappearance of all clinical and laboratory signs of the coagulopathy.[10]

The benefit of using heparin, tranexamic acid, or other anticoagulant or antifibrinolytic agents to attenuate the hemorrhagic and thrombotic risk associated with the coagulopathy before and during remission induction therapy remains questionable.

Invasive procedures such as central venous catheterization, lumbar puncture, and bronchoscopy should be avoided at diagnosis and during initial treatment as long as the coagulopathy is active.

Q11. **What is the role of allogeneic stem cell transplant in acute promyelocytic leukemia?**

Ans: A large proportion of patients with APL achieve long-term responses with available therapy, so performing a hematopoietic stem cell transplant as consolidation of first complete remission (CR) is no longer necessary.[11]

Even in the case of relapses, most patients obtain a new remission as a result of therapy with ATO and ATRA, but an effective consolidation treatment is necessary to maintain it. The experience accumulated from studies published in the last two decades shows the effectiveness of hematopoietic stem cell transplantation (HSCT) in improving the outcome of patients who achieve a new CR. At present, HSCT is the best consolidation therapy after salvage therapy for relapsed APL. Both ELN and the National Comprehensive Cancer Network (NCCN) guidelines recommend auto-HSCT as the first choice for eligible patients achieving second molecular remission, while patients failing to achieve molecular remission should undergo an allo-HSCT.

REFERENCES

1. Licht JD, Chomienne C, Goy A, Chen A, Scott AA, Head DR, et al. Clinical and molecular characterization of a rare syndrome of acute promyelocytic leukemia associated with translocation (11;17). Blood. 1995;85(4):1083-94.
2. Arber DA, Orazi A, Hasserjian R, Thiele J, Borowitz MJ, Le Beau MM, et al. The 2016 revision to the World Health Organization classification of myeloid neoplasms and acute leukemia. Blood. 2016;127(20):2391-405.

3. Sanz MA, Lo Coco F, Martín G, et al. Definition of relapse risk and role of nonanthracycline drugs for consolidation in patients with acute promyelocytic leukemia: a joint study of the PETHEMA and GIMEMA cooperative groups. Blood. 2000;96:1247.
4. Daver N, Kantarjian H, Marcucci G, Pierce S, Brandt M, Dinardo C, et al. Clinical characteristics and outcomes in patients with acute promyelocytic leukaemia and hyperleucocytosis. Br J Haematol. 2015;168:646-53.
5. Lo-Coco F, Avvisati G, Vignetti M, Thiede C, Orlando SM, Iacobelli S, et al. Retinoic acid and arsenic trioxide for acute promyelocytic leukemia. N Engl J Med. 2013;369:111-21.
6. Sanz MA, Montesinos P. How we prevent and treat differentiation syndrome in patients with acute promyelocytic leukemia. Blood. 2014;123:2777-82
7. Jimenez JJ, Chale RS, Abad AC, Schally AV. Acute promyelocytic leukemia (APL): a review of the literature. Oncotarget 2020;11:992.
8. Yilmaz M, Kantarjian H, Ravandi F. Acute promyelocytic leukemia current treatment algorithms. Blood Cancer. 2021;11(123).
9. Aribi A, Kantarjian HM, Estey EH, Koller CA, Thomas DA, Kornblau SM, et al. Combination therapy with arsenic trioxide, all-trans retinoic acid, and gemtuzumab ozogamicin in recurrent acute promyelocytic leukemia. Cancer. 2007;109:1355-9.
10. Avvisati G, Lo-Coco F, Paoloni FP, Petti MC, Diverio D, Vignetti M, et al. AIDA 0493 protocol for newly diagnosed acute promyelocytic leukemia: very long-term results and role of maintenance. Blood. 2011;117:4716-25.
11. Sanford D, Lo-Coco F, Sanz MA, Di Bona E, Coutre S, Altman JK, et al. Tamibarotene in patients with acute promyelocytic leukaemia relapsing after treatment with all-trans retinoic acid and arsenic trioxide. Br J Haematol. 2015;171:471-7.

25. Hodgkin Lymphoma

Prashant Mane

Q1. What is Hodgkin lymphoma?

Ans: Classic Hodgkin lymphoma (CHL) is a B-cell derived neoplasm, characterized by scattered neoplastic cells, Hodgkin and Reed–Sternberg cells (HRS cells), amidst the reactive inflammatory cells background.[1] The pathogenesis of CHL involves genetic alterations in the neoplastic HRS cells, their interaction with the tumor microenvironment and latent Epstein–Barr virus (EBV) infection.

Q2. What is the cell of origin of Hodgkin and Reed–Sternberg cells?

Ans: The cellular origin of HRS cells was not known for a long time, as these cells do not show a lineage specific immuno-profile. There is coexpression of immunomarkers of different cell types and lack of B-cell receptor expression. The origin of HRS cells was established, when these cells were isolated from biopsy specimens and subjected to genetic analysis by single-cell polymerase chain reaction (PCR).[1,2] The HRS cells showed immunoglobulin (Ig) heavy and light chain V gene rearrangements, which are specific for B cells,[3] indicating that these cells represent B cells. Moreover, these cells show somatic hypermutations in the *IgV* genes, a process which is seen only in germinal center B cells of the lymph nodes,[4] pointing toward germinal center B-cell derivation. The HRS cells are derived from preapoptotic germinal center B cells which has escaped apoptosis.

A minority of CHL cases show T-cell immuno-profile. Whether, these are T-cell derived CHL or "B-cell" lymphomas with aberrant T-cell expression, needs further research.

Q3. What are the genetic alterations seen in Hodgkin lymphoma?

Ans: The activation of oncogenic signaling pathways [in particular Janus kinase/signal transducer and activator of transcription (JAK/STAT) and nuclear factor kappa B (NF-κB)] by numerical chromosomal abnormalities, gene rearrangements or somatic mutations, and immune evasion, are the key factors, for survival and proliferation of HRS cells.[5]

A copy number gain of 9p24.1 (PD-L1/L2 and JAK2 locus), is the most frequent genetic alteration seen in CHL (>90% of cases), which increases PDL1 expression on HRS cells. Interaction of PD-L1 (expressed on HRS cells) with PD-1 receptor (expressed on T cells), inhibits T-cell activation and proliferation, and thereby HRS cell escape the cytotoxic T-cell activity. In addition to copy number alterations, somatic mutation of *SOCS1*, *PTPN1*, *STAT6*, *STAT3* and *CSF2RB* genes activates the *JAK/STAT* pathway and *TNFAIP3*, *NFKBIA*, and *REL* genes activates the NF-κB pathway. An inactivating mutation of the β2 microglobulin gene

(B2M), seen in up to 40% cases, limits the cell surface expression of major histocompatibility complex (MHC) class I, which helps HRS cells to escape from immune surveillance by CD8+ T cells.

Q4. What is the role of Epstein–Barr virus in the pathogenesis of Hodgkin lymphoma?

Ans: It is now well known that EBV plays a major role in the pathogenesis of EBV+ve. However, the prevalence of EBV positivity differs between the different histologic subtypes of CHL (75% in mixed cellularity CHL, 65% in lymphocyte depleted CHL, 10–25% in nodular sclerosis CHL, and 30–50% lymphocyte rich CHL).

The EBV is ubiquitous and after initial infection, EBV establishes a latent infection in the affected cell, where it remains dormant and later reactivates. During the latent phase EBV expresses different genes and depending upon the viral gene expression, the latent form of EBV is categorized into four patterns, latency 0 to latency III. EBV-infected HRS cells in CHL show a type II latency, characterized by expression of EBV-encoded small RNAs (EBERs), EBNA1 protein, latent membrane protein 1 (LMP1), and LMP2A protein.

The LMP1, interacts with CD40 receptor (tumor necrosis factor receptor family) and activates NF-κB signaling pathway. Thus, EBV+ve is not dependent on genetic alteration for the activation of NF-κB signaling pathway. HRS cells do not express functional B-cell receptor (BCR) signaling, which is essential for the B-cell survival, development, and antibody production. LMP2A, mimics BCR signaling, and thus contributes in the pathogenesis of CHL. EBV+ve shows less mutation burden, as compared to EBV-ve.[6]

Q5. What is the role of microenvironment in the pathophysiology of Hodgkin lymphoma?

Ans: The neoplastic HRS cells form very minor component of the tumor mass in CHL. The major component, tumor microenvironment, is formed by dense inflammatory cell infiltrate comprising of lymphocytes, plasma cells, eosinophils, histiocytes, neutrophils, and stromal cells. HRS cells produce different cytokines, chemokines, and growth factors, which recruit inflammatory cells and stromal cells.

The inflammatory milieu is particularly rich in CD4+ T cells. The HRS cells are surrounded by the CD4+ T cells, forming rosette. These CD4+ T cells transmit survival signals to the HRS cells and prevent interaction of HRS cells with effector CD8+ T cells. The antitumor activity of CD8+ T cells is curbed by the secretion of immunosuppressive molecules [interleukin (IL)-19, transforming growth factor-beta (TGF-B)], overexpression of programmed death (PD)L1/PDL2 and loss of MHC complex on HRS cells. Regulatory T cell (Tr1), present in the tumor microenvironment secretes IL-10, which is a strong immunosuppressive. The macrophages in the tumor microenvironment are M2 subtype, which also have immunosuppressive function.

Thus, CHL creates a tumor microenvironment which helps HRS cells to survive, proliferate, and escape immune surveillance.[7]

Q6. What is the histopathology of Hodgkin lymphoma?

Ans: CHL is characterized by sparse population (0.1–10%) of neoplastic HRS cells surrounded by non-neoplastic inflammatory background **(Fig. 1)**. The HRS cells are large, 4–5 times the size of normal lymphocytes, with abundant amphophilic cytoplasm, large nuclei, and prominent eosinophilic nucleoli. The HRS cells exhibit various forms. The pathognomic Reed–Sternberg cells are formed by incomplete cytokinesis and refusion of mononucleated Hodgkin cells.[8] The classic Reed–Sternberg cell, are binucleate with large, central eosinophilic nucleoli, and perinuclear clearing (classic owl-eye appearance). They can be multinucleated also. A Hodgkin cell is mononucleate with a prominent nucleolus. Lacunar cells, seen in nodular sclerosis CHL, have multilobated nuclei lying in empty space, created by the retraction of cytoplasm during fixation. The mummified cells are degenerated HRS cells with condensed pyknotic nuclei. The background inflammatory cell population varies with the CHL subtype. It is typically rich in T cell admixed with lymphocytes, histiocytes, neutrophils, and eosinophils. Epithelioid granulomas are not uncommon and sometimes overshadow the HRS cells.

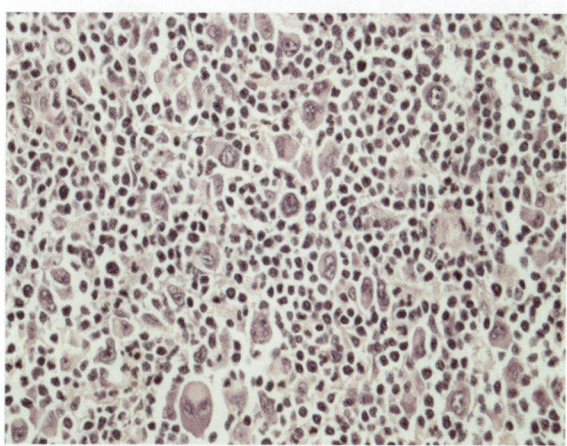

FIG. 1: Mono-nucleate and bi-nucleate HRS cells in non-neoplastic inflammatory background (H&E, magnification ×400).

Q7. What are the subtypes of Hodgkin lymphoma?

Ans: CHL is classified into four subtypes: (i) Nodular sclerosis CHL (NSCHL), (ii) mixed cellularity CHL (MCCHL), (iii) lymphocyte-rich CHL (LRCHL), and (iv) lymphocyte-depleted CHL (LDCHL). This subtyping has no therapeutic impact. But, these subtypes present with distinct clinical, morphologic, and epidemiologic characteristics.

The NSCHL shows thickened capsule and sclerotic bands surrounding the nodules composed of lacunar variant of HRS cells and inflammatory cells. Classic HRS cells are also seen. The background cells comprise lymphocytes, neutrophils, eosinophils, histiocytes, and plasma cells. Sometimes, sheets of HRS cells are seen, called syncytial variant. Necrosis can also be seen. Grading of NSCHL is obsolete now.

The MCCHL show binucleated or multinucleated Reed–Sternberg cells amidst mixed inflammatory cell infiltrate comprising of lymphocytes, histiocytes, eosinophils, and plasma cells. Epithelioid granulomas are seen.

The LRCHL shows nodular or diffuse infiltrate of small lymphocyte with scattered HRS cells. Neutrophils and eosinophils are not seen.

The LDCHL shows predominance of HRS cells amidst sparse lymphocytes in the background. Eosinophils and plasma cells are rare.

Q8. What is the immunophenotype of Hodgkin lymphoma?

Ans: CHL is characterized by loss of expression of B-cell markers and overexpression of CD30 and CD15.

The CD30 activates the NF-κB pathway and promotes HRS cells survival and proliferation. CD30 expression is seen in almost all cases, while CD15 expression is seen in majority but not all cases of CHL. The staining in CD30 and CD15 is typically membranous and Golgi zone pattern **(Figs. 2 and 3)**.

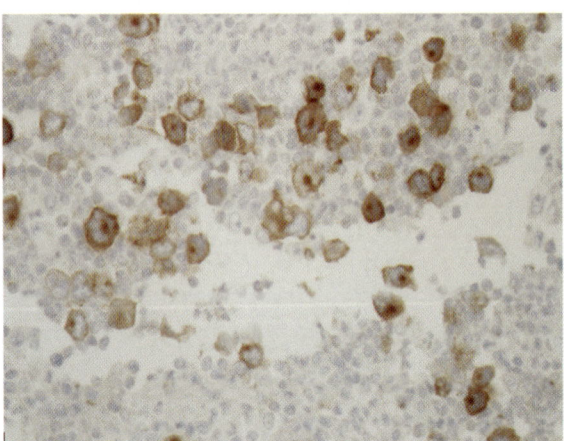

FIG. 2: CD30, HRS cells showing typical membranous and Golgi zone staining pattern.

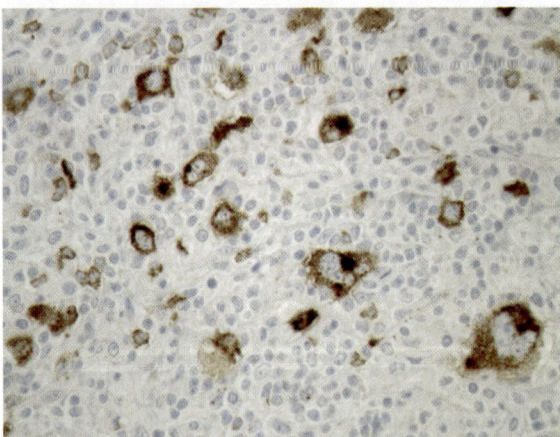

FIG. 3: CD15, HRS cells showing typical membranous and Golgi zone staining pattern.

The decreased expression of B-cell markers, except PAX5, is due to lack of expression of B-lineage–specific genes in HRS cells.[9] PAX5, is a transcriptional factor, which regulates B-cell differentiation and proliferation.[10] It is expressed in the early stages of B-cell development. The expression of PAX5 in HRS cells is typically weak, nuclear staining, compared with the background reactive B cells **(Fig. 4)**. CD20 positivity is weak, variable, and seen in minority of cells. Other transcriptional factors [octamer-binding transcription factor 2 (OCT2), B-cell octamer-binding protein 1 (BOB1), PU.1, and BCL6] are downregulated **(Fig. 5)**. Rare cases may show expression of either BOB1 or OCT2. The common leukocyte antigen (CD45) is also negative **(Fig. 6)**. Multiple myeloma oncogene 1 (MUM1), a transcriptional factor, seen in activated B cells, is strongly expressed **(Fig. 7)**.

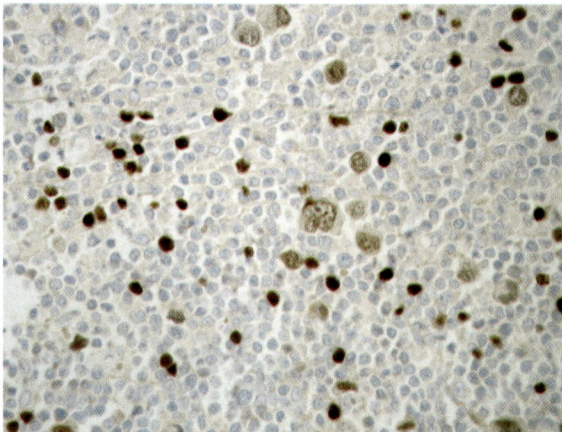

FIG. 4: PAX5, HRS cells showing typical weak nuclear staining compared to background reactive B cells.

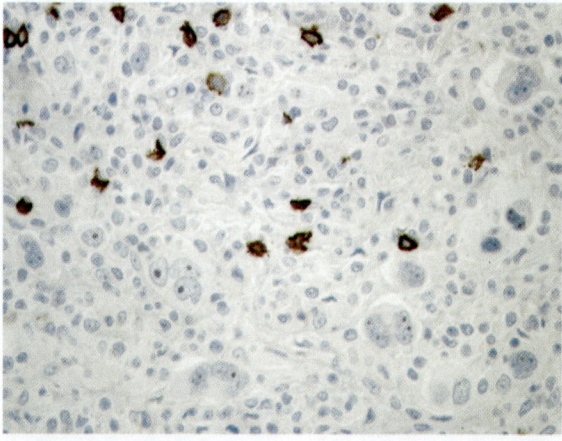

FIG. 5: CD20, negative in the HRS cells.

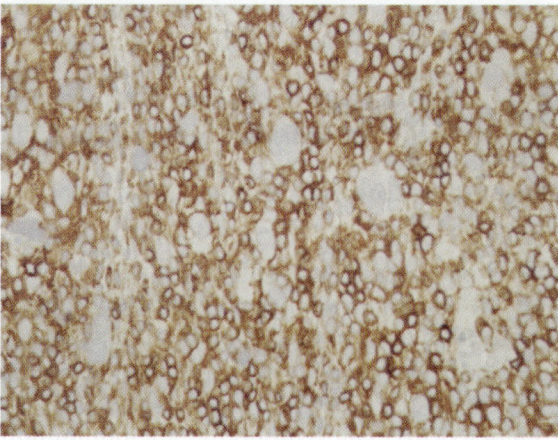

FIG. 6: CD45, negative in the HRS cells.

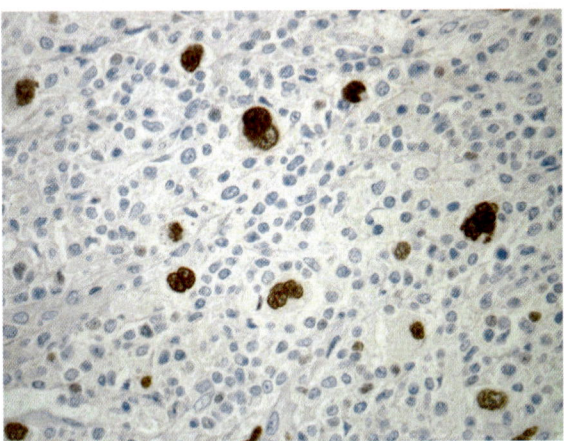

FIG. 7: MUM1 staining the HRS cells.

The EBV association is demonstrated by in situ hybridization for EBER and immunohistochemistry for LMP1 and EBNA1 proteins **(Fig. 8)**.

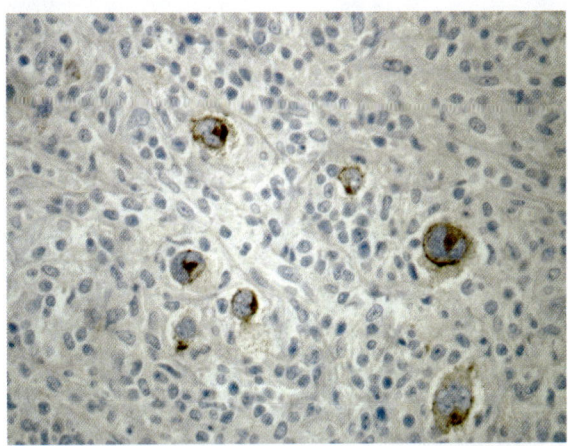

FIG. 8: EBV-LMP1, HRS cells showing typical membranous and Golgi zone staining pattern.

Other markers which are expressed in CHL are: Fascin, PD-L1, STAT6, and GATA3. These markers are rarely required, however, can be helpful in diagnostically difficult cases.

Q9. Are HRS cells diagnostic of Hodgkin lymphoma?

Ans: HRS like cells can be seen in many T-cell and B-cell non-Hodgkin lymphoma.[11] Anaplastic large cell lymphoma (ALCL) shows characteristic neoplastic "hallmark cell" which mimic HRS cells. The "hallmark cell" are also CD30+, but positivity for T-cell and cytotoxic markers and negativity for EBV and PAX5 favor, ALCL. The null cell phenotype, which is negative for T-cell markers, is a diagnostic challenge, sometimes requiring T-cell receptor rearrangement confirmation.

Nodal T-follicular helper (TFH) cell lymphoma, angioimmunoblastic type (nTFHL-AI) shows minor population of neoplastic T cells along with mixed population of reactive lymphocytes, immunoblasts, plasma cells, eosinophil, and histiocytes. There is characteristic, prominent proliferation of high endothelial venules. The scattered immunoblast in the reactive population mimic HRS cells and are EBV and CD30+. But, unlike CHL, they show strong CD20 positivity.

T-cell histiocyte rich large B-cell lymphoma (THRLBCL) is histomorphologically similar to CHL, closely resembling either MCCHL or LRCHL. THRLBCL too have scattered atypical large lymphoid cells (centroblast, immunoblast, or HRS like) amidst reactive population of T lymphocytes and histiocytes. The neoplastic cells are <10% and EBV negative. In contrast to CHL, the neoplastic cells in THRLBCL are positive for CD45 and B-cell markers (CD20, CD79a, and PAX5) while negative for CD30, CD15, and EBV.

The polymorphic subtype of EBV positive large B-cell lymphoma shows HRS like cells along with background population of reactive lymphocytes, plasma cells, and histiocytes. There is angiocentricity, angiodestruction, and extensive coagulative necrosis. The neoplastic cells are CD30 (40% cases) and EBV positive. However, they also show strong CD45 and B-cell lineage marker expression.

Mediastinal gray zone lymphoma shows intermediate features between CHL (resembling NSCHL) and primary mediastinal B-cell lymphoma. The neoplastic cells are variable positive for CD30 but uniform, strong positive for B-cell markers. They lack EBV expression.

Infectious mononucleosis shows paracortical expansion along with HRS like cells. These cells are CD30 and EBV positive but also show B-cell marker and CD45 positivity.

Q10. What is nodular lymphocyte predominant Hodgkin lymphoma?

Ans: NLPHL is characterized by scattered neoplastic B cells in the background of lymphocytes and histiocytes, similar to lymphocyte rich CHL. Hence, it is placed under the category of Hodgkin lymphoma. However, there is ample, clinical, pathological, and biological evidence suggesting that it is distinct from CHL. The recent World Health Organization (WHO) classification of hematolymphoid neoplasm, 5th edition, suggests a new terminology, "nodular lymphocyte-predominant B-cell lymphoma" for NLPHL.

The neoplastic B cells, lymphocyte-predominant cells (LP cells) have multilobated nuclei, thin nuclear membrane, fine chromatin, and one or more small nucleoli (resembling popcorn). The background reactive cell population is composed of lymphocytes and histiocytes. Neutrophils and eosinophils are not seen. LP cells are positive for B-cell markers and negative for CD30, CD15, and EBV.

REFERENCES

1. Kanzler H, Küppers R, Hansmann ML, Rajewsky K. Hodgkin and Reed–Sternberg cells in Hodgkin's disease represent the outgrowth of a dominant tumor clone derived from (crippled) germinal center B cells. J Exp Med. 1996;184(4):1495-505.
2. Marafioti T, Hummel M, Foss H-D, Laumen H, Korbjuhn P, Anagnostopoulos I, et al. Hodgkin and Reed-Sternberg cells represent an expansion of a single clone originating from a germinal center B-cell with functional immunoglobulin gene rearrangements but defective immunoglobulin transcription. Blood. 2000;95(4):1443-50.
3. Rajewsky K. Clonal selection and learning in the antibody system. Nature 1996;381(6585):751-8.
4. Küppers R, Zhao M, Hansmann ML, Rajewsky K. Tracing B cell development in human germinal centres by molecular analysis of single cells picked from histological sections. EMBO J. 1993;12(13):4955-67.
5. Brune MM, Juskevicius D, Haslbauer J, Dirnhofer S, Tzankov A. Genomic Landscape of Hodgkin Lymphoma. Cancers (Basel). 2021;13(4):682.

6. Tiacci E, Ladewig E, Schiavoni G, Penson A, Fortini E, Pettirossi V, et al. Pervasive mutations of JAK-STAT pathway genes in classical Hodgkin lymphoma. Blood. 2018;131(22):2454-65.
7. Weniger MA, Küppers R. Molecular biology of Hodgkin lymphoma. Leukemia. 2021;35(4):968-81.
8. Rengstl B, Newrzela S, Heinrich T, Weiser C, Thalheimer FB, Schmid F, et al. Incomplete cytokinesis and re-fusion of small mononucleated Hodgkin cells lead to giant multinucleated Reed-Sternberg cells. Proc Natl Acad Sci. 2013;110(51):20729-34.
9. Schwering I, Bräuninger A, Klein U, Jungnickel B, Tinguely M, Diehl V, et al. Loss of the B-lineage-specific gene expression program in Hodgkin and Reed-Sternberg cells of Hodgkin lymphoma. Blood. 2003;101(4):1505-12.
10. Horcher M, Souabni A, Busslinger M. Pax5/BSAP maintains the identity of B cells in late B lymphopoiesis. Immunity. 2001;14(6):779-90.
11. Parente P, Zanelli M, Sanguedolce F, Mastracci L, Graziano P. Hodgkin Reed-Sternberg-Like Cells in Non-Hodgkin Lymphoma. Diagnostics (Basel). 2020;10(12):1019.

26. Serum Protein Electrophoresis

Nagarjun Sai, Abhishek Purohit

Q1. What is serum protein electrophoresis?

Ans: Serum protein electrophoresis (SPEP) is a technique to separate serum proteins based on their net charge, size, and shape. It identifies normal and abnormal proteins separated by electrophoresis and is useful in evaluation of acute and chronic inflammation, various cancers, liver or kidney failure, and hereditary protein disorders. It is the most commonly used test for detecting monoclonal gammopathies seen in plasma cell dyscrasias. In this process, the patient's serum is applied to special paper treated with agarose gel and subjected to an electric current, which separates the serum proteins based on their distinct properties.[1,2] These proteins are then stained, and their density is measured to produce graphical data.

The serum contains two major types of proteins: Albumin and globulins. Albumin, the predominant protein in serum, forms the most prominent peak closest to the positive electrode during electrophoresis. Although globulins constitute a smaller fraction of total serum protein, they are the main focus of interpretation in SPEP. There are five categories of globulins: α-1, α-2, β-1, β-2, and γ, with the γ fraction being nearest to the negative electrode.

The major importance of protein electrophoresis lies in diagnosing and monitoring monoclonal and polyclonal gammopathies **(Table 1)**. Acute and chronic infections can be differentiated by their globulin patterns: Chronic infections typically show increased γ globulins without elevated α-1 and α-2 globulins and often have low albumin, whereas, acute infections present with an acute phase reaction marked by increased α-2 globulins without a polyclonal increase in γ globulins.[1,2]

- *Reference ranges:*
  - Albumin 3.3–5.7 g/dL
  - α-1 globulin 0.1–0.4 g/dL
  - α-2 globulin 0.3–0.9 g/dL
  - β-2 globulin 0.7–1.5 g/dL
  - γ globulin 0.5–1.4 g/dL

TABLE 1: Changes in serum protein electrophoresis and associated conditions.

	Increase	Decrease
Albumin	Dehydration	• Chronic disease • Chronic infections • Burns

Continued

Continued

	Increase	Decrease
		• Protein-losing enteropathies
		• Impaired liver function
		• Malnutrition
		• Nephrotic syndrome
		• Pregnancy
α-1 globulins	Pregnancy	• α-1-antitrypsin deficiency
α-2-globulins	• Adrenal insufficiency adrenocorticosteroid therapy advanced diabetes mellitus • Nephritic syndrome	• Malnutrition • Megaloblastic anemia • Protein-losing enteropathy • Severe liver disease • Wilson's disease
β-globulins	• Biliary cirrhosis • Carcinoma • Cushing's disease • Diabetes mellitus • Hypothyroidism • Iron deficiency anemia • Nephrosis • Polyarteritis nodosa • Obstructive jaundice • Third-trimester pregnancy	Protein malnutrition
γ globulins	• Amyloidosis • Chronic infections (granulomatous disease) • Chronic lymphocytic leukemia • Cirrhosis • Hodgkin lymphoma • Malignant lymphoma • Multiple myeloma • Rheumatoid and vascular diseases	• Agammaglobulinemia • Hypogammaglobulinemia

Q2. What is serum immunofixation electrophoresis, and how is it different from serum protein electrophoresis?

Ans: Monoclonal protein (M-protein) may not be detected with SPEP if its level is too low. When there is a high suspicion of a clonal plasma cell disorder, more sensitive tests like serum immunofixation electrophoresis (IFE) should be used. Additionally, specific quantitation is necessary for conditions such as α-1 antitrypsin deficiency or immunoglobulin (Ig) deficiency since SPEP lacks sensitivity for these cases.

The IFE not only separates proteins through electrophoresis but also uses specific antibodies to identify and characterize individual proteins, particularly immunoglobulins. IFE is more sensitive and specific than SPEP for detecting and characterizing monoclonal proteins **(Table 2)**. It provides detailed information about the type of immunoglobulin and its light chain (LC), essential for accurate diagnosis and treatment planning.[3]

TABLE 2: The main differences between serum protein electrophoresis and serum immunofixation electrophoresis.

Feature	Serum protein electrophoresis (SPEP)	Immunofixation electrophoresis (IFE)
Principle	Separation of protein by charge	Electrophoresis and immunoprecipitation
Method	Electrophoresis, staining, densitometry	Electrophoresis, immunofixation, staining
Protein fractions	Albumin, α-1, α-2, β, γ globulins	Specific immunoglobulins (IgG, IgA, IgM, kappa, lambda)
Uses	For screening, quantification of protein fractions	Diagnosis and characterization of monoclonal gammopathies
Sensitivity and specificity	Less specific	Highly specific and sensitive to monoclonal proteins

Q3. **What is the significance of monoclonal band in hematological diseases?**

Ans: Monoclonal proteins typically migrate into the γ region in SPEP, but they can also appear in the β or α-2 regions, especially with IgA and IgM monoclonal proteins. These bands are called M-protein or M-spike, with "M" denoting monoclonal. It is important to note that the γ region contains all immunoglobulin isotypes (IgM, IgA, IgD, and IgE), not just IgG. A monoclonal protein spike should not be mistaken for a polyclonal increase in immunoglobulins, which generally appears as a broad-based band in the γ region during inflammatory conditions.

Understanding the conditions associated with monoclonal proteins is essential. The clinical presentation can depend on the tumor burden or the monoclonal protein's toxic effects. A simple evaluation starts with identifying the type of monoclonal protein, as it can hint at the underlying disorder. For example, an IgM monoclonal protein is linked to lymphoproliferative diseases like Waldenström macroglobulinemia, while IgG is common in monoclonal gammopathy of undetermined significance (MGUS) and myeloma.

Most non-IgM monoclonal gammopathies are classified as MGUS. MGUS patients have no symptoms or lab abnormalities related to the plasma cell clone, have <3 g/dL of monoclonal protein and < 10% bone marrow plasma cells (PCs). Asymptomatic patients with higher levels are classified as smoldering multiple myeloma (SMM). Bone marrow examination can help distinguish MGUS from SMM, essential for prognosis and follow-up.

Multiple myeloma (MM) patients must meet the CRAB criteria: Hypercalcemia, renal insufficiency, anemia, or bone disease. Additional markers for myeloma include high levels of clonal PCs, specific serum-free light chain (sFLC) ratios, and focal lesions on magnetic resonance imaging (MRI). Solitary plasmacytomas need limited therapy and do not meet CRAB criteria.

In AL amyloidosis, misfolded monoclonal proteins deposit in organs, causing dysfunction. Symptoms vary based on organ involvement, such as cardiomyopathy, neuropathy, proteinuria, hepatomegaly, or gastrointestinal issues. Light chain deposition diseases (LCDD) involve LCs in organs, primarily the kidneys.

The IgM monoclonal gammopathy usually indicates a B-cell disorder, with true IgM myeloma being rare. Most IgM gammopathies are IgM MGUS or Waldenström macroglobulinemia, the latter presenting with cytopenias, hyperviscosity, and organomegaly. Diagnosis involves clinical, radiologic, and laboratory findings, with the MYD88 mutation common in Waldenström macroglobulinemia.

Other conditions such as POEMS (polyneuropathy, organomegaly, endocrinopathy, monoclonal plasma cell disorder, skin changes) syndrome, scleromyxedema, Schnitzler syndrome, and TEMPI (telangiectasias, erythrocytosis with elevated erythropoietin, monoclonal gammopathy, perinephric fluid collections, intrapulmonary shunting) syndrome should be considered based on specific symptoms. VEXAS (vacuoles, E1 enzyme, X-linked, autoinflammatory, somatic) syndrome, a male-specific autoinflammatory disease, is associated with monoclonal gammopathy in some cases.[4,5]

Q4. How are light chains quantified?

Ans: Immunoglobulins are made up of heavy chains and LCs, which are usually bound together as "intact immunoglobulins." PCs produce more LCs than heavy chains, and these unbound LCs circulate freely in the blood. These "free" LCs are present in healthy individuals and patients with myeloma. These patients often have negative protein electrophoresis and serum immunofixation results. The sFLC assay detects these disorders. It measures free kappa (κ) and lambda (λ) LC concentrations, which depend on production rates from PCs and renal clearance. In clonal plasma cell disorders, one type of LC is overproduced, causing an abnormal κ/λ ratio. Renal failure can affect these levels and ratios.

The International Myeloma Working Group (IMWG) defines an involved/uninvolved free light chain (FLC) ratio of 100 or greater, with an involved FLC level of at least 100 mg/L, requiring therapy. The serum FLC test is vital for evaluating and monitoring amyloidosis, replacing urine protein electrophoresis and immunofixation in initial screenings. If a monoclonal plasma cell disorder is detected, a 24-hour urine collection with electrophoresis and immunofixation is recommended to assess disease progression and therapy response.

The FLC assay predicts prognosis in MGUS, smoldering myeloma, AL amyloidosis, and solitary plasmacytoma, and monitors oligosecretory MM, light-chain MM, and AL amyloidosis.

For years, detecting sFLCs was challenging because no analytical method could distinguish between LCs bound to intact immunoglobulins and FLCs. However, in the early 2000s, an assay was developed that targets an epitope hidden in intact immunoglobulins but visible in FLCs. This assay uses both polyclonal and monoclonal antibody-based immuno-chemical methods to quantify FLCs.

Polyclonal antihuman FLC antisera are created by immunizing rabbits or sheep with a mix of Bence Jones proteins (BJPs) and then adsorbing the product with IgG or Cohn fraction II to remove antibodies that react with bound immunoglobulin LCs. The FLC antibodies must specifically recognize epitopes hidden in intact immunoglobulins to avoid false positives from cross-reaction. Ideally, these polyclonal antibodies target the constant domain of the LCs, which has minimal structural variation and have enough specificity and affinity to bind to individual monoclonal FLCs.

Monoclonal antibody-based FLC methods require antibodies that target the LC domains present in Cκ allotypes and Cλ isotypes on the FLCs and must have consistent immunoreactivity for all variable region (VL) subgroups. Enzyme-linked immunosorbent assay (ELISA)-based assays offer high sensitivity and can detect low concentrations of FLCs in serum. Additionally, automated ELISA platforms enable the simultaneous analysis of multiple serum sample dilutions, facilitating the detection of antigen excess, and nonlinear FLC immunoreactivity.[6-8]

Q5. How are plasma cells identified?

Ans: Plasma cells are the terminally differentiated nondividing B cells. They constitutively secrete antibodies at a high rate and persist in niches of the bone marrow, thus maintaining serum antibody levels constant.

The morphology ranges from mature-appearing PCs to immature, plasmablastic, and pleomorphic variants, including multinucleated and multilobated forms. Mature PCs are oval-shaped with an eccentric nucleus, spoke-wheel or clock-face chromatin, and no nucleolus. They feature abundant basophilic cytoplasm with a perinuclear hof.

In contrast, immature forms display more dispersed nuclear chromatin, a higher nuclear-to-cytoplasmic (N:C) ratio, and a prominent nucleolus. Because nuclear immaturity and pleomorphism are rarely seen in reactive PCs, they are reliable indicators of malignancy. MM cells have abundant endoplasmic reticulum, which may contain condensed or crystallized cytoplasmic immunoglobulin, resulting in various distinctive morphological features. These include multiple pale bluish-white, grape-like accumulations (Mott cells, morula cells), cherry-red refractile round bodies (refractile bodies), vermilion-staining glycogen-rich IgA (flame cells), overstuffed fibrils (Gaucher-like cells, thesaurocytes), and crystalline rods. However, these changes are not pathognomonic of MM.[9]

Q6. How is amyloid detected in a specimen? How is primary amyloid differentiated from secondary amyloid?

Ans: Amyloidosis is a rare disorder where insoluble amyloid proteins build up in organs, leading to dysfunction and death. Diagnosis typically requires a tissue biopsy to detect amyloid deposits, except for cardiac transthyretin amyloidosis, which can sometimes be diagnosed without a biopsy if strict criteria are met. Identifying the type of amyloid is crucial to avoid inappropriate treatment, particularly distinguishing non-AL amyloidosis from AL amyloidosis.

Histologically, amyloid appears as amorphous, eosinophilic deposits on hematoxylin and eosin (H&E)-stained sections and is confirmed with Congo red staining, showing red or salmon-pink deposits under light microscopy and apple-green birefringence under polarized light. Sections should be at least 5 μm thick to avoid missing deposits.

The amyloid subtype must be determined after detection. While clinical presentation or genetic testing can suggest the type, definitive diagnosis requires identifying the amyloid fibril protein. Methods include antibody-based techniques such as immunohistochemistry (IHC), immunofluorescence, immunoelectron microscopy, and mass spectrometry-based proteomic analysis. Laser capture microdissection of amyloid deposits followed by tandem mass spectrometry (LCM-MS), involving laser dissection and tandem mass spectrometry, is a recent and effective method for protein identification, detecting not only the fibrillogenic protein but also other constituent proteins, confirming the presence of amyloid.[10]

Differentiation of Primary and Secondary Amyloid

- *Clinical context and history:*
  - *Primary amyloidosis (AL amyloidosis):* Often associated with plasma cell disorders such as MM. Patients may have symptoms related to monoclonal gammopathy and organ involvement, like renal, cardiac, and neurological manifestations.
  - *Secondary amyloidosis (AA amyloidosis):* Typically associated with chronic inflammatory conditions such as rheumatoid arthritis, tuberculosis, or familial Mediterranean fever. The presence of a long-standing inflammatory or infectious condition is a key differentiator.

- *Protein typing:*
  - *AL amyloidosis:* Amyloid deposits are composed of LCs (either κ or λ). IHC and mass spectrometry can be used to identify these LCs.
  - *AA amyloidosis:* Amyloid deposits are composed of serum amyloid A (SAA) protein. This can be identified using specific antibodies against SAA protein in IHC or mass spectrometry.
- *Laboratory tests:*
  - *Serum and urine protein electrophoresis and immunofixation:* These tests can detect monoclonal proteins (M proteins) in blood and urine, which are indicative of AL amyloidosis.
  - *Serum amyloid A levels:* Elevated SAA levels in the blood are typically associated with AA amyloidosis and chronic inflammatory conditions.
- *Genetic testing:* In cases of hereditary amyloidosis, genetic testing can identify mutations in genes known to cause familial amyloid syndromes, helping to differentiate them from acquired forms of amyloidosis.[11]

Q7. What are the histological features of renal amyloidosis?

Ans: Amyloidosis can be localized or systemic and may impact any organ, with the kidneys being the most commonly affected in systemic cases. Over 25 amyloid precursor proteins have been identified, with the two most common types of renal amyloidosis being immunoglobulin-derived amyloidosis secondary to plasma cell dyscrasia, and reactive AA amyloidosis, associated with SAA from chronic inflammatory conditions. Renal amyloidosis should be considered in patients with proteinuria, with or without nephrotic syndrome, and especially If they exhibit other systemic symptoms such as heart failure, orthostatic hypotension, gastrointestinal issues, or neuropathy. A kidney biopsy is typically necessary for a definitive diagnosis.[12,13]

Characteristic histologic findings of renal amyloidosis on kidney biopsy include:
- *Light microscopy:* Reveals diffuse glomerular deposition of amorphous hyaline material that is Congo red-positive, initially in the mesangium and then along the capillary loops. These nodules stain weakly with periodic acid-Schiff and methenamine silver stain, indicating they are primarily composed of amyloid fibrils rather than extracellular matrix, as seen in diabetes mellitus. In some patients, amyloid is mainly deposited in the interstitium, along the tubular basement membranes, or in the small arteries and arterioles.
- *Immunofluorescence:* It is negative for immunoglobulins and complement in non-AL amyloidosis, but positive for λ or κ LCs in AL amyloidosis. The presence of only one LC type (λ or κ) confirms AL amyloidosis. When immunofluorescence results are equivocal, additional IHC is needed to identify other types of amyloid. The gold standard for amyloid typing is laser microdissection with mass spectrometry-based proteomic analysis.
- *Electron microscopy:* It shows straight, solid, and nonbranching fibrils that are randomly arranged and measure 8–12 nm in diameter, typically found in the mesangium and along the glomerular capillary walls. The fibril size differentiates renal amyloidosis from other kidney diseases with organized immunoglobulin deposits, such as fibrillary glomerulonephritis. While immunoelectron microscopy has a high diagnostic accuracy for typing amyloidosis, it is not widely available.

Q8. How is renal amyloidosis different from monoclonal gammopathy of renal significance?

Ans: Monoclonal gammopathy of renal significance (MGRS) is a plasma cell or B-cell neoplasm that does not meet the accepted criteria for malignancy or initiation of treatment but secretes a monoclonal immunoglobulin or immunoglobulin fragment resulting in kidney injury.[9]

The term MGRS was proposed in 2012 by the International Kidney and Monoclonal Gammopathy Research Group to collectively describe patients who would otherwise meet the criteria for MGUS but demonstrate kidney injury attributable to the underlying monoclonal protein.

Renal amyloidosis and MGRS are both conditions involving abnormal protein deposition in the kidneys, but they have distinct differences in their pathophysiology, clinical presentation, and management.[14,15]

Renal Amyloidosis

Pathophysiology
- Caused by the deposition of amyloid fibrils in the kidney.
- Amyloid fibrils are abnormal, misfolded proteins that form β-pleated sheet structures.
- The most common types affecting the kidneys are AL (LC) amyloidosis and AA (SAA) amyloidosis.

Etiology
- *AL amyloidosis:* Associated with plasma cell dyscrasias, like MM.
- *AA amyloidosis:* Secondary to chronic inflammatory conditions such as rheumatoid arthritis, chronic infections, or familial Mediterranean fever.

Clinical Presentation
- Proteinuria, often in the nephrotic range.
- Progressive renal dysfunction.
- May present with symptoms of the underlying disease (e.g., MM in AL amyloidosis).

Diagnosis
- Renal biopsy showing apple-green birefringence under polarized light after staining with Congo red.
- Immunohistochemistry or mass spectrometry to identify the type of amyloid protein.

Treatment
- Targeting the underlying disease (e.g., chemotherapy for plasma cell dyscrasia in AL amyloidosis).
- Supportive care for renal dysfunction (e.g., dialysis).

Monoclonal Gammopathy of Renal Significance

Pathophysiology
- A spectrum of kidney disorders caused by a monoclonal immunoglobulin produced by a nonmalignant or indolent B-cell clone.
- The monoclonal protein can cause kidney damage through various mechanisms, such as forming immune complexes or directly depositing in kidney tissues.

Etiology
Associated with a variety of plasma cell or B-cell disorders, such as MGUS, indolent lymphomas, or smoldering myeloma.

Clinical Presentation
- Proteinuria, hematuria, and varying degrees of renal dysfunction.
- Can present with different histopathologic patterns, such as monoclonal immunoglobulin deposition disease (MIDD), light chain proximal tubulopathy (LCPT), or C3 glomerulopathy.

Diagnosis
- Detection of a monoclonal protein in serum or urine by electrophoresis and immunofixation.
- Renal biopsy with immunofluorescence and electron microscopy to identify specific patterns of monoclonal protein deposition.

Treatment
- Targeting the underlying monoclonal B-cell clone with therapies similar to those used for plasma cell dyscrasias but adjusted to the specific condition and patient's renal function.
- Supportive care for renal dysfunction.

Key Differences
- *Nature of deposits:*
  - *Renal amyloidosis:* Amyloid fibrils.
  - *MGRS:* Monoclonal immunoglobulins or their fragments.
- *Pathophysiological mechanism:*
  - *Renal amyloidosis:* Misfolded proteins forming amyloid fibrils.
  - *MGRS:* Various mechanisms, including direct deposition of immunoglobulins, immune complex formation, or complement activation.
- *Associated conditions:*
  - *Renal amyloidosis:* Often linked to plasma cell dyscrasias or chronic inflammatory diseases.
  - *MGRS:* Associated with a broader range of monoclonal gammopathies, including MGUS and indolent B-cell disorders.
- *Histopathology:*
  - *Renal amyloidosis:* Characteristic Congo red-positive amyloid deposits.
  - *MGRS:* Diverse histopathologic patterns depending on the type of monoclonal protein and mechanism of kidney injury.

Q9. **What is the role of CD138, CD56, and light chain immunohistochemistry in the diagnosis of myeloma?**

Ans: Plasma cells are mature, antibody-secreting B-cells that can increase in the bone marrow in both reactive and neoplastic conditions. Numerous malignant PC disorders exist and are further classified into plasmacytoma, MGUS, asymptomatic PC myeloma (PCM), symptomatic myeloma, and primary amyloidosis. Accurate enumeration of PCs is crucial for diagnosing these disorders and distinguishing them from each other. Typically, a threshold of 10% clonal PCs is used to differentiate MGUS from both symptomatic and asymptomatic PCM.

The method used to count PCs on well-stained bone marrow aspirate smears might not provide an accurate count, often showing fewer PCs compared to a bone marrow biopsy due to several reasons: (i) Marrow involvement might be focal and not present at the aspirate site; (ii) PCs express various adhesion molecules such as CD138 and CD56, causing them to adhere to one another and the marrow stroma; (iii) PCs' lipophilic nature can cause them to stick in marrow particles; (iv) Bone marrow aspirate samples are prone to hemodilution. Therefore, evaluating bone marrow biopsy is essential in myeloma diagnosis.

In H&E stained marrow biopsy sections, small foci of PCs may be missed, leading to an underestimation of PC percentage. IHC on bone marrow biopsy is superior for identifying PCs, with Syndecan-1/CD138 expression specifically marking polyclonal and clonal PCs. Using CD138 in combination with κ and λ LCs aids in differentiating reactive from clonal PCs.

The use of CD138, CD56, and LC IHC is crucial in the diagnosis and evaluation of MM. These markers help identify and characterize PCs, assess the clonality of PCs, and distinguish myeloma from other plasma cell disorders.[16-18]

Role of CD138 (Syndecan-1)

- *Identification of PCs:* CD138 is a transmembrane heparan sulfate proteoglycan expressed on the surface of PCs. It is a reliable marker for identifying normal and malignant PCs in tissue biopsies and bone marrow aspirates.
- *Tumor burden assessment:* CD138 staining helps in quantifying the plasma cell burden in bone marrow, which is important for the diagnosis and staging of MM.
- *Sample preparation:* CD138 can also be used to isolate PCs for further genetic and molecular studies, improving the accuracy of myeloma diagnostics.
- CD138 is also used as a target of CAR T cells in MM.

Role of CD56 (Neural Cell Adhesion Molecule)

- *Differentiation marker:* CD56 is expressed in a subset of PCs in MM. Its presence helps to differentiate malignant PCs from normal PCs and other hematologic malignancies.
- *Prognostic marker:* CD56 expression is often associated with a more aggressive disease course in MM. Its absence can be a marker of extramedullary disease and is linked to poor prognosis.
- *Diagnostic utility:* CD56 is not expressed in normal PCs, and its detection on PCs supports the diagnosis of MM.

Role of Light Chain Immunohistochemistry (κ and λ Light Chains)

- *Clonality assessment:* LC IHC helps determine the clonality of PCs by assessing the expression of κ and λ LCs. In MM, there is typically a monoclonal population of PCs expressing either κ or λ LCs.
- *Diagnosis of MM:* The presence of a monoclonal LC population (i.e., either κ or λ, but not both) supports the diagnosis of MM or other monoclonal gammopathies.
- *Detection of LC restriction:* LC restriction (overrepresentation of one type of LC) in PCs indicates a clonal process, distinguishing MM from reactive plasmacytosis (which shows a polyclonal pattern).

Summary

- *CD138:* Identifies and quantifies PCs.
- *CD56:* Differentiates malignant PCs and provides prognostic information.
- *Light chains (κ and λ):* Assesses clonality to confirm monoclonal plasma cell populations.

Together, these markers are essential in diagnosing MM, differentiating it from other plasma cell disorders, and providing prognostic information to guide treatment decisions.

REFERENCES

1. Vavricka SR, Burri E, Beglinger C, Degen L, Manz M. Serum protein electrophoresis: an underused but instrumental test. Digestion. 2009;79(4):203-10.
2. Sheffield H, Jeon-Slaughter H, Chowattukunnel N, Haque W, Lim M. Optimizing the utility of serum protein electrophoresis. J Cli Med Dia Res. 2024;2(1):01-6.
3. Csako G. Immunofixation Electrophoresis for Identification of Proteins and Specific Antibodies. In: Kurien B, Scofield R (Eds). Electrophoretic Separation of Proteins. Methods in Molecular Biology, Volume 1855. New York, NY: Humana Press; 2019.
4. Ríos-Tamayo R, Paiva B, Lahuerta JJ, López JM, Duarte RF. Monoclonal gammopathies of clinical significance: A critical appraisal. Cancers (Basel). 2022;14(21):5247.
5. Bird J, Behrens J, Westin J, Turesson I, Drayson M, Beetham R, et al. UK Myeloma Forum (UKMF) and Nordic Myeloma Study Group (NMSG): guidelines for the investigation of newly detected M-proteins and the management of monoclonal gammopathy of undetermined significance (MGUS). Br J haematol. 2009:147(1):22-42.
6. Tate J, Bazeley S, Sykes S, Mollee P. Quantitative serum free light chain assay-analytical issues. Clin Biochem Rev. 2009;30(3):131-40.
7. Tosi P, Tomassetti S, Merli A, Polli V. Serum free light-chain assay for the detection and monitoring of multiple myeloma and related conditions. Ther Adv Hematol. 2013;4(1):37-41.
8. Rajkumar SV, Dimopoulos MA, Palumbo A, Blade J, Merlini G, Mateos MV, et al. International Myeloma Working Group updated criteria for the diagnosis of multiple myeloma. Lancet Oncol. 2014;15(12):e538-48.
9. WHO Classification of Tumours Editorial Board. Haematolymphoid tumours. WHO Classification of tumours series, 5th edition; volume 11. Lyon (France): International Agency for Research on Cancer; 2024.
10. Wisniowski B, Wechalekar A. Confirming the diagnosis of amyloidosis. Acta Haematol. 2020;143(4):312-21.
11. Picken MM. The pathology of amyloidosis in classification: A review. Acta Haematol. 2020;143(4):322-34.
12. Said SM, Sethi S, Valeri AM, Leung N, Cornell LD, Fidler ME, et al. Renal Amyloidosis: Origin and Clinicopathologic Correlations of 474 Recent Cases. Clin J Am Soc Nephrol. 2013;8(9):1515-23.
13. von Hutten H, Mihatsch M, Lobeck H, Rudolph B, Eriksson M, Röcken C. Prevalence and origin of amyloid in kidney biopsies. Am J Surg Pathol. 2009;33(8):1198-205.
14. Leung N., Bridoux F, Batuman V, Chaidos A, Cockwell P, D'Agati VD, et al. The evaluation of monoclonal gammopathy of renal significance: a consensus report of the International Kidney and Monoclonal Gammopathy Research Group. Nat Rev Nephrol. 2019;15(1):45-59.
15. Vaxman I, Dispenzieri A, Muchtar E, Gertz M. New developments in diagnosis, risk assessment and management in systemic amyloidosis. Blood Rev. 2020;40:100636.
16. Riccardi F, Tangredi C, Dal Bo M, Toffoli G. Targeted therapy for multiple myeloma: an overview on CD138-based strategies. Front Oncol. 2024;14:1370854.
17. Rawstron AC, Orfao A, Beksac M, Bezdickova L, Brooimans RA, Bumbea H, et al. Report of the European Myeloma Network on multiparametric flow cytometry in multiple myeloma and related disorders. Haematologica. 2008;93(3):431-8.
18. Kumar SK, Callander NS, Adekola K, Anderson L, Baljevic M, Campagnaro E, et al. Multiple myeloma, version 3.2021, NCCN clinical practice guidelines in oncology. J Natl Compr Canc Netw. 2020;18(12):1685-717.

27

Light Chain Myeloma

Gurleen Oberoi

Q1. What are Bence Jones proteins? What are its characteristic features?

Ans: Bence Jones proteins are free light chains (FLCs) of immunoglobulins found in the urine. They are associated with multiple myeloma and other plasma cell disorders. These proteins are produced by malignant plasma cells and can be identified through specific diagnostic tests. Bence Jones protein was first described in 1845 in a patient admitted to St. George's Hospital in London with vague continuous pain in the chest, back, and pelvis. Dr Henry Bence Jones tested the patient's urine and found a substance precipitated by adding nitric acid. The term Bence Jones protein was coined by Dr Fleischer in 1880.[1] At least 60% of patients with classical myeloma have Bence Jones protein in their urine. More importantly, 20% of patients with multiple myeloma produce only Bence Jones proteins without heavy chains.[2]

Key characteristics of Bence Jones protein are:
- *Composition:* Bence Jones proteins represent a homogeneous population of kappa (κ) or lambda (λ)-type light chains produced in excess in conditions like multiple myeloma. They lack the heavy chains found in whole immunoglobulins.[3]
- *Urine detection:* These proteins are small enough to pass through the kidneys and be excreted in the urine. Their presence is indicative of certain plasma cell disorders.[4]
- *Heat solubility:* Bence Jones proteins are notable for their heat solubility. When urine containing these proteins is heated to 50–60°C, the proteins become soluble. Upon cooling, they precipitate out. This property is used diagnostically.[5]
- *Clinical significance:* Testing for Bence Jones proteinuria is indicated when plasma cell disorders such as multiple myeloma are suspected and warrants referral to hematology clinic. The presence of these proteins in the urine can aid in confirming the diagnosis and assessing the disease's progression, severity, and treatment response. Monitoring these proteins over time helps assess treatment efficacy and detect disease relapse.[6] With the availability of better tests such as serum and urine FLC assays (κ and λ) the utility of Bence Jones proteinuria has reduced.

Q2. What is Bence Jones protein test?

Ans: Test for Bence Jones proteins is done by conventional high-resolution electrophoresis or capillary zone electrophoresis followed by confirmation through immunofixation electrophoresis (IFE) (preferable) or immunoelectrophoresis.

Urine sample collection: A 24-hour urine sample is collected. This method is preferred to capture a representative quantity of urine proteins over a full day, increasing the likelihood of detecting Bence Jones proteins if present.[4]

Techniques

- *Urine protein electrophoresis:* Proteins in urine is separated based on their size and charge. Bence Jones proteins are small with low molecular weight, usually identified in the β and γ regions of the electrophoretic pattern.[4]
- *Immunofixation electrophoresis:* This method provides more specific identification by using antibodies to detect and quantify light chains. It can differentiate between κ and λ light chains, which is essential for accurate diagnosis.[7]
- *Heat precipitation test:* Historically, Bence Jones proteins were identified by heating the urine sample to 50–60°C (122–140°F). Proteins in the urine that are Bence Jones proteins will become soluble at these temperatures and precipitate out upon cooling. This test takes advantage of their unique thermal properties.[6]
- *Quantitative analysis:* The concentration of Bence Jones proteins can be measured using various immunoassays, which helps in monitoring disease activity and therapeutic response. Quantitative testing provides a more accurate assessment of proteinuria related to plasma cell disorders.[8]

Q3. What are the immunoassays for free light chains? Compare various serum free light chain (sFLC) assays?

Ans: The Freelite assay can accurately detect and quantify both κ and λ FLC through polyclonal antibodies recognizing a variety of FLC epitopes. The ratio of κ/λ FLC is a sensitive marker of monoclonality, which is key to the clinical utility of the assay. It is well established for aiding in the diagnosis, prognosis, and monitoring of plasma cell proliferative disorders.

Immunoassays for Free Light Chains

Enzyme-linked Immunosorbent Assay

Enzyme-linked immunosorbent assay (ELISA) is a common method used to quantify FLCs in serum and urine for diagnosis and monitoring of multiple myeloma and light chain amyloidosis. This assay uses antibodies specific to either κ or λ light chains that are attached to a solid phase (e.g., microplate). After binding of FLCs from the sample, a secondary enzyme-linked antibody is added, which binds to the FLCs. A substrate is then added that reacts with the enzyme to produce a measurable signal, typically a color change.

Immunoturbidimetry

Immunoturbidimetry provides a reliable assessment of light chain levels and assisting in the diagnosis and management of plasma cell disorders involves the use of antibodies specific to κ or λ light chains that, when mixed with a patient sample, form immune complexes. These complexes cause a decrease in the intensity of transmitted light through the sample, which is measured as a change in turbidity.[9]

Mass Spectrometry-based Assays

- Advanced mass spectrometry techniques can accurately measure the concentration of FLCs and provide information about their molecular weights and structures. This

high-resolution method helps differentiate between FLCs and bound light chains, offering precise quantification and characterization.[10]
- *Application:* Although less commonly used than ELISA and immunoturbidimetry, mass spectrometry provides highly detailed information and is used in specialized laboratories for research and detailed clinical diagnostics.[8]

Comparison of Various Free Light Chain Assays

- *FreeLite™ assay:* Utilizes nephelometric technology to quantify free κ and λ light chains. It measures light scatter caused by the antigen-antibody complexes formed between the light chains and specific antibodies. It is most widely used, provides reliable results, and is validated for routine clinical use. It is effective for diagnosing and monitoring multiple myeloma and other plasma cell disorders.
- *N-latex FLC assay:* Employs nephelometric technology using latex particles coated with antibodies specific to κ and λ light chains. The assay measures the change in light scattering caused by the formation of immune complexes. It may be influenced by sample interference and requires specific instrumentation.
- *Seralite™ FLC assay:* Uses a proprietary immunoassay technology for the quantification of free κ and λ light chains. It combines capture antibodies with detection methods to measure light chains in serum or urine. It provides good sensitivity and specificity as well as is easy to use and integrate into clinical practices. Widespread availability and standardization can be an issue.
- *Sebia FLC assay:* Combines immunofixation with electrophoresis to separate and quantify FLCs. This method separates proteins by size and charge before detection with specific antibodies. It provides detailed information about light chain types and quantities, useful for identifying and characterizing monoclonal gammopathies, however, it is more complex and time-consuming than nephelometric assays. Requires specialized equipment and expertise.[11]

Comparison between the various FLC assays showed significant absolute differences in FLC concentrations in individual patients, particularly at higher FLC concentrations. Studies have demonstrated that up to 10-fold differences in sFLC concentration between the sFLC assays in individual sera can be observed. An international reference method for sFLC quantification is not available, it is challenging to assess which of the four sFLC assays is most accurate. Overall, it can be concluded that the involved FLC (iFLC) concentrations measured by the sFLC assays were significantly higher compared to serum protein electrophoresis (SPEP) in a vast majority of the samples. The absolute differences in iFLC concentration between SPEP and the sFLC assays were highest for Freelite. Mass spectrometry methods appear to be promising in overcoming the analytical problems of immunoassays and have the potential to improve both diagnostic accuracy and sensitivity. As such mass spectrometry could in the future be a potential candidate as FLC reference method.[12,13]

Q4. Which instruments are used for measuring FLCs?

Ans: Serum FLC assays are used to measure FLCs in the blood, and they are particularly important for diagnosing and monitoring diseases such as multiple myeloma and light chain amyloidosis. Several instruments and platforms are available for measuring FLCs, each with its own methodology **(Table 1)**.

TABLE 1: Advantages and limitations of instrument for serum free light chain (FLC) assays.

Instrument type	Principle	Advantages	Limitations
Nephelometers	Measures light scattered by immune complexes	High sensitivity, rapid results, standardized methods	Interference, cost, complex calibration
Turbidimeters	Measures turbidity from light scattering	Sensitive detection, ease of use	Interference, limited versatility
Immunoassay platforms	Uses antibodies to produce detectable signals	Versatility, high specificity, integration	Cross-reactivity, variability, cost
Mass spectrometry	Measures mass-to-charge ratio of ions	High specificity and sensitivity, quantitative analysis	Complexity, cost, time-consuming
Chemiluminescent assays	Uses light emission from chemical reactions	High sensitivity, automation, rapid results	Background noise, cost, interference

Nephelometers

Principle

Nephelometry measures the scattered light produced when light interacts with particles (such as immune complexes) in a solution. In the context of FLC assays, a specific antibody is used to bind to the FLCs, forming immune complexes that scatter light. The amount of scattered light is proportional to the concentration of FLCs in the sample.[12,13]

Advantages

- *High sensitivity:* Capable of detecting low concentrations of FLCs.
- *Rapid results:* Provides quick results, beneficial for clinical decision-making.
- *Standardized protocols:* Established methods and protocols ensure consistency across laboratories.

Limitations

- *Interference:* Presence of other proteins or substances in the serum can cause false positives or negatives.
- *Cost:* High initial investment and maintenance costs.
- *Complex calibration:* Requires regular calibration and maintenance for accurate results.

Example of Instruments

- Beckman Coulter Immage 800
- Siemens BN II

Turbidimeters

Principle

Turbidimetry measures the turbidity (cloudiness) of a sample, which occurs when light is scattered by particles in the solution. In FLC assays, light scattering is caused by the formation of immune complexes between FLCs and specific antibodies. The degree of turbidity is used to determine the concentration of FLCs.

Advantages

- *Sensitive detection:* Effective at detecting low levels of FLCs.
- *Ease of use:* Generally straightforward operation and maintenance.

Limitations
- *Interference:* Turbidity from other serum components can affect measurement accuracy.
- *Limited versatility:* Less commonly used compared to nephelometry.

Example of Instruments
- Thermo Scientific™ Cascadion™

Immunoassay Platforms
Principle
Immunoassays use antibodies that specifically bind to the target FLCs. There are different types of immunoassays, such as ELISA and chemiluminescent immunoassays (CLIA). In these assays, the FLCs are detected by their binding to antibodies, and a detectable signal (color change in ELISA or light emission in CLIA is produced that correlates with the concentration of FLCs.[9]

Advantages
- *Versatility:* Can be adapted for various target proteins and conditions.
- *High specificity:* Specific antibodies ensure accurate detection of FLCs.
- *Integration:* Can be part of automated testing systems.

Limitations
- *Cross-reactivity:* Potential for cross-reactivity with other proteins or antibodies.
- *Variability:* Results may vary based on the assay and platform used.
- *Cost:* High cost of instruments and reagents.

Example of Instruments
- Freelite™ by the binding site
- Roche Cobas® 6000

Mass Spectrometry
Principle
Mass spectrometry measures the mass-to-charge ratio of ions. In the context of FLC assays, proteins are ionized, and then sorted by their mass-to-charge ratio. The resulting data provides detailed information about the molecular weight and structure of the FLCs, allowing for precise quantification and identification.

Advantages
- *High specificity and sensitivity:* Capable of providing detailed molecular information and precise quantification.
- *Quantitative analysis:* Offers exact measurements and structural details of proteins.

Limitations
- *Complexity:* Requires specialized knowledge and complex sample preparation.
- *Cost:* High initial investment and ongoing operational costs.
- *Time-consuming:* Generally, longer processing times compared to other methods.

Example of Instruments
- Agilent 6495B triple quadrupole LC/MS

Chemiluminescent Immunoassays

Principle
Chemiluminescence involves a chemical reaction that emits light when FLCs bind to specific antibodies. The emitted light is measured and correlated with the concentration of FLCs in the sample. This method can use various chemiluminescent substrates that react with the detection antibody to produce light.

Advantages
- *High sensitivity:* Capable of detecting very low concentrations of FLCs.
- *Automation:* Often integrated into high-throughput automated systems.
- *Rapid results:* Provides fast results, enhancing clinical efficiency.

Limitations
- *Background noise:* Light emission can be affected by background noise or interference.
- *Cost:* Instruments and reagents can be expensive.
- *Interference:* Other substances in the serum can impact the accuracy of the results.

Example of Instruments
Siemens Immulite® 2000

Q5. What are the normal serum half-lives of immunoglobulin G and free light chains?

Ans: The normal serum half-lives of immunoglobulin G (IgG) and FLCs are important for understanding their behavior in the body, especially in the context of plasma cell disorders and other conditions.
- *Immunoglobulin G:* The serum half-life of IgG is approximately 21–23 days. This relatively long half-life is due to its ability to bind to the neonatal Fc receptor (FcR) in the endothelial cells, which protects it from degradation and extends its duration in the bloodstream.[14] The long half-life of IgG is beneficial for providing prolonged immunity and is a key factor in the use of IgG-based therapies and monitoring of conditions affecting IgG levels.[9]
- *Free light chains:* The serum half-life of FLCs is considerably shorter than that of IgG, approximately 2–4 hours. This short half-life is due to their rapid filtration and metabolism by the kidneys.[15] The short half-life of FLCs makes them useful for monitoring changes in plasma cell disorders, as their levels can fluctuate more quickly compared to longer-lived immunoglobulins.[9]

Q6. What is the role of urine protein electrophoresis?

Ans: Urine protein electrophoresis (UPEP) is a diagnostic test used to analyze and separate proteins in urine based on their size, charge, and other properties. This test plays a significant role in diagnosing and monitoring various conditions, including kidney disorders, monoclonal gammopathies, and multiple myeloma. Up to 20% of multiple myeloma patients present with light-chain-only multiple myeloma (LCMM), which is not detectable using SPEP testing. 24-hour urinalysis may be the guideline-endorsed method for monitoring LCMM, but impracticalities can limit its use.

Role of Urine Protein Electrophoresis

Diagnosis of Proteinuria

Urine protein electrophoresis separates urinary proteins into different fractions, such as albumin, α-1 globulins, α-2 globulins, β-globulins, and γ-globulins. This separation helps in identifying abnormal protein patterns that may indicate various plasma cell disorders and renal disorders, such as nephrotic syndrome, glomerulonephritis, or tubular disorders. For example, a predominance of low-molecular-weight proteins like β-2 microglobulin or light chains can suggest damage to the renal tubules.[16]

- *Detection of monoclonal proteins (Bence Jones proteins):* In conditions like multiple myeloma or other monoclonal gammopathies, UPEP can detect monoclonal light chains (Bence Jones proteins) that are produced in excess. These proteins are not typically present in normal urine and are indicative of plasma cell dyscrasia.[3,4]
- *Monitoring disease progression and treatment response:* UPEP is used to monitor the progression of diseases and the effectiveness of treatment. In patients with multiple myeloma, regular UPEP can track changes in the level of Bence Jones proteins or other abnormal proteins, providing insights into the response to therapy.[17] By comparing electrophoresis patterns over time, clinicians can assess whether treatment is effectively reducing the abnormal protein levels or if the disease is relapsing.[9]
- *Differentiation of protein types*
  - *Description:* The test helps in differentiating between different types of proteins and identifying specific abnormal proteins. This can aid in distinguishing between different types of kidney diseases and guiding further diagnostic or therapeutic interventions.
  - *Application:* For instance, distinguishing between albuminuria (high levels of albumin) and light chain proteinuria (presence of Bence Jones proteins) helps in diagnosing the specific underlying condition affecting the kidneys.

The 24-hour urine tests for UPEP are not used often in routine clinical practice.

Performing UPEP in addition to sFLC regularly may be the ideal practice for monitoring LCMM, impracticalities such as issues with collection technique and proper storage of urine samples may be hindering its regular use in the real world. The sFLC test may present a more realistic alternative for evaluation of disease status in patients with LCMM, and its ease of use could facilitate more frequent serial testing. This in turn could improve the measurement of progression at more regular intervals, potentially reducing patient exposure to therapies that are no longer effective. A number of studies have assessed the use of sFLC analysis in the detection of plasma cell disorders. Most studies have found that sFLC testing has superior diagnostic sensitivity to UPEP for detecting plasma cell dyscrasias, particularly AL amyloidosis, light chain deposition disease (LCDD), and nonsecretory multiple myeloma.[16]

Q7. What is the correlation between serum and urine concentrations of monoclonal FLCs?

Ans: The correlation between serum and urine concentrations of monoclonal FLCs is significant in the diagnosis and monitoring of plasma cell disorders, such as multiple myeloma.

Correlation between Serum and Urine Concentrations of Monoclonal FLCs

In multiple myeloma and related disorders, plasma cells produce an excess of monoclonal light chains, which can be either κ or λ. These light chains can be detected in both serum and urine.[3]

- *Serum levels:* Monoclonal FLCs are usually present at elevated levels in the serum due to their overproduction. However, the serum concentration of FLCs can be influenced by factors such as renal function, as the kidneys filter these light chains from the bloodstream.[15]
- *Urine levels:* Urine concentrations of FLCs, particularly Bence Jones proteins, are often used for diagnostic purposes. In patients with normal renal function, high levels of monoclonal light chains in the serum typically correlate with high levels in the urine. However, in patients with renal impairment, urine levels may not always correlate well with serum levels due to impaired filtration and excretion.[17]

Clinical Significance

- *Diagnostic utility*: The correlation between serum and urine FLC concentrations is used to confirm the presence of monoclonal gammopathy and to differentiate between different types of light chains. A high serum concentration of FLCs coupled with detectable urine levels can support a diagnosis of multiple myeloma.[17]
- *Monitoring disease progression*: Tracking both serum and urine FLC levels provides insight into the effectiveness of treatment and disease progression. An increase in serum FLC levels with corresponding changes in urine levels can indicate disease progression or relapse.[15]
- *Renal function impact*: In patients with renal impairment, the correlation between serum and urine FLC levels may be less straightforward. Decreased renal function can lead to reduced excretion of FLCs, resulting in higher serum levels and lower or normal urine levels, even if the disease activity is high.[9]

Q8. Why is ratio of serum free light chains considered more appropriate? Is it a better modality than difference in free light chain concentration?

Ans:

Differentiation between Monoclonal and Polyclonal Production

- *Ratio of FLCs:* The ratio of κ-to-λ light chains in the serum is used to distinguish between monoclonal (pathological) and polyclonal (normal) production of light chains. In multiple myeloma and other monoclonal gammopathies, the ratio is typically skewed due to the excessive production of one type of light chain (κ or λ) by malignant plasma cells.[6] A significantly abnormal κ-to-λ ratio can indicate a monoclonal gammopathy, whereas a normal ratio, despite the presence of elevated light chain levels, may suggest a polyclonal increase due to inflammation or other conditions.[15]
- *Diagnostic specificity: Ratio versus difference*—measuring the ratio of κ-to-λ FLCs provides a more specific diagnostic tool compared to the difference in their concentrations. The ratio helps identify whether the light chain abnormality is due to a single clone of plasma cells producing excessive light chains or due to other conditions where both types of light chains are increased but remain in balance.[6]

Example: In a patient with multiple myeloma, the κ-to-λ ratio might be markedly abnormal (e.g., >100 or <0.01), reflecting the predominance of one type of light chain. In contrast, a difference in FLC concentrations alone might not differentiate between monoclonal and polyclonal increases effectively.[17]

Monitoring and Prognosis

- *Treatment response:* The FLC ratio is valuable in monitoring disease progression and response to treatment. A normalization of the κ-to-λ ratio often indicates a favorable response to therapy, whereas persistent abnormalities may suggest ongoing disease activity or relapse.[9]
- *Prognostic value:* The FLC ratio provides prognostic information, with certain ratios correlating with disease severity and prognosis. For example, a very high or very low ratio might be associated with more aggressive disease or poorer prognosis.[8]

Comparison with Difference in Free Light Chain Concentrations

- *Sensitivity to renal function:* The ratio is less affected by changes in renal function compared to the absolute concentrations of FLCs. Renal impairment can alter the serum concentrations of FLCs, making the ratio a more reliable indicator of disease status.[15]
- *Standardization:* The ratio is a standardized measure that allows for more consistent interpretation across different laboratories and patients, whereas differences in concentrations can be influenced by various factors, including assay methodologies and individual patient variability.[9]

Q9. How are serum free light chains useful for monitoring myeloma? Do sFLCs have independent predictive power for outcome irrespective of heavy chains?

Ans: Serum FLCs are increasingly recognized as a valuable tool for monitoring multiple myeloma. Utility of sFLCs in monitoring multiple myeloma are:

Early Detection of Disease Progression and Relapse

- *Sensitivity to disease activity:* sFLCs are sensitive markers of disease activity in multiple myeloma. Elevated levels of sFLCs can reflect active disease and are useful in detecting relapse earlier than other markers, such as SPEP or imaging.[3]
- *Monitoring trends:* Regular measurement of sFLCs allows for monitoring trends in disease activity over time. A rise in sFLC levels may indicate disease progression or relapse, even before clinical symptoms or other diagnostic tests show changes.[15]

Assessment of Treatment Response

- *Early indicator of response:* sFLC levels often normalize more quickly than other markers of disease, such as heavy chain immunoglobulin levels or bone marrow involvement. This rapid response can be used to gauge the effectiveness of therapy, including chemotherapy, immunotherapy, or targeted treatments.[3]
- *Quantitative monitoring:* The absolute levels and ratios of sFLCs (κ-to-λ ratio) provide quantifiable data that helps in evaluating how well the disease is controlled. A decrease in the abnormal sFLC ratio and levels generally indicates a positive response to treatment.[6]

Prognostic Value

- High sFLC levels at diagnosis or persistently high levels despite treatment are associated with a poorer prognosis. Studies have shown that elevated sFLC levels can independently predict outcomes and overall survival, providing prognostic information beyond what is available from heavy chain measurements alone.[8]
- Elevated sFLC levels often correlate with tumor burden and disease severity. Thus, changes in sFLC levels can reflect variations in disease burden and help tailor individual patient management strategies.[15]
- *Independent predictive power of sFLCs:* Research has demonstrated that sFLCs have independent predictive power for patient outcomes, irrespective of heavy chain status. For example, elevated sFLC levels and an abnormal κ-to-λ ratio are strong predictors of adverse outcomes, even when heavy chain levels are not significantly abnormal.[9]
- *Clinical implications:* This independent predictive power is particularly useful in cases where heavy chain measurements may not fully capture disease activity or in patients with nonsecretory myeloma, where heavy chains may be undetectable or not informative.[7]

CASE STUDY

A 56-year-old male patient presented with bone pain, fatigue, and anemia. Laboratory tests revealed elevated serum calcium, renal impairment, and a monoclonal spike in SPEP suggesting a monoclonal gammopathy. A bone marrow biopsy confirmed multiple myeloma.

Ans:

Initial Diagnostic Workup

- *Serum FLCs:* Initial sFLC measurements showed a high serum κ light chain concentration of 400 mg/L and a λ light chain concentration of 10 mg/L. The κ-to-λ ratio was 40:1 (normal range is 0.26–1.65).
- *Heavy chains:* The initial heavy chain immunoglobulin levels were also elevated, consistent with the multiple myeloma diagnosis.

Treatment and Monitoring

- *Initial treatment:* He was started on a regimen including bortezomib, lenalidomide, and dexamethasone.
- *Follow-up testing:* Regular follow-up involved monitoring sFLCs, SPEP, and heavy chain levels.

Monitoring with Serum Free Light Chains

- *Early response to treatment:* After one cycle of treatment, Mr Smith's sFLCs showed a significant decrease. Kappa light chains dropped to 150 mg/L, λ light chains remained stable at 10 mg/L, and the κ-to-λ ratio decreased to 15:1. This early reduction in sFLCs suggested an initial positive response to the treatment.
- *Assessment of disease progression:* Despite a decrease in sFLCs, his sFLC ratio remained elevated. He reported new symptoms of bone pain, and imaging revealed a progression of bone lesions. Follow-up tests showed that while the sFLC levels decreased, the ratio remained abnormal, indicating persistent disease activity despite treatment.

- *Treatment adjustment:* Treatment was adjusted based on the continued elevation of the sFLC ratio and progression symptoms. New therapy options were introduced, and sFLC monitoring was intensified.
- *Long-term monitoring:* After adjusting the treatment regimen, his κ light chain concentration normalized to 25 mg/L, λ light chain levels remained at 10 mg/L, and the κ-to-λ ratio normalized to 2:1. This significant improvement in the ratio indicated a favorable response to the new treatment.

Analysis of Serum Free Light Chains and Prognostic Power

- *Early detection of disease progression:* The persistent elevation of the κ-to-λ ratio despite an initial drop in sFLC concentrations helped identify that the disease was not adequately controlled. This allowed for timely intervention before more severe complications arose.[17]
- *Predictive power independent of heavy chains:* Throughout Mr Smith's treatment, the sFLC ratio provided valuable information beyond what was obtained from heavy chain measurements. For instance, at times when heavy chain levels were not markedly abnormal, the sFLC ratio continued to reflect the underlying disease activity, indicating its independent prognostic value.[3]
- *Adjustment of treatment:* The sFLC measurements allowed for adjustments to Mr Smith's treatment plan. By focusing on the κ-to-λ ratio, clinicians could make informed decisions about the efficacy of the therapy and whether a change in treatment was needed.[6]

In this case study, the use of sFLCs provided critical insights into the patient's disease activity, response to treatment, and prognosis. The κ-to-λ ratio was particularly useful for early detection of disease progression and for making informed treatment decisions. The independent predictive power of sFLCs, regardless of heavy chain measurements, highlighted their importance in managing multiple myeloma effectively.

Q10. Why are serum free light chain measurements used as an early marker of relapse in multiple myeloma?

Ans: Serum FLC measurements are used as an early marker of relapse in multiple myeloma due to their sensitivity to changes in disease activity and their ability to detect disease progression before other clinical signs become apparent.

Reasons why sFLC measurements are used as early markers of relapse:
- *Sensitivity to disease activity:*
  - *Early detection of relapse:* sFLC levels can change rapidly in response to disease activity. Unlike other markers that might reflect more stable aspects of disease, sFLCs can increase quickly when the disease becomes active again. This makes them sensitive indicators of early relapse.[3]
  - *High turnover rate:* Monoclonal light chains produced by plasma cells are released into the bloodstream and filtered by the kidneys. Elevated sFLCs can occur with minimal increases in disease burden, thus providing an early signal of relapse even when other tests, such as SPEP or imaging studies, may not yet show significant changes.[15]
- *Prognostic value and predictive power:*
  - The κ-to-λ ratio is particularly useful in detecting relapse. An abnormal ratio often reflects an imbalance in the production of light chains due to the predominance of malignant plasma cells. A deviation from the previously normal ratio can signal disease recurrence.[17]

- *Independent predictor:* Studies have shown that changes in sFLC levels and ratios are independent predictors of relapse and progression, providing prognostic information beyond what is available from other tests. This predictive power is useful for identifying patients at risk of relapse even before symptomatic or imaging-based evidence emerges.[6]
- *Rapid response to treatment changes:*
  - *Monitoring treatment response:* sFLC levels typically decrease more rapidly in response to effective treatment compared to other markers. Conversely, if sFLC levels begin to rise, it may indicate that the treatment is no longer effective or that the disease is relapsing. This rapid feedback allows for timely adjustments in therapy.[8]
  - *Example case:* In multiple myeloma patients, a rise in sFLC levels before clinical symptoms or increases in other markers can prompt early intervention. For instance, if a patient's κ-to-λ ratio begins to deviate from the baseline, it may indicate emerging disease activity even if the patient remains asymptomatic.[9]

Q11. **What are the limitations of serum free light chain analysis?**

Ans: Serum FLC analysis is a valuable tool for diagnosing and monitoring multiple myeloma and other plasma cell dyscrasias. Primary limitations of sFLC analysis include:

- *Variability in reference ranges:* There is a significant variability in sFLC levels among healthy individuals, which can complicate the interpretation of results. Normal reference ranges can vary between different laboratories and populations, making it challenging to standardize results across different settings.[3] Factors such as age and renal function can influence sFLC levels. For example, impaired renal function can lead to elevated sFLC levels, potentially complicating the interpretation in patients with concurrent renal disease.[13]
- *Limited specificity:* Elevated sFLC levels can occur in conditions other than multiple myeloma, such as LCDD, light chain amyloidosis, chronic inflammation, renal impairment, and other malignancies. This lack of specificity can lead to false positives and requires careful interpretation alongside other clinical and diagnostic findings.[6]
- *Lack of standardization and variability in assays:* Different laboratories may use different methods for measuring sFLCs. These variations in analytical techniques and calibration standards between different immunoassay platforms can affect the comparability of results across laboratories and studies. Standardization of assays is crucial for ensuring consistent and accurate measurements.[17]
- *Interpretation challenges:* Interpreting abnormal κ-to-λ ratios can be challenging. For example, patients with a balanced increase in both κ and λ light chains may have a normal ratio despite having a plasma cell disorder.[9] Patients may have normal or near-normal sFLC levels despite significant disease activity. This can be particularly true in patients with nonsecretory myeloma or those with a low tumor burden.[15]
- *Sensitivity issues:* While sFLC measurements are sensitive, they may not detect very low levels of monoclonal light chains, particularly in early stages of the disease or in cases where the light chain production is minimal.[6]

Q12. **Why is the short half-life of sFLCs clinically useful?**

Ans: The short half-life of sFLCs provides various advantages in the management of multiple myeloma and other plasma cell dyscrasias.

Clinical Utility of the Short Half-life of Serum Free Light Chains

- *Rapid detection of disease activity:* The short half-life of sFLCs (approximately 2–6 hours) means that their levels can fluctuate quickly in response to changes in disease activity. This sensitivity allows for rapid detection of increases in FLC production, which may indicate disease progression or relapse.[3] For instance, if a patient's myeloma becomes more active, sFLC levels will rise quickly, providing an early signal of worsening disease before other clinical signs or imaging results become apparent.[17]
- *Early monitoring of treatment response:* Due to their short half-life, sFLC levels decrease rapidly in response to effective treatment. This allows for early monitoring of treatment efficacy. For example, if a new therapy is effective, sFLC levels will fall quickly, giving clinicians prompt feedback on how well the treatment is working.[6] This rapid response helps in adjusting treatment strategies in a timely manner.
- *Detection of minimal residual disease (MRD):* The short half-life enhances the ability to detect MRD. Even small numbers of malignant plasma cells producing FLCs will cause detectable changes in sFLC levels due to their rapid turnover. This makes sFLC measurements a sensitive marker for identifying residual disease that might not be apparent through other methods such as imaging.[8]
- *Improved disease management:* The rapid turnover of sFLCs supports dynamic monitoring of disease status.[15]
- *Predictive power for relapse:* The ability of sFLCs to change quickly means they can serve as an early indicator of relapse. If sFLC levels begin to rise, it may signal emerging relapse even before other clinical symptoms or imaging results confirm it. This allows for earlier intervention and adjustment of treatment to address relapse promptly.[9]

Q13. **Why are monoclonal free light chains nephrotoxic?**

Ans: Monoclonal FLCs are nephrotoxic primarily due to their direct toxic effects on renal tubular cells and their impact on kidney function.

Mechanisms of Nephrotoxicity of Monoclonal Free Light Chains

Direct Tubular Toxicity

- Monoclonal FLCs can cause direct injury to renal tubular cells. These light chains can accumulate in the tubular cells, leading to cellular dysfunction and death. The accumulation of these proteins is toxic to the renal tubules due to their high molecular weight and inherent chemical properties, which can lead to oxidative stress and inflammation.[9]
- *Cast formation:* Monoclonal light chains can precipitate in the renal tubules, forming casts. These casts can obstruct tubular lumens, leading to increased intratubular pressure, reduced glomerular filtration rate (GFR), and ultimately, acute kidney injury (AKI).[15] The formation of light chain casts is a hallmark of light chain nephropathy, a condition associated with multiple myeloma.

Effects on Renal Hemodynamics

High levels of monoclonal FLCs can affect renal hemodynamics by altering renal blood flow. The toxicity can lead to constriction of afferent arterioles and decreased glomerular filtration pressure, thereby impairing kidney function.[17] This reduction in blood flow can exacerbate renal damage and contribute to progressive renal impairment.

Proteinuria and Tubular Dysfunction

The presence of monoclonal FLCs in the urine can lead to significant proteinuria. This increased excretion of light chains in the urine can contribute to tubular damage and further renal injury due to chronic exposure. The excessive protein load can overwhelm the reabsorption capacity of the renal tubules, leading to tubular dysfunction, secondary kidney damage, and contributing to chronic kidney disease (CKD).[9]

Inflammation and Fibrosis

The accumulation of monoclonal FLCs can trigger an inflammatory response within the kidneys. This inflammation can lead to further renal damage and fibrosis. Prolonged inflammation and fibrosis can impair renal function and contribute to the progression of kidney disease.[8]

Q14. **Why are serum tests preferable to urine tests?**

Ans: Monoclonal FLCs are critical biomarkers in diagnosing and managing plasma cell disorders, such as multiple myeloma and light-chain (AL) amyloidosis. Both serum and urine tests can measure FLCs, but serum tests are generally preferred for several reasons.

Advantages of Serum Tests

- *Ease of collection and processing:* Serum collection is simpler and less cumbersome compared to 24-hour urine collection. Obtaining a serum sample typically involves a straightforward blood draw at a single point in time, which is less time-consuming than requiring patients to collect 24-hour urine samples. A 24-hour urine collection can be problematic, leading to potential errors or incomplete collections. This can result in inaccurate measurement of urine FLC levels and complicate interpretation.[18,19]
- *Stability of serum samples:* Serum samples are generally more stable than urine. Serum samples can be stored for longer periods without significant degradation of the analytes, whereas urine samples may degrade more rapidly, potentially affecting the accuracy of FLC measurements. Serum samples are less affected by variations in hydration status or renal function, which can impact urine concentration and complicate interpretation.
- *Higher sensitivity and specificity:* Serum FLC assays tend to have higher sensitivity and specificity compared to urine assays. This is particularly important for detecting low levels of monoclonal FLCs and monitoring MRD in multiple myeloma.
- *Clinical relevance and diagnostic value:*
  - *Disease monitoring:* Serum FLC measurements are a key component in monitoring disease progression and response to treatment in multiple myeloma and other plasma cell disorders. They provide real-time information about the clonal plasma cell burden and are critical for assessing treatment efficacy.
  - *Prognostic value:* Elevated serum FLC levels have well-established prognostic significance in multiple myeloma and AL amyloidosis. Serum assays are widely used in clinical practice to guide therapeutic decisions and predict outcomes.[17]
- *Reduced risk of artifacts:*
  - Urine samples are more susceptible to technical artifacts such as contamination, changes in urine pH, and variations in specific gravity, which can affect FLC measurements. Serum assays are less prone to these issues, providing more reliable and reproducible results.

○ *Quality control:* Serum testing methodologies generally benefit from more standardized quality control procedures compared to urine testing, enhancing the accuracy and reliability of the results.

While urine FLC measurements can be useful in certain conditions, such as light chain cast nephropathy, they are less commonly used in routine clinical practice compared to serum FLC assays. The diagnostic and monitoring value of urine FLCs is often secondary to that of serum FLCs.[20,21]

Serum tests for measuring monoclonal FLCs are generally preferred over urine tests due to their ease of collection, stability, higher sensitivity and specificity, and reduced risk of artifacts. Serum assays provide reliable and clinically relevant information for diagnosing and managing plasma cell disorders, making them the preferred method in most clinical scenarios. While urine tests can be useful in specific situations, the advantages of serum testing make it the standard choice for assessing monoclonal FLC levels in routine practice.

Q15. **What is the frequency of abnormal serum free light chains in solitary plasmacytoma?**

Ans: Solitary plasmacytoma is a type of plasma cell neoplasm characterized by the presence of a single mass of clonal plasma cells, usually in bone or extramedullary sites, without the widespread disease seen in multiple myeloma. sFLCs are components of immunoglobulins and are measured to assess the presence of clonal plasma cell disorders. An abnormal κ-to-λ light chain ratio or elevated levels of one type of light chain can indicate an underlying monoclonal plasma cell proliferation.

- In solitary plasmacytoma, the frequency of abnormal sFLCs is generally lower compared to multiple myeloma. Some patients with solitary plasmacytoma may exhibit abnormal sFLC levels, many have normal sFLC measurements. A study by Palumbo et al. (2001) indicated that about 40% of patients with solitary plasmacytoma showed abnormal sFLC levels, which is lower than the frequency observed in multiple myeloma.[17] This variability can be influenced by the extent and location of the disease, as well as the individual patient's response to disease.
- The frequency of abnormal sFLCs can be influenced by whether the plasmacytoma is solitary and localized or if there is an additional disease burden not apparent at initial diagnosis. Localized plasmacytomas, especially in solitary bone lesions, may not always produce detectable levels of abnormal sFLCs.[18] In solitary plasmacytoma, the burden of clonal plasma cells is typically lower than in multiple myeloma. This lower plasma cell burden can contribute to less pronounced abnormalities in serum FLC levels.[19]

Diagnostic and Prognostic Implications

- Abnormal sFLC levels are less frequently observed in solitary plasmacytoma, they can still provide useful diagnostic information. Elevated or abnormal FLCs might indicate more extensive disease or progression to multiple myeloma.[20]
- *Prognosis:* The presence of abnormal sFLC levels in solitary plasmacytoma can have prognostic significance. Patients with abnormal FLCs may be at higher risk for progression or relapse and might require more intensive monitoring and management.[21]

Normal sFLC levels do not rule out solitary plasmacytoma, and abnormal sFLC levels may suggest disease progression or transformation. Regular monitoring and comprehensive evaluation remain essential for effective management.

Q16. What is the mechanism of increased serum free light chain levels in renal impairment?

Ans: Serum FLCs are components of immunoglobulins that can be used to diagnose and monitor plasma cell disorders, such as multiple myeloma and light chain amyloidosis which has elevated sFLC levels. However, renal impairment can further complicate the interpretation of these levels.

Mechanism of Increased Serum Free Light Chain Levels in Renal Impairment

Normal Renal Clearance of Free Light Chains

In healthy individuals, FLCs are filtered by the kidneys and excreted in the urine. The kidneys play a crucial role in clearing excess FLCs from the bloodstream. Approximately, 90% of FLCs are filtered through the glomeruli and reabsorbed in the proximal tubular cells, where they are catabolized.[19]

Impact of Renal Impairment on Free Light Chain Clearance

- In renal impairment, the GFR decreases, which reduces the kidney's ability to filter FLCs from the blood. This results in elevated sFLC levels due to impaired clearance.[22]
- *Tubular dysfunction:* Beyond glomerular filtration, proximal tubular reabsorption and catabolism of light chains can be impaired. Tubular dysfunction further exacerbates the accumulation of FLCs in the serum, as they are not adequately reabsorbed and broken down in the tubules.[21]

This is particularly evident in CKD and end-stage renal disease (ESRD), where substantial elevations in sFLCs are commonly observed.[23] It is essential to consider renal function when interpreting FLC results to avoid misdiagnosis or overestimation of disease activity.

Clinical Management and Adjustments

- *Adjusting FLC measurements:* In patients with renal impairment, it may be necessary to adjust the interpretation of sFLC levels by taking renal function into account. Some laboratories provide FLC reference ranges adjusted for renal function to better reflect the clinical situation in such patients.
- *Monitoring disease progression:* Elevated FLC levels in the context of renal impairment should be monitored alongside other clinical indicators and diagnostic tests to assess disease progression and treatment response accurately.

Q17. Why do serum free light chains provide rapid assessment of response compared to immunofixation electrophoresis?

Ans: Serum FLCs and IFE are both diagnostic tools used in the management of plasma cell disorders, including multiple myeloma and light chain amyloidosis. sFLCs are particularly valued for their ability to provide rapid assessment of disease response, whereas IFE is often used for more detailed analysis.

Mechanisms of Serum Free Light Chains Rapid Response Assessment

- *Sensitivity and specificity of sFLCs:* sFLCs assays are highly sensitive and specific for detecting subtle changes in the levels of FLCs in the blood. Elevated sFLC levels typically indicate increased disease activity, while decreased levels suggest therapeutic response

or disease control and thus allows for early detection of response to therapy. This direct correlation allows for a straightforward assessment of treatment efficacy.[21]
- *Rapid turnaround time:* FLC assays, including the Freelite assay by The Binding Site, are designed for rapid processing by automation and can provide results within a few hours to a day. This quick turnaround is beneficial for monitoring treatment response and making timely clinical decisions.[22]
- *Quantitative measurement helps in continuous monitoring:* sFLC levels are measured quantitatively, providing precise information about the extent of disease burden and response to treatment. Regular monitoring of these levels can show trends over time, helping clinicians evaluate the effectiveness of therapeutic interventions quickly.[23]
- *Comparison with IFE:* IFE is a method used to identify and characterize monoclonal proteins (M-proteins) by separating them through electrophoresis and then applying specific antisera to identify the light and heavy chain types. IFE is excellent for confirming the presence of monoclonal proteins and their type but it is less sensitive in detecting small changes in protein levels.[19]
  - IFE is less sensitive compared to sFLC assays in detecting MRD or very early responses to treatment. This lower sensitivity means IFE may not reflect small but clinically significant changes in disease status as quickly as sFLCs.[15]
  - Due to its quick processing time and ease of use, sFLC levels can be monitored frequently, allowing for rapid adjustments in treatment based on the latest results. IFE requires more time for sample processing and interpretation, which can delay the availability of results. This extended processing time can make it less practical for routine or frequent monitoring of treatment response.[24] IFE is valuable for detailed characterization of the type of monoclonal proteins and for confirming the presence of abnormal bands. It is used to verify the presence of M-proteins and to assist in diagnosis and staging rather than for frequent monitoring.[25]

Clinical Implications

- *Treatment monitoring:* The rapid assessment provided by sFLC assays allows clinicians to make timely adjustments to treatment plans based on the latest data. This is particularly important in managing aggressive or relapsing forms of plasma cell disorders.
- *Prognostic information:* Changes in sFLC levels can provide prognostic information about the likelihood of relapse or progression, helping guide long-term management strategies.[26]

Serum FLC assays offer a rapid and sensitive means of assessing response to treatment in plasma cell disorders due to their high sensitivity, quick turnaround times, and quantitative nature. In contrast, IFE, while valuable for detailed characterization of monoclonal proteins, is less sensitive and slower in providing information about early treatment responses.

Q18. **Can conditions causing hypergammaglobulinemia produce increases in serum free light chains?**

Ans: Hypergammaglobulinemia is characterized by elevated levels of immunoglobulins in the blood and can lead to increased sFLCs. Mechanisms involved are:
- *Increased production of immunoglobulins:* Conditions with hypergammaglobulinemia, such as chronic infections, autoimmune diseases, and lymphoproliferative disorders, often lead to an increase in immunoglobulin production. Immunoglobulins consist of two heavy

chains and two light chains (either κ or λ). An excess production of immunoglobulins results in an increased release of FLCs into the bloodstream.[27]

- *Monoclonal or polyclonal expansion:*
  - In diseases like multiple myeloma, a single clone of plasma cells produces large quantities of a specific type of immunoglobulin and its corresponding FLCs. This monoclonal proliferation results in significantly elevated levels of sFLCs.[28]
    - Conditions such as chronic infections or autoimmune diseases result in broad increases in immunoglobulin production. This polyclonal expansion also leads to elevated sFLCs as the overall immunoglobulin production and FLC release are increased.[29]
- *Renal dysfunction:* The kidneys play a critical role in filtering and excreting FLCs. In cases of renal dysfunction, the ability to clear these chains is impaired, resulting in elevated sFLC levels.[30] Hypergammaglobulinemia can exacerbate this issue by increasing the load of FLCs in the bloodstream.
- *Altered light chain metabolism:* Conditions associated with hypergammaglobulinemia can affect the metabolism and clearance of FLCs. When the production of FLCs exceeds their clearance capacity, serum levels rises.[31]

Clinical Implications

- Elevated sFLCs in the context of hypergammaglobulinemia can complicate the differentiation between true monoclonal gammopathies (e.g., multiple myeloma) and conditions causing polyclonal hypergammaglobulinemia. This necessitates a comprehensive diagnostic approach combining sFLC levels with other tests.[32]
- In conditions associated with hypergammaglobulinemia, sFLC levels can be used to assess disease activity and response to treatment. However, accurate interpretation requires considering the broader clinical picture and additional diagnostic information.[33]
- Elevated sFLCs provide prognostic information regarding disease progression or response to therapy but the specificity of sFLC levels for diagnosing specific conditions can be limited, requiring integration with other diagnostic findings.[9]

Q19. What is the role of free light chains in the diagnosis and management of AL amyloidosis?

Ans: AL amyloidosis is characterized by the deposition of amyloid fibrils derived from monoclonal light chains in various organs. The diagnosis and management of AL amyloidosis also rely on the measurement of FLCs in serum and urine.

Diagnostic and Prognostic Role of Free Light Chains

- Serum FLC assays are pivotal in the initial diagnosis of AL amyloidosis. Elevated levels of monoclonal FLCs are indicative of the clonal plasma cell dyscrasia underlying the amyloidosis. The presence of a monoclonal FLC peak, in conjunction with other diagnostic criteria, helps confirm the diagnosis.[20] Thus, sFLC ratio can provide additional diagnostic information. In AL amyloidosis, a significantly abnormal FLC ratio often supports the diagnosis of a clonal plasma cell disorder.[17]
- Monitoring sFLC levels is essential for assessing response to treatment in AL amyloidosis. Regular FLC measurements allow clinicians to adjust treatment strategies based on the patient's response.[20]

- Serum FLC levels serve as a critical prognostic marker. Higher baseline FLC levels are associated with worse outcomes and may correlate with more aggressive disease. Monitoring changes in FLC levels over time helps in evaluating the disease course and predicting prognosis.[17] It is important to note that patients with high levels of FLCs and bone marrow plasma cells and severe end-organ involvement are more likely to experience treatment failure and diminished survival.[33]
- The use of the iFLC level and FLC ratio was pioneered by the Mayo group. They further advocated for analysis of the difference in FLC (dFLC). dFLC is the difference between involved and uninvolved FLCs. Higher levels of dFLC at the time of diagnosis are associated with an increased plasma cell burden, greater severity of gastrointestinal disease, and greater likelihood of renal insufficiency and cardiac involvement as well as greater severity of heart disease. It can be used to monitor AL amyloidosis.[34]

The FLCs play a central role in the diagnosis and management of AL amyloidosis. They are crucial for confirming the diagnosis, differentiating AL amyloidosis from other conditions, and assessing disease involvement. sFLC measurements are also vital for monitoring response to treatment, guiding therapeutic decisions, and long-term disease surveillance.

Q20. What is light chain deposition disease?

Ans: Monoclonal immunoglobulin deposition disease (MIDD) occurs from nonamyloid deposition of monoclonal immunoglobulin in tissue secondary to a plasma cell neoplasm or rarely B-cell neoplasm. It has three subtypes based on the monoclonal immunoglobulin deposits. LCDD is the most common and makes up 80% of cases, followed by heavy chain deposition disease and light and heavy chain deposition disease.

The most common monoclonal immunoglobulin detected in the serum is IgG followed by monoclonal light chain, IgA and IgM. The tissue immunoglobulin deposits can differ from the monoclonal immunoglobulin in the blood. In patients with LCDD, only the monoclonal immunoglobulin light chain is deposited even if the entire immunoglobulin is detected in the serum.

Light chain deposition disease is a rare condition characterized by the deposition of monoclonal light chains in various tissues and organs, leading to organ dysfunction.[35] It is associated with monoclonal gammopathies, such as multiple myeloma or other plasma cell dyscrasias, but differs from other light chain-related disorders such as AL amyloidosis and myeloma cast nephropathy.

Pathophysiology

- *Monoclonal light chains:* In LCDD, monoclonal light chains produced by clonal plasma cells deposit in tissues as amorphous or granular deposits. These deposits can cause tissue damage and organ dysfunction.
- *Organs affected:* The kidneys are most commonly affected, leading to a form of nephropathy that resembles CKD. Other organs can also be involved, including the heart, liver, and skin, though less frequently.
- *Mechanism of deposition:* The deposition of light chains is due to their abnormal production and reduced clearance. In LCDD, monoclonal light chains in the family of VκIV are overrepresented. These light chains aggregate and deposit in tissues, disrupting normal cellular functions and causing inflammation and fibrosis.

Clinical Presentation

- *Renal involvement:* The most common presentation of LCDD is renal impairment. Patients often present with nephrotic syndrome, which includes symptoms such as proteinuria, edema, and hypoalbuminemia.
- *Systemic symptoms:* In addition to renal symptoms, patients may experience systemic symptoms such as fatigue, weight loss, and generalized weakness. Extrarenal manifestations are less common but can include cardiac and hepatic involvement.
- *Diagnostic challenges:* LCDD can be difficult to diagnose due to its clinical and histological similarities with other light chain-related disorders. It is essential to differentiate it from AL amyloidosis and myeloma cast nephropathy.

Serum and Urine Tests

- *Serum FLC assay:* Elevated sFLCs with an abnormal κ-to-λ ratio may suggest a clonal plasma cell disorder.
- *24-hour urine collection:* Increased urinary light chain excretion can support the diagnosis, although it is not specific to LCDD.

Histopathology

- *Kidney biopsy:* The definitive diagnosis of LCDD often relies on kidney biopsy. Histological examination reveals light chain deposits within the glomeruli, tubules, or interstitium, often without the characteristic Congo red staining which is seen in amyloidosis. The deposits are most frequently found in tubular basement membranes, glomerular basement membranes, vascular walls, and in the interstitium of the kidney.[36]
- *Immunofluorescence microscopy:* Immunofluorescence microscopy can identify the light chain deposits, which may show a granular pattern.
- *Bone marrow biopsy:* A bone marrow biopsy may be performed to assess the presence of clonal plasma cells and quantify their proportion. This helps confirm an underlying plasma cell disorder.

Imaging Studies

Imaging studies can evaluate the extent of renal damage and guide management decisions.

Essential Diagnostic Criteria

- *Essential:* Demonstration of monoclonal immunoglobulin deposition in tissue.
- *In the kidney:* This should be demonstrated by immunohistochemistry and electron microscopy.
- *In cases where there is coexistence of light chain cast nephropathy:* MIDD may be demonstrated by immunohistochemistry only.
- Diagnosis in other tissues relies on immunohistochemistry, as electron microscopy is not commonly used. Besides light chain cast nephropathy, AL amyloidosis and light chain proximal tubulopathy have been found to coexist with MIDD in the same kidney.

Q21. Should serum free light chain tests be used as a screen for monoclonal proteins instead of serum protein electrophoresis?

Ans: Both tests play important roles in the diagnostic process, and each has its strengths and limitations. Even though sFLC tests offer significant advantages in detecting and monitoring monoclonal proteins, they are not necessarily a replacement for SPEP but rather a complementary tool. SPEP remains important for its broad screening capabilities and for identifying the overall protein profile. Combining both tests can provide a more comprehensive diagnostic approach.

REFERENCES

1. Sewpersad S, Pillay TS. Historical perspectives in clinical pathology: Bence Jones protein-early urine chemistry and the impact on modern day diagnostics. J Clin Pathol. 2021;74(4):212-5.
2. Smith D, Yong K. Multiple myeloma. BMJ. 2013;346:3863.
3. Kyle RA, Rajkumar SV. Multiple myeloma. N Engl J Med. 2004;351(18):1860-73.
4. Tietz NW, Burtis CA, Ashwood ER, Bruns DE. Tietz Fundamentals of Clinical Chemistry and Molecular Diagnostics, 8th edition. St. Louis, USA: Elsevier; 2014.
5. Abbas AK, Aster JC, Aster JC, Kumar V. Robbins and Cotran Pathologic Basis of Disease, 10th edition. Amsterdam: Elsevier; 2018.
6. Dispenzieri A, Kyle RA. Diagnosis and management of light chain (amyloid) AL amyloidosis. J Am Soc Nephrol. 2013;24(5):691-5.
7. Kyle RA, Gertz MA. Light-chain multiple myeloma. In: Doyle LA, Colgan JP, (Eds). Hematology/Oncology Clinics of North America. 2006;20(6):1017-31.
8. Rawstron AC, Davies F, Palumbo A, et al. Flow cytometric analysis of multiple myeloma: the role of monoclonal antibodies in the diagnosis of Bence-Jones myeloma. Haematologica. 2007;92(1):99-103.
9. Kyle RA, Rajkumar SV. Multiple myeloma and other monoclonal gammopathies. Hematology: Basic Principles and Practice, 7th edition. USA: Elsevier; 2018. pp. 2221-60.
10. Farrar WB, Knight S, et al. Use of mass spectrometry to quantify free light chains in multiple myeloma. J Mass Spectrom. 2010;45(5):493-502.
11. Davis T, McNally J. Comparative evaluation of free light chain assays. Am J Clin Pathol. 2019;152(1):55-61.
12. Jacobs JF, Tate JR, Merlini G. Is accuracy of serum free light chain measurement achievable? Clin Chem Lab Med. 2016;54(6):1021-30.
13. VanDuijn MM, Jacobs JF, Wevers RA, Engelke UF, Joosten I, Luider TM. Quantitative measurement of immunoglobulins and free light chains using mass spectrometry. Anal Chem. 2015;87(16):8268-74.
14. Dall'Acqua WF, Kiener PA, Wu H. Pharmacokinetics and pharmacodynamics of IgG. In: Dall'Acqua WF, Kiener PA, Wu H (Eds). Immunoglobulins in Clinical Medicine. New York USA: Academic Press; 2017. pp. 267-80.
15. Gertz MA, Dispenzieri A. Free light chain measurement in multiple myeloma. In: Gertz MA, Dispenzieri A (Eds). Multiple Myeloma: Current Treatment Options. USA: Springer; 2018. pp. 135-48.
16. Kher KK, Sharma AP. Urinary protein electrophoresis: a useful test for the diagnosis of kidney disease. Am J Kidney Dis. 2004;43(1):12-9.
17. Palumbo A, Anderson K. Multiple myeloma. N Engl J Med. 2011;364(11):1046-60.
18. Dimopoulos MA, Palumbo A. The role of serum and urine free light chains in the diagnosis and management of multiple myeloma. Eur J Haematol. 2018;101(3):336-46.
19. Rajkumar SV, Kumar S. Multiple myeloma: Current treatment algorithms. Blood Can J. 2020;10(9):94.
20. Kumar S, Dispenzieri A. Diagnosis and management of light-chain amyloidosis. J Clin Oncol. 2014;32(22):2436-45.
21. Gertz MA, Comenzo RL. The treatment of AL amyloidosis. Blood. 2015;126(4):490-9.
22. Muchtar E, Dispenzieri A. The role of serum free light chains in diagnosing and monitoring plasma cell disorders. Hematology/Oncology Clinics of North America. 2018;32(5):887-907.
23. Palladini G, Merlini G. Management of light-chain (AL) amyloidosis. Blood Can J. 2014;4(11):e234.
24. Dimopoulos MA, Moreau P. Management of patients with solitary plasmacytoma. Hematology/Oncology Clinics of North America. 2014;28(3):651-60.
25. Gertz MA, Rajkumar SV. Diagnosis and treatment of solitary plasmacytoma. Am J Hematol. 2017;92(8):845-52.
26. Kumar S, Dispenzieri A. Diagnosis and management of AL amyloidosis. J Clin Oncol. 2018;32(22):2436-45.

27. Rajkumar SV, Palumbo A. Multiple Myeloma: Current Treatment Algorithms. Blood Can J. 2019;9(5):52.
28. Kumar S, Paiva B, Anderson KC, van Duin M, Sonneveld P, Mateos MV, et al. Multiple Myeloma. Nat Rev Dis Primers. 2017;3:17046.
29. Gertz MA. Hypergammaglobulinemia: A Comprehensive Review. Hematology/Oncology Clinics of North America. 2021;35(1):1-15.
30. Palladini G, Merlini G, Seldin DC. Systemic Light Chain Amyloidosis: Current Treatment Algorithms. Hematology/Oncology Clinics of North America. 2013;27(6):1301-12.
31. Mead GP, Carr-Smith HD, Drayson MT, Morgan GJ, Child JA, Bradwell AR. Serum free light chains for monitoring multiple myeloma. Br J Haematol. 2004;126(3):348-54.
32. Dimopoulos MA, Moreau P, Palumbo A. Multiple Myeloma: Current Treatment Algorithms. Clinical Lymphoma Myeloma & Leukemia. 2016;16(5):245-58.
33. Baker KR. Light Chain Amyloidosis: Epidemiology, Staging, and Prognostication. Methodist Debakey Cardiovasc J. 2022;18(2):27-35.
34. Kumar S, Dispenzieri A, Katzmann JA, Larson DR, Colby CL, Lacy MQ, et al. Serum immunoglobulin free light-chain measurement in primary amyloidosis: prognostic value and correlations with clinical features. Blood. 2010;116(24):5126-9.
35. Gertz MA, Dispenzieri A. Diagnosis and treatment of light-chain deposition disease. Hematology/Oncology Clinics of North America. 2016;30(6):1017-31.
36. Shimamura Y, Ogawa Y, Takizawa H, Hayashi T, Sakurai Y. Light chain deposition disease diagnosed using computed tomography-guided kidney biopsy. Cureus. 2021;13(5):e15102.

28. Basics of Transfusion Medicine

Rasika Dhawan Setia, Mitu Dogra

Q1. How is blood grouping and pretransfusion testing done?

Ans: The term "blood group" refers to the red blood cell (RBC) antigens whose specificity is controlled by genes. Karl Landsteiner discovered the first human blood group system, ABO and later many other blood group systems were identified including Rh, Kell, Lewis, MNS, Duffy, Kidd, etc.[1] ABO Rh grouping is the most frequently performed test in the blood centers and is the most immunogenic and clinically important.

Both ABO forward and reverse grouping tests must be performed on all donors and patients as there is an inverse reciprocal relationship between the forward and reverse type; thus, one serves as a check on the other **(Table 1)**. Example, if the individual has B antigens only on their RBCs, there will be an "expected" naturally occurring anti-A antibody in their plasma since they lack the A antigen.

TABLE 1: ABO forward and reverse grouping.

Forward grouping						Reverse grouping			
Anti A*	Anti B*	Anti AB*	Anti D1*	Anti D2*	A cell$	B cell$	O cell$		Result
+	0	+	+	+	0	+	0		A+
0	+	+	+	+	+	0	0		B+
+	+	+	+	+	0	0	0		AB+
0	0	0	+	+	+	+	0		O+

*Test run with the commercially available antisera.
$Test run either with the commercially available reagent red cells or in house freshly prepared reagent red cells.

Techniques for blood grouping are:[2]
- *Tube test:* This test is considered as gold standard especially in cases of ABO discrepancies as it gives you a lot of flexibility in terms of incubation at different temperatures, changing cell:plasma ratio, etc.
- *Microplate test:* Microplate techniques can be used to test for antigens on red cells and antibodies in serum. A microplate can be considered as a matrix of 96 "short" test tubes. The principles that apply to hemagglutination in tube tests also apply to tests in microplates.
- *Column agglutination test:* This test is performed in a microcolumn in which the red cell agglutinates are trapped in the glass bead matrix during centrifugation, and unagglutinated cells form a pellet at the bottom of the column.
- *Molecular typing:* Used commonly in cases of ABO discrepancies or medicolegal cases.

Pretransfusion Testing

Pretransfusion testing can be defined as the use of serologic principles and tests to ensure compatibility and prevent an immune-mediated hemolytic transfusion reaction.[3] If the antigens on a donor's red cells are not an identical match to those of the recipient, transfused red blood is capable of inducing an antibody response in the recipient. Thus, it is important to identify the antigenic substances on both the donor's red cells and those of the intended recipient.

Steps in Pretransfusion Testing

- Written request for transfusion.
- Identification of transfusion recipient and collection of blood specimen.
- *Testing of transfusion recipient's blood specimen*:
  - Evaluation of specimen for testing suitability.
  - ABO group
  - Rh type (weak D testing is optional when testing the patient)
  - Screening for unexpected antibodies to red cell antigens
  - Antibody identification if unexpected antibodies are detected.
  - Comparison of current and previous test results, and any discrepancies shall be investigated and appropriate action taken before a unit is issued for transfusion.
- *Donor RBC unit testing*:
  - ABO group confirmation and Rh type confirmation for Rh-negative RBC units
- *Donor RBC unit selection*:
  - Selection of components of ABO group and Rh type that are compatible with the transfusion recipient and with an unexpected allogeneic antibodies.
- *Compatibility testing (crossmatch)*:
  - Serologic
  - Computer or electronic
- Labeling of blood or blood components with the recipient's identifying information and issue.

Compatibility Testing (Crossmatch)

Immediate spin crossmatch: Recipient plasma is mixed with cells from the donor unit, immediately centrifuged, and observed for agglutination and/or hemolysis. Absence of either indicates ABO compatibility, whereas positive results require further investigation.[3]

Antiglobulin crossmatch: The antiglobulin crossmatch consists of an immediate spin crossmatch with the recipient's plasma and red cells from the donor unit. The test system is then incubated at 37°C and completed with the antiglobulin test. Antiglobulin crossmatching may be performed in tube tests, typically with the addition of low-ionic saline solutions (LISS) or polyethylene glycol (PEG) enhancements or in column agglutination and solid-phase red cell adherence tests. Observable reactivity and/or hemolysis at any phase of testing indicate incompatibility.

Computer crossmatch: ABO compatibility can be done electronically via a validated, on-site computer system. Electronic crossmatching eliminates the need for a serologic crossmatch, thereby reducing sample volume and turnaround time. Two determinations of the recipient's ABO grouping at different time must be on file, one of which is from the current specimen collection. The confirmatory ABO grouping may be from historical records or from an additional collection. The recipient must not have detectable clinically significant antibodies or a history of antibodies. The laboratory information system (LIS) must contain donor unit information to include the donation identification number, component name, ABO group, Rh type, donor confirmation typing, and the interpretation of compatibility with the recipient. A method must be in place to verify that data entry is correct before the release of blood components. In addition, the LIS must contain logic that sound the user of any discrepancies between recipient records and the donor unit.

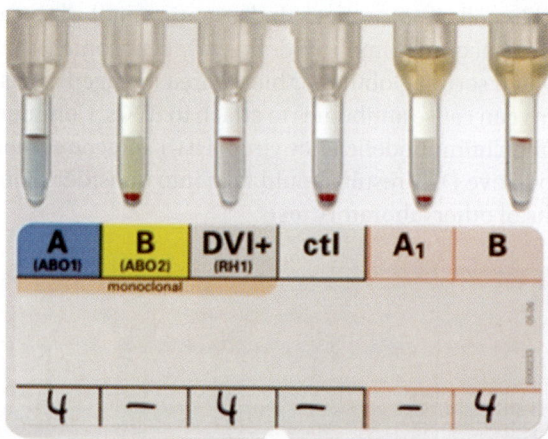

FIG. 1: ABO Rh grouping cards.

Q2. What is direct Coombs test and what is its significance?

Ans: The direct antiglobulin test (DAT) detects in vivo sensitization of RBCs with immunoglobulin (Ig)G or complement components.[4] The DAT is performed by testing freshly washed red cells directly with antiglobulin reagents containing anti-IgG and anti-C3d (polyspecific DAT). If it is positive, monospecific DAT (IgG, IgM, IgA, C3d, and C3b) is done to appropriately characterize the immune process involved. Once IgG is confirmed, they are further categorized into IgG subclass and finally, titer of the responsible subclass is done.

Although any red cells may be tested, ethylenediaminetetraacetic acid (EDTA) anticoagulated blood samples are preferred. The EDTA prevents in vitro fixation of complement by chelating the calcium that is needed for C1 activation. If red cells from a clotted blood sample have a positive DAT result due to complement, the results should be confirmed on red cells from freshly collected blood kept at 37°C or an EDTA-anticoagulated specimen if these results are to be used for diagnostic purposes

The DAT should be performed when:
- Autocontrol is found positive in antibody identification studies.
- Hemolysis has been established in a patient and we want to distinguish immune from nonimmune cause.

Clinical conditions that can result in in vivo coating of RBCs with antibody or complement are the following:
- Hemolytic disease of the fetus and newborn (HDFN)
- Hemolytic transfusion reaction (HTR)
- Autoimmune and drug-induced hemolytic anemia (AIHA)
- Drug-induced antibodies
- Antibodies produced by passenger lymphocytes (e.g., in transplanted organs or hematopoietic components)
- Nonspecifically adsorbed proteins (e.g., hypergammaglobulinemia, high-dose intravenous immune globulin.
- The DAT can also be positive for IgG or complement without a clear correlation with anemia in patients with sickle cell disease, beta thalassemia renal disease, multiple myeloma, autoimmune disorders, acquired immunodeficiency syndrome (AIDS), or other. Diseases associated with elevated serum globulin or blood urea nitrogen levels.
- Sometimes, infections can cause antibodies to attach to RBCs. Common infections that cause this are: Malaria, human immunodeficiency virus (HIV), infectious mononucleosis, etc.

Interpretation of a positive DAT result should take into consideration the patient's history, clinical data, and results of other laboratory tests.

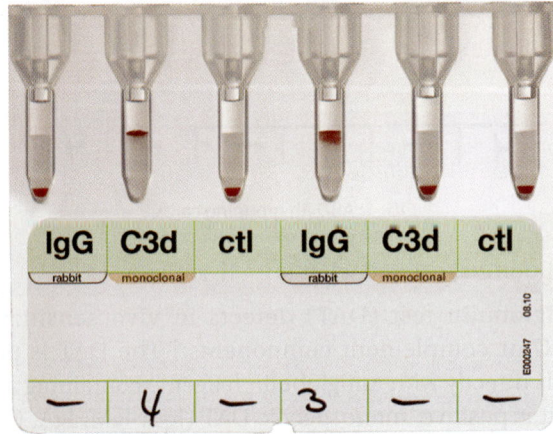

FIG. 2: Direct antiglobulin test.

Q3. What is monospecific direct antiglobulin test?

Ans: A positive DAT with polyspecific antihuman globulin (AHG) generally indicates that the red cells are coated in vivo with immunoglobulin and/or complement. To differentiate the reaction, monospecific AHG reagents are used, such as anti-IgG, -IgA, -IgM, -C3, -C3b, -C3c, -C3d, and -C4.[4,5]

Differential or monospecific DAT is performed to appropriately characterize the immune process involved and determine the diagnosis.

The EDTA anticoagulated blood samples are preferred. If cold reacting autoantibodies are suspected the sample is collected at 37°C, transported, and kept at 37°C till tests are completed. Antibodies dependent for their detection upon the binding of complement may not be detected if aged serum or plasma from an anticoagulated sample is used.

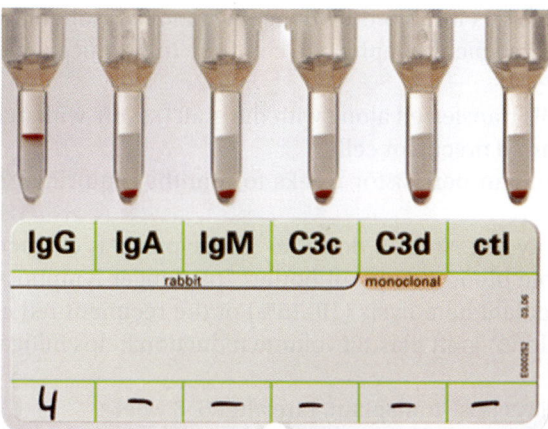

FIG. 3: Monospecific direct antiglobulin test.

Q4. What is forward and reverse typing?

Ans: *Forward grouping* (cell type) is defined as using known sources of commercial antisera (anti-A, anti-B) to detect antigens on an individual's RBCs.

Reverse grouping (serum type) is defined as detecting ABO antibodies in the patient's serum by using known reagent RBCs, namely A1 and B cells.

Both ABO forward and reverse grouping tests must always be performed on donors and patients.[6] There is always an inverse reciprocal relationship between the forward and reverse type; thus, one serves as a check on the other. For example, if the individual has A antigens only on their RBCs, there will be an "expected" naturally occurring anti-B antibody in their serum since they lack the B antigen.

Antibodies against ABO antigens are known as "naturally occurring" because they occur without any exposure of blood transfusion/transplant and are present from birth (0–6 months) however, it has been postulated that certain bacteria, pollen particles, and other substances present in nature are chemically similar to A and B antigens, which constantly exposes individuals to A-like and B-like antigens. This exposure serves as a source of stimulation of anti-A and anti-B.

All other defined blood group systems do not regularly have "naturally occurring" antibodies expected in their serum to antigens they lack on their RBCs. Antibody production in most other blood group systems requires the introduction of foreign RBCs by either transfusion or pregnancy, although some individuals can occasionally have antibodies present that are not related to the introduction of foreign RBCs.

Q5. How is blood group affected by stem cell transplant?

Ans: ABO incompatible hematopoietic stem cell transplantation (HSCT) is classified as either major, minor, or bidirectional.[7]

Major incompatible HSCT (e.g., from A donor to O recipient) is characterized by the presence of antidonor blood group antibodies in recipient plasma. Major incompatibilities may result in delayed RBC engraftment, clinically characterized by diminished reticulocyte counts and a corresponding increase in RBC transfusion requirements. In pure red cell aplasia (PRCA), conversion to donor hematopoietic progenitor cells (HPC) RBC production takes place, but

the reconstituting marrow is inhibited by the persistence of isohemagglutinins secreted by recipient plasma cells. Recipient lymphocyte continue to produce antidonor IHAs for about 3-4 months.
- Hemolysis of red cells transferred along with the graft (severe with marrow than HPC-A).
- Destruction of erythroid precursor cells.

The RBC chimerism can persist for weeks to months requiring prolonged transfusion requirement.

Minor incompatibility (e.g., from B donor to AB recipient) is characterized by the passive transfer of incompatible blood group antibodies "passenger lymphocytes" from the donor to the recipient. Immediate hemolysis (10-15%) of the recipient red cells. Because of ABO isohemagglutinins in donor graft plasma volume reduction helps mitigate the adverse effects (AEs).
- Can manifest 5-15 days post-transplant, rare after 6-8 weeks.
- Monitoring of the antibody titer is required.
- In bidirectional ABO incompatibility (e.g., from B donor to A recipient), both major and minor incompatibilities are present.

After a successful stem cell transplant, the recipient's blood type will be gradually converted to the donor's blood type. Patients who have received stem cells from a donor with a different blood type will display a mixed blood type until full engraftment occurs. As we know, ABO blood typing is determined by the presence of blood group antigens on the surface of RBCs (forward typing, FT) as well as by the presence of blood group antibodies in the plasma (reverse typing, RT), inconsistency or discrepancy may be seen between FT and RT. Many times we may find mixed field reactions suggesting presence of two population of cells.

When to Switch to Donor Type Blood Components?
- Cell and serum grouping only of donor type (no mixed field pattern).
- No transfusion for 90-120 days or as per institutional protocol.
- No incompatible isoagglutinins against newer red cell phenotype.
- Consistency and persistent blood group—minimum of two samples and occasions.
- Negative DAT report.

Q6. **What are the blood transfusion reactions?**

Ans: Transfusion reactions are undesirable signs and symptoms in recipients of blood transfusions, which can occur from minutes to even weeks after administration of blood components.[8] Noninfectious transfusion-related adverse events may happen due to a wide variety of reasons, which may be specific to a blood component, amount of transfusion, or even human error. It is important for any medical professionals involved with blood transfusions to understand the pathophysiology of these reactions.

Classification of Noninfectious Complications of Blood Transfusion

Noninfectious complications of blood transfusion are broadly classified as acute and delayed reactions based on time of occurrence and are further subclassified based on etiology, whether it is immune or nonimmune.

Acute Reaction (<24 Hours)

- *Immune-mediated reactions:*
  - Acute hemolytic transfusion reaction (AHTR)
  - Febrile nonhemolytic transfusion reaction (FNHTR)
  - Allergic reactions
  - Anaphylactic reactions
  - Transfusion-related acute lung injury (TRALI)
  - Transfusion associated dyspnea (TAD)
- *Nonimmune mediated reactions:*
  - Air embolism
  - Transfusion-associated circulatory overload (TACO)
  - Nonimmune hemolysis

Delayed Reaction (>24 Hours)

- *Immune-mediated reactions:*
  - Delayed hemolytic transfusion reaction (DHTR)
  - Alloimmunization:
    - To human leukocyte antigen (HLA) antigens
    - To platelet antigens
    - To red cell antigens
  - Transfusion-related immunomodulation (TRIM)
  - Transfusion-associated graft versus host disease (TA-GVHD)
  - Post-transfusion purpura (PTP)
- *Nonimmune reaction:*
  - Iron overload

Acute hemolytic transfusion reaction is caused by immunologic incompatibility between donor and recipient.
- Seen most often after transfusion of incompatible red cell components.

Diagnosis is based on presence of signs and symptoms and their temporal association with the transfusion, which include presence of fever during or within hours of cessation of transfusion. Fever is associated with mild-to-severe pain located in flanks, back, abdomen, chest, or infusion site shortly after initiation of transfusion, hypotension that may progress to shock, disseminated intravascular coagulation (DIC) that can present as microvascular leakage to uncontrollable bleeding along with red or dark urine and oliguria that may progress from elevated blood urea nitrogen (BUN) to acute kidney injury (AKI).

Acute hemolytic transfusion reaction [Center for Disease Control (CDC)] diagnostic criteria:
- *Definitive:*
  - Reaction occurs during or within 24 hours of cessation of transfusion and is associated with any of the following:
    - Back, flank, or intravenous (IV) site pain
    - Fever, chills, or rigors
    - DIC
    - Hypotension
    - Hemoglobinuria, oliguria, or AKI

- Two or more laboratory findings:
    - Low haptoglobin, elevated bilirubin, and elevated lactate dehydrogenase (LDH)
    - Pink-to-red plasma color consistent with hemolysis, increased plasma hemoglobin
    - Spherocytes on blood smear
    - Positive DAT and positive elution test (antibody present on transfused RBCs)

Febrile Nonhemolytic Transfusion Reaction
- Suspect febrile nonhemolytic transfusion reaction (FNHTR) when:
    - Fever associated with transfusion cannot be explained by other causes.
    - Chills or rigors are present in afebrile patient.
  The FNHTR CDC diagnostic criteria
- *Definitive*:
    - Reaction occurs during or within 4 hours of cessation of transfusion and is associated with either:
        - Fever [38°C (100.4°F) oral or higher and a change of at least 1°C (1.8°F) from baseline], or
        - Chills and/or rigors are present.

Allergic Reaction
- Suspect allergic reaction if skin rash:
    - Is a maculopapular rash that occurs during or within 4 hours following transfusion.
    - Is associated with itching, flushing, or erythema.
    - Is associated with hives.

Severe Allergic Reaction (Anaphylaxis)
- Severe allergic reaction is suspected (anaphylaxis) if hypotension is associated with:
    - Other findings suggestive of allergic reaction such as urticaria, pruritus, flushing, or angioedema.
    - Respiratory symptoms such as hoarseness, stridor, wheezing, chest tightness, or cough.

Severe Allergic Reaction (Anaphylaxis) Center for Disease Control Criteria
- *Definitive:*
    - Occurs during or within 4 hours of cessation of transfusion and two or more of the following are present:
        - Urticaria (hives), flushing, maculopapular rash, pruritus
        - Lip, tongue, periorbital, or uvula erythema, and edema, and
        - Airway symptoms (e.g., hoarseness, stridor, and wheezing), or
        - Hypotension, cardiac arrhythmias, or syncope.

Transfusion-related Acute Lung Injury
- Suspect TRALI if fever is associated with:
    - Acute onset of dyspnea, cyanosis, hypoxemia, or other findings of acute respiratory distress syndrome (ARDS).
    - Hypotension that does not respond to administration of IV fluids.
    - Bilateral pulmonary edema on chest radiograph or computed tomography (CT) scan.

Transfusion-related Acute Lung Injury Center for Disease Control Criteria
- *TRALI type I*:
  - Patients with no risk factors for ARDS who meet the following criteria:
    - Acute onset of:
      - *Hypoxemia:* PaO_2/FiO_2 <300 mm Hg or SpO_2 <90% on room air.
      - Bilateral pulmonary edema on chest radiograph or CT.
      - No evidence of circulatory overload (e.g., elevated pulmonary capillary wedge pressure).
      - Onset during or within 6 hours of cessation of transfusion.
      - No temporal relationship to other risk factors for ARDS.
- *TRALI type II*:
  - Patients with risk factors for ARDS (but no current diagnosis of ARDS), or
  - Patients with mild ARDS (PaO_2/FiO_2 of 200–300 mm Hg) but who deteriorate as a result of transfusion, determined by:
    - Acute onset
      - *Hypoxemia:* PaO_2/FiO_2 < 300 mm Hg or O_2 saturation < 90% on room air.
      - Bilateral pulmonary edema on chest radiograph or CT scan.
      - No evidence of circulatory overload (e.g., elevated pulmonary capillary wedge pressure).
      - Onset during or within 6 hours of cessation of transfusion.
  - Stable respiratory findings 12 hours before transfusion.

Transfusion-associated Circulatory Overload
- Suspect TACO when ARDS occurs during or shortly after transfusion and is associated with:
  - Dyspnea, orthopnea, and hypoxemia.
  - S3 gallop, jugular venous distension, and hypertension.
  - Radiographic findings of pulmonary edema and widened cardiothoracic ratio.
  - Fluid overload that responds to diuretic therapy.

Transfusion-associated Circulatory Overload Center for Disease Control Criteria
Minimum of three required:
- Acute or worsening respiratory distress
  - Dyspnea, tachypnea, cyanosis, decreased O_2 saturation, and chest tightness
- Radiographic or clinical evidence of worsening pulmonary edema
  - Crackles, orthopnea, and cough
  - S3 gallop on heart auscultation
- Elevated brain natriuretic peptide (BNP) or N-terminal pro-BNP (NT-pro BNP)
  - Post/pretransfusion NT-proBNP ratio > 1.5 can aid in the diagnosis of TACO.
  - Post-transfusion levels of BNP < 300 or NT-proBNP < 2,000 pg/mL, drawn within 24 hours of the reaction, make TACO unlikely.
- Cardiovascular changes not explained by an underlying medical condition are:
  - Elevated central venous pressure
  - Tachycardia
  - Hypertension
  - Widened pulse pressure

- Left heart failure
  - Enlarged cardiac silhouette on chest imaging
  - Peripheral edema
- *Fluid overload*: Time to onset of symptoms
  - Up to 12 hours after cessation of transfusion

Delayed Hemolytic Transfusion Reaction

- Significant drop in hemoglobin within 21 days after transfusion and one or more of the following:
  - New RBC alloantibody
  - Hemoglobinuria
  - Reticulocytosis
  - Increase in LDH levels

Cutaneous Rash During or Following Transfusion

Suspect TA-GVHD if a skin rash during or after a transfusion.
- *Definitive*:
  - Occurs 2 days and up to 6 weeks after cessation of transfusion with:
    - Erythematous rash that spreads to extremities
    - Diarrhea
    - Fever
  - Hepatomegaly
  - Elevation of aspartate aminotransferase (AST), alanine transaminase (ALT), and alkaline phosphatase
  - Pancytopenia
  - Compatible histologic findings on skin or liver biopsy

Post-transfusion Purpura Center for Disease Control Criteria

Thrombocytopenia typically occurs 5–12 days after the transfusion of cellular blood components, characterized by the presence of antibodies in the patient directed against the human platelet antigen (HPA) system.

Definitive: Alloantibodies in the patient directed against HPA or other platelet specific antigen detected at or after development of thrombocytopenia.
And

Thrombocytopenia: A decrease in platelets to less than 20% of pretransfusion count.

Probable: Alloantibodies in the patient directed against HPA or other platelet specific antigen detected at or after development of thrombocytopenia.
And
Decrease in platelets to levels between 20 and 80% of pretransfusion count.

Possible: PTP is suspected, but laboratory findings and/or information are not sufficient to meet defined criteria above. For example, the patient has a drop in platelet count to less than 80% of pretransfusion count but HPA antibodies were not tested or were negative. Other, more specific adverse reaction definitions do not apply.

Q7. What is dimethyl sulfoxide (DMSO) and how stem cells are preserved in DMSO?

Ans: Dimethyl sulfoxide or DMSO is an organic solvent that is used as a cryoprotectant when cells are frozen down for cryostorage.[9] This polar solvent penetrates the cell membrane, reduces intracellular ice formation, and prevents cell damage due to dehydration during freezing. As a component of cell freezing media, DMSO protects cells by preventing the formation of both extracellular and intracellular ice crystals. It is currently the gold standard for cell cryopreservation of hematopoietic progenitor cell. It increases cellular permeability by affecting membrane dynamics in a concentration dependent manner. At lower concentrations (5%), evidence suggests that DMSO decreases membrane thickness increasing membrane permeability. At higher concentrations of 10%, it induces water pore formation in biological membranes and allows intracellular water to be more readily replaced by cryoprotectants that promote vitrification. At high concentrations, DMSO is known to produce severe AEs during infusion. AEs related to DMSO are dose-dependent and cumulative when multi-dose cell therapies are given. They are usually mild-to-moderate but can be severe including blood pressure alterations and even severe arrhythmia.

Q8. What is cryoprecipitate and how is it prepared?

Ans: Cryoprecipitate (cryo) is cold-insoluble protein that precipitates when fresh frozen plasma (FFP) is thawed. Cryoprecipitated antihemophilic factor (AHF), or simply "cryoprecipitate" is a concentrated cryoglobulin fraction that is prepared from FFP. FFP can be thawed to prepare cryoprecipitated.[10]

The AHF by placing the FFP in a refrigerator (at 1–6°C) overnight or in a circulating waterbath at 1–6°C. Cold-insoluble protein that precipitates when FFP is thawed to 1–6°C is collected by centrifugation, and the supernatant plasma is transferred into a satellite container. The precipitate is resuspended in a small amount of residual plasma, generally 15 mL and the precipitate is refrozen. The cryoprecipitated AHF is placed in a freezer within an hour of removal from the refrigerated centrifuge and can be stored at less than –30°C for 12 months from the original collection date. Cryoprecipitate contains factor VIII, factor XIII, von Willebrand factor (vWF), fibrinogen, and fibronectin. The antihemophiliac activity (factor VIII) in the final product should not be < 80 units/bag and fibrinogen at least 150 mg/bag.

Q9. What precautions should be taken while thawing fresh frozen plasma?

Ans: The following precautions should be taken:
- FFPs should be thawed in a plasma bath or other equipment designed for the purpose, within a vacuum-sealed overwrap bag according to a validated procedure.
- The optimal temperature at which the component should be thawed is 37°C; temperatures between 33 and 37°C are acceptable.
- Protocols must be in place to ensure that the equipment is regularly cleaned and maintained to minimize the risk of bacterial contamination.
- After thawing, and at the time of administration, the content should be inspected to ensure that no insoluble precipitate is visible and that the container is intact.

Q10. How is fresh frozen plasma prepared?

Ans: Fresh frozen plasma is prepared by extracting the noncellular portion of blood and freezing it within 6 hours of donation. It is prepared by separating whole blood and extracting the liquid portion (plasma).[11]

This can be carried out in two ways:
1. *Centrifugation*
    - For the harvest of packed red blood cell (PRBC) and platelet-rich plasma (PRP), centrifuge whole blood using light spin (2,000 × g for 3 minutes plus deceleration time).
    - For the harvest of PRBC and fresh frozen plasma (FFP), centrifuge whole blood using a heavy spin (5,000 × g for 5 or 7 minutes plus deceleration time at a temperature of 4°C).

    The spinning forces the heavier components, such as RBCs to separate from the plasma and collect at the bottom of the bag. The plasma separated on the top can be collected in a satellite bag either by using a manual plasma extractor or an automated plasma extractor.

2. *Plasmapheresis*
    Blood is extracted from a donor, plasma is then removed and the rest of the blood is returned to the donor.

Plasma collected must be rapidly frozen either using a snap freezer or deep freezer maintaining a temperature between −75 and −80°C. Once frozen, FFP should be stored in a deep freezer, maintaining the temperature between −30 and −40°C. Ideally, the time taken to freeze the plasma to a core temperature less than −30°C should not exceed 1 hour from the time freezing is commenced. Core temperature refers to the temperature in the center of the unit—the warmest part of the plasma pack during the freezing process. FFP contains normal amounts of all coagulation factors, antithrombin, and ADAMTS13, and it has a shelf life of 1 year when stored at a temperature less than −30°C. PVC bags used for storing plasma have a glass transition temperature of about −25 to −30°C. Hence, the containers should be handled with care to prevent breakage during handling and transport, as they are brittle at such low temperatures.

Q11. How are random donor platelets prepared?

Ans: Random donor platelets concentrates (RDPs/PCs) are prepared either from whole blood donations (random donor/recovered platelets).[12]

The RDPs from whole blood can be prepared by two methods:
1. Platelet rich plasma (PRP) method
2. Buffy coat (BC) method

The PRP method involves a soft spin followed by a hard spin, while in the BC method RDPs are prepared by a hard spin followed by a soft spin. BC method causes less platelet activation during processing as PCs are centrifuged against the cellular elements of whole blood compared to the PRP preparation method, where platelets are centrifuged against the platelet bag. PCs are usually suspended in 50–70 mL of plasma. However, the volume of plasma for resuspension of platelets is determined by the maintenance of pH of not <6 during the storage period. Once prepared, PCs should be stored between 20° and 24°C with continuous gentle agitation throughout storage for a period of 5 days.

REFERENCES

1. Mitra R, Mishra N, Rath GP. Blood groups systems. Indian J Anaesth. 2014;58(5):524-8.
2. Li HY, Guo K. Blood Group Testing. Front Med (Lausanne). 2022;9:827619.
3. British Committee for Standards in Haematology; Milkins C, Berryman J, Cantwell C, Elliott C, Haggas R, Jones J, et al. Guidelines for pre-transfusion compatibility procedures in blood transfusion laboratories. British Committee for Standards in Haematology. Transfus Med. 2013;23(1):3-35.

4. Parker V, Tormey CA. The Direct Antiglobulin Test: Indications, Interpretation, and Pitfalls. Arch Pathol Lab Med. 2017;141(2):305-10.
5. Zantek ND, Koepsell SA, Tharp DR Jr, Cohn CS. The direct antiglobulin test: A critical step in the evaluation of hemolysis. Am J Hematol. 2012;87(7):707-9.
6. Qiu H, Wang X, Shao Y. Forward and reverse typing discrepancy and crossmatch incompatibility of ABO blood groups: cause analysis and treatment. Hematology. 2023;28(1):2240146.
7. Booth GS, Gehrie EA, Bolan CD, Savani BN. Clinical Guide to ABO-incompatible allogeneic stem cell transplantation. Biol Blood Marrow Transplant. 2013;19(8):1152-8.
8. Hendrickson JE, Hillyer CD. Noninfectious serious hazards of transfusion. Anesth Analg. 2009;108(3):759-69.
9. Awan M, Buriak I, Fleck, Fuller B, Goltsev A, Kerby J, et al. Dimethyl Sulfoxide: a central player since the dawn of cryobiology, is efficacy balanced by toxicity? Regen Med. 2020;15(3):1463-91.
10. Callum JL, Karkouti K, Lin Y. Cryoprecipitate: The current state of knowledge. Transfus Med Rev. 2009;23(3):177-88.
11. Liumbruno G, Bennardello F, Lattanzio A, Piccoli P, Rossettias G; Italian Society of Transfusion Medicine and Immunohaematology (SIMTI). Recommendations for the transfusion of plasma and platelets. Blood Transfus. 2009;7(3):132-50.
12. Sloand EM, Yu M, Klein HG. Comparison of random-donor platelet concentrates prepared from whole blood units and platelets prepared from single-donor apheresis collections. Transfusion. 1996;36(11-12):955-59.

29. Blood Banking Procedures

Kriti Batni, Satyam Arora

Q1. What do you understand by secretor and soluble ABH antigens?

Ans: *Secretor:* This refers to an individual who has the ability to secrete blood group antigens (ABH antigens) into body fluids, such as saliva, mucus, and other secretions.[1] This ability is determined by the presence of the *Se* gene, which encodes an enzyme that adds blood group antigens to glycoproteins and glycolipids in secretions. Approximately 80% of people are secretors. The *Se* gene (Secretor gene) is located on chromosome 19.
- *Secretors:* Individuals with at least one dominant Se allele (usually SeSe or Sese) can secrete blood group antigens into their saliva and other bodily fluids.
- *Nonsecretors:* Individuals who are homozygous recessive for the secretor gene (sese) do not have this enzyme and thus cannot secrete blood group antigens into their saliva or other secretions.

Soluble ABH antigens: These are blood group antigens (A, B, and H) that are found in body fluids and secretions when they are released from the surfaces of cells into the surrounding fluid. These antigens are present in the secretions of secretors and can be detected in saliva, urine, and other bodily fluids. In contrast, nonsecretors do not have these antigens in their secretions because they lack the *Se* gene.

Utility in transfusion medicine: Blood group discrepancies occur when there is a mismatch between the expected and actual blood group results obtained from blood typing tests. These discrepancies can arise for various reasons, including technical errors, physiological factors, or biological variations. Saliva grouping can sometimes help resolve or understand certain types of discrepancies. Here's how:
- *Confirming secretor status:* If there is a discrepancy between the blood group determined by serological testing and the blood group inferred from other tests (e.g., historical data or patient records), saliva grouping can help confirm whether the individual is a secretor. This can be relevant if discrepancies involve the presence or absence of specific antigens that are known to be secreted into body fluids.
- *Antigen variation:* Discrepancies might occur due to rare antigen variations or weak expression of antigens. Saliva grouping can help confirm the presence of ABH antigens in body fluids, which can sometimes provide clues about the strength of antigen expression or the presence of antigens that might not be evident in standard blood tests.
- *Confirming consistency:* If there are inconsistencies in blood typing results, such as unexpected reactions in the blood typing panels, saliva grouping can provide additional

confirmation about the presence or absence of specific antigens, helping to rule out or confirm potential technical errors in blood testing.

Q2. How is antibody identification done?

Ans: Antibody identification involves detecting and characterizing antibodies present in a patient's serum that may react with specific antigens on red blood cells (RBCs).[2] This process is crucial for ensuring compatibility between donor and recipient blood.
- *Preparation of the sample*:
  - *Sample collection:* Blood samples are collected from the patient, usually in a tube without anticoagulant (serum separator tube).
  - *Serum separation:* The blood sample is centrifuged to separate the serum from the RBCs.
- *Screening for unexpected antibodies*:
  - *Antibody screen [indirect antiglobulin test (IAT)]:* The patient's serum is tested against a panel of RBCs with known antigenic profiles by antibody screen (indirect Coombs test). Cell panels comprise specific cells of group O and maybe of varying numbers (screening panel; 2-cell panel, 3-cell panel, etc.). They may be in-house prepared or commercially available.
  - *Antibody panel testing:* If the antibody screen is positive, further testing uses a more comprehensive panel of RBCs covering a wide range of known antigens (identification panel; 11-cell panel or 16-cell panel, etc.).
- *Analyzing reaction patterns*:
  - *Pattern analysis:* The pattern of reactions (positive or negative) with the panel cells help identify the specific antibodies present. For example, if the patient's serum reacts with RBCs expressing antigen A but not with cells lacking antigen A, it suggests an antibody against antigen A.
  - *Cross-out method:* The reactions are compared against known antibody profiles to determine the specific antibody. This often involves using reference charts or databases that match reaction patterns with specific antibodies. Record the reactions (positive or negative) of the patient's serum with each panel cell on the antigram chart. This will create a pattern of reactivity. Cross out or eliminate the antigens associated with the positive reactions. This helps narrow down the list of potential antibodies. Compare the pattern of positive reactions against the antigen profiles of the panel cells. Antigens that are consistently present in cells that react positively with the patient's serum are indicative of the antibody specificity.
- *Additional testing*:
  - *Elution studies:* In some cases, if the antibody is not identified with the panel, an elution study might be done to remove (elute) the antibody from the RBCs and then test it again. This is only performed when the direct antiglobulin test (DAT) is positive.
  - *Phenotyping:* Testing the RBCs for specific antigens to confirm the absence or presence of those antigens which can help in identifying the antibodies.

Q3. What is hemolytic disease of newborns?

Ans: Hemolytic disease of the newborn (HDN), also known as erythroblastosis fetalis, is a condition where the baby's RBCs are destroyed by antibodies from the mother's blood. This condition typically arises when there is an incompatibility between the blood types of the mother and the fetus, leading to severe anemia and other complications in the newborn.[3]

Causes and Mechanisms

Blood group incompatibility:
- *Rh incompatibility:* The most common cause of clinically significant HDN is due to Rh incompatibility. This occurs when an Rh-negative mother has developed antibodies against Rh-positive blood cells, usually from a previous pregnancy or transfusion. If the fetus is Rh-positive, these antibodies [immunoglobulin (Ig)G type] can cross the placenta and attack the fetus's RBCs. This is the most common form of HDN and the antibody implicated in majority cases is anti D.
- *ABO incompatibility:* This usually occurs when the mother has type O blood and the fetus has type A, B, or AB blood. Although less severe than Rh incompatibility, ABO incompatibility can still lead to HDN.

Pathophysiology

- The mother's antibodies (IgG type) against fetal RBC antigens cross the placenta and bind to the RBCs of the fetus.
- This binding activates the immune response, leading to the destruction of fetal RBCs (hemolysis).
- The destruction of RBCs leads to anemia, and the fetus may also develop jaundice due to the accumulation of bilirubin from the breakdown of hemoglobin.

Symptoms and Effects

- *In utero symptoms:*
  - *Hydrops fetalis:* Severe form of HDN can cause fluid buildup in the fetal tissues and organs, leading to swelling and heart failure.
  - *Anemia:* Reduced RBC count may lead to poor oxygen delivery to tissues and organs.
- *At birth:*
  - *Jaundice:* Yellowing of the skin and eyes due to high bilirubin levels.
  - *Anemia:* Low RBC count can cause pallor and lethargy.
  - *Hepatosplenomegaly:* Organs may become enlarged due to increased work from clearing damaged RBCs.
  - *Kernicterus:* Severe jaundice can lead to bilirubin deposits in the brain, potentially causing neurological damage.

Diagnosis

Prenatal Testing
- Maternal IAT, maternal and cord blood group.
- *Ultrasound:* To monitor fetal growth, check for signs of hydrops fetalis (peak systolic velocity of the middle cerebral artery is >1.5MOM—indicative of anemia), and assess the condition of the fetus.

At Birth
- IAT and DAT of baby
- Serum bilirubin

Prevention

For Rh HDN—Rh immunoglobulin [Rho(D) immune globulin]: Administered to Rh-negative mothers during and after pregnancy to prevent the development of antibodies against Rh-positive RBCs. This is usually given around the 28th week of pregnancy and within 72 hours after delivery if the baby is Rh-positive.

Treatment

- Phototherapy
- *Exchange transfusion:* In severe cases, this procedure may be used to replace the baby's blood with donor blood to remove antibodies and excess bilirubin.
- *Intravenous immunoglobulin (IVIG):* Can be used to reduce hemolysis and bilirubin levels in some cases.

Q4. What are the minimum requirements for starting a blood bank?

Ans: Starting a blood bank in India involves complying with several regulations, including those stipulated in the Drugs and Cosmetics Act, 1940, and its amendments, particularly the Drugs and Cosmetics (Amendment) Act, 2020. These regulations ensure that blood banks operate safely, maintain high standards, and provide quality service.[4]

- *Licensing and registration*:
    - *License requirement (XIIB):* Blood banks must obtain a license from the Drug Control Authority. This includes both the initial registration and renewal of the license. License is valid for a period of 5 years after which it needs to be renewed. Each blood bank has a unique license number. The license mentions each component being prepared at the blood center.
    - *Eligibility criteria:* The premises must meet specific criteria related to space, equipment, and personnel as outlined in the regulations.
- *Infrastructure and facilities*:
    - *Building and space:* The facility should be spacious and designed to maintain cleanliness and sterility. It should include areas for blood collection, processing, testing, and storage—a minimum of 150 m^2.
    - *Equipment:* Adequate and properly maintained equipment for blood collection, separation, testing, and storage is mandatory.
    - *Storage requirement for the component:* Blood and its components must be stored in appropriate conditions, including refrigerators and freezers to maintain the required temperatures.
- *Staffing and personnel*:
    - *Qualified staff:* The blood bank must employ qualified personnel, including a Medical Officer, Blood Bank Technologist, nursing staff, and other supporting staff. The eligibility and experience of doctors, technicians, and staff should be as per the Drugs and Cosmetics Act, 1940, and its amendments.
    - *Training:* Staff must undergo regular training to stay updated on best practices and safety protocols.
- *Quality control and assurance*:
    - *Standard operating procedures (SOPs):* The blood bank must have SOPs for all processes including collection, testing, processing, and storage.

- Quality assurance: Regular quality checks and audits must be conducted to ensure compliance with standards.
- Testing and screening:
  - Testing: Blood must be mandatorily tested for infectious diseases, including human immunodeficiency virus (HIV), hepatitis B and C, malaria, and syphilis.
  - Donor screening: Proper screening of donors to ensure the safety and suitability of blood is essential.
- Documentation and records:
  - Record keeping: Accurate records of blood donations, testing results, and inventory must be maintained and should be kept for at least 5 years.
  - Reporting: Regular reports must be submitted to regulatory authorities as required the External Quality Assessment Scheme (EQAS).
- Regulatory compliance:
  Compliance with amendments: Adherence to the latest amendments in the Drugs and Cosmetics Act, including those introduced by the Drugs and Cosmetics (Amendment) Act, 2020, which may update requirements related to blood bank operations.

Q5. How are blood components screened for viral infections? What is nucleic acid testing (NAT)?

Ans: Testing for transfusion-transmitted infections (TTIs) is crucial for ensuring the safety of blood components. The main testing modalities include serological tests based on enzyme-linked immunosorbent assay (ELISA) or chemiluminescence principle whereas nucleic acid-based tests (NATs) are an additional test on donated blood in India.[5] As per the Drugs and Cosmetics Act, 1940, and its amendments it is mandatory to test using a serological test. Each has specific uses, advantages, and limitations.

- Serological tests:
  - Enzyme-linked immunosorbent assay—detects antibodies or antigens in the blood. Common infections tested—HIV 1 and 2, hepatitis B virus (HBV), hepatitis C virus (HCV), syphilis. Sensitivity—high (70–100%) and specificity—High (90–100%).
  - Chemiluminescence—involves detecting light emitted from a chemical reaction to identify specific antibodies or antigens. Purpose—detects antibodies or antigens using light emission. Infections tested—HIV 1 and 2, HBV, HCV, and syphilis. Sensitivity—high (90–100%), specificity—high (90–100%).
  - Rapid diagnostic tests (RDTs)—provides quick screening results. Common infections tested—HIV, malaria (in some cases). Techniques—lateral flow immunoassays for rapid screening. Sensitivity—moderate (70–90%), specificity—moderate (80–95%).
- Nucleic acid-based tests: Nucleic acid-based tests detect the genetic material of pathogens, offering high sensitivity and early detection. This test is not yet mandatory as per the Drugs and Cosmetics Act, 1940, and its amendments and it can be adopted as an additional layer of safety.
  - Polymerase chain reaction (PCR)—detects and quantifies specific deoxyribonucleic acid (DNA) or ribonucleic acid (RNA) sequences. Infections tested—HIV, HBV, and HCV. Techniques—real-time PCR, nested PCR. Sensitivity—very high (95–100%), specificity—very high (95–100%).
  - Transcription-mediated amplification (TMA)—amplifies RNA for detection of viral RNA. Infections tested—HIV and HCV. Techniques—TMA for RNA amplification. Sensitivity—very high (95–100%), specificity—very high (95–100%).

- Hybrid capture—detects specific RNA or DNA through hybridization and amplification, techniques—hybrid capture assays, sensitivity—high (80–95%), specificity-high (85–95%).

Q6. How is peripheral blood stem cell harvest done? What are the various machines available for stem cell harvest?

Ans: Peripheral blood stem cell (PBSC) harvest is a procedure used to collect stem cells from the bloodstream, which can then be used for transplantation or other therapeutic purposes.[6] Here is a detailed overview of how PBSC harvest is done and the various machines available for this process.

Peripheral Blood Stem Cell Harvest Procedure

- *Preharvest preparation:*
  - *Donor assessment:* A thorough evaluation of the donor's health and suitability for the procedure including human leukocyte antigens (HLAs) antigen typing and recipient anti HLA antibody typing.
  - *Mobilization:* The donor receives medications to increase the number of stem cells in the bloodstream. This is typically achieved using growth factors such as granulocyte colony-stimulating factor (G-CSF) administered via daily injections for 4–5 days before the collection or plerixafor which is sometimes used in combination with G-CSF to enhance stem cell mobilization.
- *Collection procedure:*
  - *Apheresis:* This is the primary method used for collecting stem cells from peripheral blood. The process involves the following steps:
    - *Placement of a central venous catheter:* A catheter is usually inserted into a large vein, often in the femoral or jugular, to facilitate venous access. Blood is drawn from the donor's body and passed through a cell separator machine. The machine separates stem cells from other blood components (RBCs, platelets, and plasma) and the remaining blood components are returned to the donor's body through the same catheter. Using peripheral access using a large bore cannula is preferred in cases of an allogenic harvest.
    - Harvesting from pediatric age group of patients is often very challenging and needs extra care and should only be done by trained apheresis physicians.
- *Postharvest care:*
  - *Monitoring:* The donor is monitored for any adverse reactions or complications.
  - *Recovery:* The donor may experience some fatigue or discomfort but generally recovers quickly. Regular follow-up ensures that the donor's blood counts return to normal.

Machines Available for Stem Cell Harvest

Several types of apheresis machines are used to collect peripheral blood stem cells. These machines utilize different methods of separation and collection.
- Continuous flow apheresis machines—use continuous flow of blood to separate components using centrifugal force. Efficient for collecting large volumes of stem cells in a single session. Examples: Cobe Spectra, Fenwal Amicus, Terumo Optia.

- Intermittent flow apheresis machines—use intermittent or pulsatile flow of blood for component separation. Blood is drawn in cycles, processed, and returned in stages. Allows for collection of stem cells in multiple cycles, often used when continuous flow is not ideal. Examples: Baxter CS 3000 plus, Terumo blood and cell technologies (BCT) mononuclear cell (MNC).

Q7. What is donor lymphocyte harvest? How donor lymphocytes are harvested?

Ans: Donor lymphocyte harvest involves collecting lymphocytes from a donor for therapeutic purposes, such as boosting the immune response in patients with cancer specifically chronic myelogenous leukemia (CML). This process is particularly important in the context of adoptive immunotherapy and hematopoietic stem cell transplantation.[7]

Indications for Donor Lymphocyte Harvest
- *Post-transplantation immunotherapy:* To enhance the graft-versus-leukemia (GVL) effect in patients who have undergone stem cell or bone marrow (BM) transplantation. This helps in targeting residual cancer cells.
- *Adoptive cell therapy:* For treating cancers like leukemia or lymphoma by transferring donor-derived immune cells to the patient.
- *Treatment of viral infections:* In cases where the patient is immunocompromised, donor lymphocytes can help fight off viral infections.

Harvesting Donor Lymphocytes
- *Preharvest preparation:*
  - *Donor assessment and mobilization (only if required):* Donors are given medications to increase the number of lymphocytes in the blood. This may include the use of growth factors like granulocyte colony-stimulating factor (G-CSF).
- *Collection procedure:*
  - *Apheresis:* Lymphocytes are collected using apheresis, a procedure where blood is drawn from the donor, processed to separate lymphocytes from other blood components, and then returned to the donor. The apheresis machine separates lymphocytes from other blood components using a centrifugation process. The remaining blood components are returned to the donor's body through the same catheter.

Machines Used for Donor Lymphocyte Harvest
- Continuous flow apheresis machines
- Intermittent flow apheresis machines

Types of Donor Lymphocyte Infusion
- *Standard donor lymphocyte infusion (DLI):* Involves infusing a standard dose of donor lymphocytes into the patient. It is used to boost the immune response against residual cancer cells or infections.
- *Escalated DLI:* Involves administering progressively higher doses of donor lymphocytes if the initial infusions do not achieve the desired effect.
- *Adoptive T-cell therapy:* A specialized form of DLI where specific T-cells from the donor are selected, expanded, and infused into the patient.

Q8. What precautions should be taken when there is a major blood group mismatch between the donor and the stem cell transplant recipient? How much red blood cell contamination is allowed in stem cell products in bone marrow and peripheral blood stem cell harvest?

Ans: A major ABO mismatch is a condition when the donor for hematopoietic stem cell transplant (HSCT) possesses an A and/or B antigen and the recipient has the corresponding isoagglutinin against the same.[8] For example the donor is A and the recipient is O or B. A major blood group mismatch between the donor and recipient in stem cell transplantation can lead to significant complications, such as hemolytic reactions.

Precautions and Management Strategies

Pretransplant Compatibility Testing
- *Blood group typing and crossmatch:* Thorough pretransplant blood group and antibody screening and crossmatching. Crossmatching between donor and recipient to detect any immediate reactions.
- *Human leukocyte antigen matching:* While blood group compatibility is important, HLA matching is also crucial for minimizing the risk of graft-versus-host disease (GVHD).

Desensitization Protocols
- *Blood group antigen removal:* In cases of ABO incompatibility, techniques such as red cell reduction may be used to reduce the red cell content of the stem cell harvested from the donor.
- *Antibody reduction by plasma exchange:* In cases of ABO incompatibility, techniques may be used to reduce the recipient's antibodies against the donor's blood group antigens. In some cases, plasma exchange may be used to remove antibodies from the recipient's blood.

Post-transplant Monitoring
- *Monitor for reactions:* Close monitoring for signs of hemolytic reactions, including fever, chills, and jaundice.
- Special monitoring for possible complications such as pure red cell aplasia, passenger lymphocyte syndrome, etc.
- *GVHD surveillance:* Regular monitoring for signs of GVHD, including skin rash, liver dysfunction, and gastrointestinal symptoms.

Supportive care: Immunosuppressive therapy—use immunosuppressive medications as prescribed to prevent GVHD and manage any immune reactions.

Graft manipulation techniques: Red cell depletion—techniques such as red cell depletion may be employed [using sedimenting agents like hydroxyethyl starch (HES)] to reduce the risk of hemolysis and reactions caused by RBC antigens.

Red Blood Cell Contamination Limits in Stem Cell Products

In stem cell products, RBC contamination can affect the safety and efficacy of the transplant. The limits for RBC contamination [according to American Society for Transplantation and Cellular Therapy (ASTCT) and the European Society for Blood and Marrow Transplantation

(EBMT)] are defined to ensure the quality and safety of the stem cell product. The specific acceptable levels may vary based on the type of stem cell product:

Marrow—donor hematopoietic progenitor cells (HPCs) may be obtained from BM [(HPC(M)], apheresis-derived peripheral blood progenitor cells [(HPC(A)], or umbilical cord blood [(HPC(C)] which differ concerning the volume of RBCs, plasma, and the number and maturity of lymphocytes present. For example, RBCs comprise 25-35% of the total volume of HPC(M), thus, HPC derived in this manner may contain the equivalent of 1-2 units of RBCs; resulting in an increased risk for acute hemolysis, particularly in the setting of a major ABOi HPC transplantation.

Apheresis—in comparison, HPC(A) possesses characteristically small numbers of RBCs (hematocrit ~2-3% or <10 mL RBCs) and thus, the risk of acute hemolysis is thought to be less; however, it contains a 10-fold greater number of lymphocytes.

Cord—in contrast, while HPC(C) initially contains proportionally large volumes of RBCs [similar to HPC(M)], it usually undergoes processing prestorage to reduce total volume and RBC content; further, lymphocytes from HPC(C) have not yet been immunized to RBC antigens, therefore, transfusion of HPC(C) is associated with a reduced risk of delayed hemolytic transfusion reactions and pure red cell aplasia (PRCA).

Q9. **What are the kinetics of blood group transition post-ABO-mismatched allogeneic stem cell transplant?**

Ans:
- *Day 0-7:* Initial phase
  - *Transplant day (Day 0):* The stem cell transplant is performed, introducing donor hematopoietic stem cells into the recipient. At this point, the recipient's blood primarily consists of their existing autologous blood cells.[9]
  - *Early days (Day 1-7):* The recipient's blood still predominantly reflects their original blood group. The donor's stem cells begin to engraft, but the existing recipient's blood cells continue to circulate.
- *Day 8-14:* Early engraftment
  - *Engraftment begins:* Donor stem cells start to proliferate and begin producing new blood cells. The first cells to engraft are platelets and neutrophils. This phase may show early signs of transition, but the recipient's blood type is still largely reflective of their original type due to the presence of their preexisting cells.
  - *Mixed field reactions:* The blood group may show mixed-field reactions where both the donor's and recipient's blood group antigens are present. This is common as the donor's cells begin to populate but have not yet completely taken over.
- *Day 15-21:* RBC engraftment
  - *Red blood cell engraftment:* Typically, around day 21, the donor's RBCs begin to dominate as the engraftment process progresses. By this time, the recipient's blood group starts to shift more noticeably toward that of the donor.
- *Day 22-30:* Stabilization
  - *Complete transition:* By approximately day 30.
  - The recipient's blood group should generally reflect that of the donor, assuming successful engraftment. Most of the recipient's blood cells are now produced by the donor's stem cells.

Stabilized Blood Group

Immunoglobulin (Ig) levels seem to recover in parallel to B-cell reconstitution, in which recovery of Ig subclasses usually occurs in a distinctive order. As a reflection of normal ontogeny, IgM production will reconstitute relatively early and, on average, reaches normal levels within the first 6 months after HSCT. Similar to IgM, IgG generally reaches normal levels in the second half of the first year. Due to this variability in B-cell engraftment and functionality, isohemagglutinins in ABO-compatible HSCT cases usually start to appear within 1–3 months post-transplant, but this can vary based on individual circumstances and immune system recovery. Regular monitoring is essential to detect and manage any potential issues early.

Q10. **What is the pathophysiology of pure red cell aplasia following ABO mismatched allogeneic stem cell transplant?**

Ans: PRCA happens in a background of an ABO mismatched stem cell transplant which involves a donor and recipient with different ABO blood groups.[10] This mismatch can cause several complications, including blood group-specific immune reactions.

The presence of prolonged erythroid aplasia with myeloid, lymphoid, and megakaryocyte engraftment in BM biopsies and prolonged transfusion dependency for > 90 days after HSCT in the absence of relapse, infections, or drug-related toxicity was noted to determine the occurrence of PRCA after HSCT.

Immune mechanisms leading to PRCA are:
- *Alloimmunization and immune reaction:* During and after an ABO mismatched transplant, the recipient's immune system can recognize the donor's blood group antigens as foreign. This immune recognition can trigger an alloimmune *response.*
- *Antibody production:* The recipient's immune system may produce antibodies against the donor's blood group antigens. These antibodies primarily target RBC precursors in the BM.
- *Direct destruction:* The antibodies can directly bind to and destroy RBC precursors (erythroblasts) in the BM, leading to reduced RBC production.
- *Graft-versus-host disease (GVHD):* In some cases, PRCA can be related to GVHD, where donor T-cells attack the recipient's tissues, including the BM.
- *Immune cell attack:* Donor T-cells may attack and damage the erythroid progenitor cells in the BM, further exacerbating the reduction in RBC production.

Bone marrow impact: In PRCA, the BM is typically normocellular or hypercellular with a significant decrease in erythroid precursors. This contrasts with other types of anemia where the BM may be less cellular or depleted. The specific inhibition of erythropoiesis (RBC production) occurs while other hematopoietic lineages (e.g., granulocytes, platelets) remain relatively unaffected.

Clinical Manifestations

Anemia with low reticulocyte count indicates ineffective erythropoiesis. Prolonged RBC transfusion support beyond 30 days of infusion.

Diagnostic and Therapeutic Considerations

- PRCA is diagnosed based on clinical presentation, BM examination, and exclusion of other causes of anemia.

- *Bone marrow biopsy:* Shows an adequate number of RBC precursors but a decrease in mature RBCs.
- *Antibody testing:* To identify any donor-specific or recipient-specific antibodies that may be contributing to the destruction of RBC precursors.

Treatment

Management focuses on treating the underlying cause and alleviating anemia, use of immunosuppressive therapies to suppress the immune response if related to GVHD or alloimmunization. Blood transfusions are often necessary to manage anemia. In cases where antibodies are identified, transfusions with RBCs lacking the specific antigen can help prevent further destruction of transfused cells.

Q11. What is passenger lymphocyte syndrome?

Ans: Passenger lymphocyte syndrome (PLS) is indeed more commonly associated with solid organ transplants than with stem cell transplants. The presence of donor-derived lymphocytes in the transplanted organ can lead to a variety of immune-related reactions specifically hemolytic anemia with a positive direct Coombs test.[11]

Clinical context and presentation: Fever, skin rash—often a maculopapular rash and patients may present with anemia. Hemolytic anemia—a notable presentation of PLS can be hemolytic anemia. This occurs due to the production of antibodies by donor lymphocytes against recipient RBCs. The hemolysis can lead to symptoms such as fatigue, pallor, jaundice, and an elevated reticulocyte count.

Direct Coombs test (DCT): In PLS, the DCT may be positive due to the presence of donor-derived antibodies or complement components attached to recipient RBCs. This is indicative of an immune-mediated hemolysis.

Pathophysiology of hemolytic anemia in PLS: Donor lymphocytes, present in the transplanted organ, may produce antibodies against the recipient's RBC antigens. These antibodies can destroy RBCs. The antibodies bind to the recipient's RBCs, leading to their destruction in the spleen and liver and complement activation. The hemolytic anemia associated with PLS is generally transient and resolves as the donor lymphocytes are cleared from the recipient's system. This occurs over weeks to months.

Diagnosis and Management

Diagnosis is based on the clinical presentation of symptoms and laboratory findings.
   Hemolytic anemia—low hemoglobin, elevated reticulocyte count, increased indirect bilirubin, and positive DCT. Other causes of hemolysis or anemia must be excluded.

Management

Supportive care: Treatment typically involves supportive care, including blood transfusions to manage anemia.

Immunosuppressive therapy: In severe or persistent cases, immunosuppressive therapy may be used to manage the immune response, though this is less common.

REFERENCES

1. Harmening DM, Firestone D. The ABO blood group system. In: Harmening DM (Ed). Modern Blood Banking & Transfusion Practices, 7th edition. Philadelphia: F.A. Davis Company; 2019.
2. Harmening DM, Firestone D. Detection and identification of antibodies. In: Harmening DM (Ed). Modern Blood Banking & Transfusion Practices, 7th edition. Philadelphia: F.A. Davis Company; 2019.
3. Jennifer Webb, Wen Lu, Meghan Delaney. Hemolytic disease of the fetus and newborn In: Simon TL, Gehrie EA, McCullough J, Roback JD (Eds). Rossi's principles of transfusion medicine, 6th edition. Oxford: Wiley-Blackwell; 2022.
4. Ministry of Health and Family Welfare, Government of India. Drugs and Cosmetics Act 1940 and Rules 1945. [online] Available from https://cdsco.gov.in/opencms/opencms/system/modules/CDSCO.WEB/elements/download_file_division.jsp?num_id=NTc2MQ==) [Last accessed April, 2025].
5. Directorate General of Health Services. Ministry of Health and Family Welfare, Government of India. Transfusion medicine technical manual, 3rd edition. India: DGHS, MoHFW, GoI; 2022.
6. Booth GS. Hematopoietic stems cells and transplantation. In: Simon TL, Gehrie EA, McCullough J, Roback JD (Eds). Rossi's Principles of transfusion medicine, 6th edition. Oxford: Wiley-Blackwell; 2022.
7. Fesnak AD, Siegel DL. Chimeric antigen receptor T cells and other cellular immunotherapies. In: Simon TL, Gehrie EA, McCullough J, Roback JD (Eds). Rossi's Principles of transfusion medicine, 6th edition. Oxford: Wiley-Blackwell; 2022.
8. Staley EM, Schwartz J, Pham HP. An update on ABO incompatible hematopoietic progenitor cell transplantation. Transfus Apheres Sci. 2016;54(3):337-44.
9. Van der Maas NG, Berghuis D, van der Burg M, Lankester AC. B Cell reconstitution and influencing factors after hematopoietic stem cell transplantation in children. Front Immunol. 2019;10:782.
10. Mangla A, Hamad H. Pure red cell aplasia. In: StatPearls. Treasure Island (FL): StatPearls Publishing; 2024.
11. Dubey A, Pandey H, Sonker A, Chaudhary RK. A case of passenger lymphocyte syndrome following minor ABO incompatible renal transplantation. Asian J Transfus Sci. 2014;8(1):56-8.

CAR T-cell Therapy

Sanjeev Kumar Sharma, Divya Doval

Q1. What is CAR T-cell therapy?

Ans: Chimeric antigen receptor (CAR) T-cell therapy is called "immunotherapy" because it uses a patient's own T cells (lymphocytes that are part of the immune system) to recognize and attack cancer cells.[1] Deoxyribonucleic acid (DNA) is introduced into the T cells to produce CARs on the surfaces of the cells. Genetic modification is done outside the body: The modified cells are then reproduced in large numbers before they are reintroduced into patients' body. This is vital in treating leukemias, which have already damaged the body's immune cell "factories." CAR T-cells are, therefore, considered "living drugs" that can become more potent after they are administered.[2,3] Lentiviral gene transfer is the most frequently applied procedure to engineer CAR T-cells for clinical use.

Q2. How is CAR T-cell therapy done?

Ans: In autologous CAR T-cell therapy, T cells are collected by leukapheresis and sent to a laboratory.[4] This is similar to stem cell collection before autologous transplantation (but involves collection of CD3 cells rather than CD34 cells). As CD3 cells are present in the blood no mobilizing medication is needed. In the lab, T cells are engineered to express the CAR, and the number of these engineered CAR T-cells is expanded. This process may take 2–4 weeks depending upon the product. Then these modified cells are frozen and sent to the patient's treatment center. Meanwhile the patient receives some lymphodepletion chemotherapy. Then, these modified cells are reinfused into the patient's bloodstream, where they can seek and kill cancer cells.

Q3. What are the side effects of CAR T-cell therapy?

Ans: Early recognition and appropriate management is the key for effective management of complications. The incidence and severity of complications may depend upon the type of cellular product used and also the type of tumor and disease burden. The complications of CAR T-cell therapy include:
- *Cytokine release syndrome (CRS)*: This potentially serious side effect is frequently associated with CAR T-cell therapy. When the CAR T-cells encounter their antigen targets, they are rapidly activated. At this point, numerous inflammatory cytokines, including interleukin-6 (IL-6), tumor necrosis factor-alpha (TNF-α) and interferon gamma (IFN-γ), are released. These cytokines cause acute systemic inflammatory syndrome characterized by fever and multiorgan dysfunction syndrome. Clinical manifestations may range from

mild flu like symptoms to potentially life-threatening signs and symptoms (systemic inflammatory response syndrome). Tocilizumab (IL-6 antagonist) is approved for patients who develop CAR T-cell-induced severe or life-threatening CRS.[5] Besides this, Anakinra (IL-1 antagonist), Siltuximab (IL-6 antagonist), Emapalumab (IFN-γ blocking antibody) and other supportive care is needed.
- *Immune effector cell-associated neurotoxicity syndrome (ICANS)*: This refers to the neurological complications, which develop as a result of CAR T-cells infusion. The underlying cause of ICANS is unclear. It is thought to be driven by proinflammatory cytokines entering the central nervous system even if the CAR T-cells themselves do not. It often presents with subtle word finding difficulties followed by confusion or seizures. Levetiracetam may be used as prophylaxis and corticosteroids are the mainstay of ICANS management along with neurology team support.
- *Hemophagocytic lymphohistiocytosis (HLH)*: This resembles CRS but is characterized by hyperferritinemia, transaminitis, and coagulopathy (hypofibrinogenemia and thrombocytopenia). Anakinra (IL-1 antagonist) along with steroids may be used for management.
- *B-cell aplasia*: CAR T-cell therapy that targets antigens found on the surface of B cells destroys not only cancerous B cells but also normal B cells. Killing healthy B cells along with cancer cells is worthwhile for patients with otherwise incurable blood cancers (whereas natural immune systems would not make this calculated sacrifice). Therefore, B-cell aplasia is an expected result of successful CD19-specific CAR T-cell treatment, and it has served as a useful indicator of ongoing CAR T-cell activity.
- *Other complications of CAR T-cell therapy include*: Tumor lysis syndrome, anaphylaxis, and infections.
- Allogeneic "off-the-shelf" CAR T-cells are engineered by genetically eliminating the T-cell receptor alpha (TCR-α) constant (TRAC) locus and/or human leukocyte antigen (HLA) from the T-cell surface, reducing the risk of graft versus host disease (GVHD) and allograft rejection. As the name suggests they are readily available and can be administered as needed without having to wait for 2–4 weeks of manufacturing and are potentially cheaper.

Q4. What should be the properties of a tumor antigen for recognition by a CAR T-cell?

Ans:
- The antigen should be expressed on the cell surface and readily accessible.
- It should have a uniform expression on all malignant cells.
- The antigen should not undergo down regulation or deletion (i.e., no escape variants).
- It should not be expressed on normal tissue cells.
- It should be easy to reproduce it in laboratory.

Q5. How tumor cells escape CAR T-cells?

Ans:
- Antigen loss represents the ultimate adaptation of a cancer cell to the selective pressure of targeted immunotherapy. Complete target loss is a phenomenon typically occurring after T-cell-based therapy, such as CAR T-cell. In B-cell malignancies, CD19 loss has been noted in up to 40% of patients with B-cell acute lymphoblastic leukemia treated with different

CAR 19 products.[6] Antigen loss is the key mechanism of resistance to novel immunotherapies targeting CD19, CD20, and CD22.
- *Exhaustion of CAR T-cells*: It was shown that tumor-infiltrating CAR T-cells undergo rapid loss of functionality, limiting their therapeutic efficacy. This hyporesponsiveness appears to be reversible when the T cells are isolated away from the tumor.[7]
- *Microenvironment-mediated tumor resistance*: The bone marrow tumor microenvironment is known to upregulate antiapoptotic mechanisms in tumor cells through tight cross—talk of mesenchymal stromal cells (MSCs) and tumor cells.

Q6. Is bridging therapy necessary before CAR T-cell therapy?

Ans: Bridging therapy can be given after leukapheresis and before lymphodepletion during CAR T-cell manufacturing. The primary goal of bridging therapies is to prevent uncontrolled progression of the underlying disease during the manufacturing period before CAR T-cell infusion. Several studies indicate that a high tumor burden is associated with an increased risk of complications after CAR T-cell infusion.[8] Therefore, controlling the disease and even possibly decreasing the tumor burden is critical during the manufacturing period. The choice of bridging therapies is essential for the success of the procedure. It can be either chemotherapy or radiation.

CAR T-cells have been evaluated in patients with refractory and early relapsed non-Hodgkin lymphoma. Being refractory to the last line of chemotherapy was not a significant prognostic factor in these studies. Therefore, in contrast to autologous or allogeneic stem cell transplant (SCT), being in remission is not a prerequisite for the application of CAR-T therapy. The primary challenge limiting the use of CAR T-cells in myeloid malignancies is the absence of an ideal antigen. Myeloid antigens are often coexpressed on normal hematopoietic stem/progenitor cells (HSPCs).

Q7. What are the current indications for CAR T-cell therapy?

Ans: CAR T-cells can recognize antigens on the surface of cancer cells without human major histocompatibility complex (MHC) molecules unlike normal T cells. Therefore, CAR T-cells can distinguish a wider range of targets than natural T cells. The indications of CAR T-cell therapy include:[9]
- Refractory/relapsed B-cell precursor acute lymphoblastic leukemia.
- Relapsed or refractory diffuse large B-cell lymphoma (DLBCL).
- Adult patients with relapsed or refractory follicular lymphoma.
- Adult patients with relapsed or refractory mantle cell lymphoma.
- Relapsed or refractory multiple myeloma.

REFERENCES

1. Gill S, Maus MV, Porter DL. Chimeric antigen receptor T-cell therapy: 25 years in the making. Blood Rev. 2016;30(3):157-67.
2. Moretti A, Ponzo M, Nicolette CA, Tcherepanova IY, Biondi A, Magnani CF. The past, present, and future of non-viral CAR T cells. Front Immunol. 2022;13:867013.
3. Brudno JN, Maus MV, Hinrichs CS. CAR T cells and T-Cell therapies for cancer: A translational science review. JAMA. 2024;332(22):1924-35.
4. Levine BL, Miskin J, Wonnacott K, Keir C. Global manufacturing of CAR T Cell Therapy molecular therapy. Methods & clinical development. 2017;4:92-101.

5. Brudno JN, Kochenderfer JN. Recent advances in CAR T-cell toxicity: mechanisms, manifestations and management. Blood Rev. 2019:34;45-55.
6. Orlando EJ, Han X, Tribouley C, Wood PA, Leary RJ, Riester M, et al. Genetic mechanisms of target antigen loss in CAR19 therapy of acute lymphoblastic leukemia. Nat Med. 2018;24(10):1504-6.
7. Moon EK, Wang LC, Dol DV, Wilson CB, Ranganathan R, Sun J, et al. Multifactorial T-cell hypofunction that is reversible can limit the efficacy of chimeric antigen receptor-transduced human T cells in solid tumors. Clin Cancer Res. 2014;20(16):4262-73.
8. Cohen AD, Garfall AL, Stadtmauer EA, Melenhorst JJ, Lacey SF, Lancaster E, et al. B cell maturation antigen-specific CAR-T cells are clinically active in multiple myeloma. J Clin Invest. 2019;129(6):2210-21.
9. Chen YJ, Abila B, Mostafa Kamel Y. CAR-T: What Is Next? Cancers (Basel). 2023;15(3):663.

31 Clinical Case Studies

Kundan Mishra

Q1. A 65-year-old male presented with progressively increasing weakness, pedal edema, and bleeding from nose for last 4 weeks. On examination, he was found to have enlarged tongue and hepatomegaly. He also had proteinuria. His echocardiography revealed left ventricular ejection fraction (LVEF) of 40%.
  a. How will you evaluate this patient?
  b. How will you confirm the diagnosis of amyloidosis?
  c. What are the prognostic risks markers of amyloidosis?
  d. What is the survival of this patient?
  e. How will you treat this patient?

Ans:
  1a. A patient presenting with unexplained pedal edema, epistaxis, macroglossia, hepatomegaly, proteinuria, restrictive cardiomyopathy, should be evaluated for AL amyloidosis. The evaluation includes serum and urine protein electrophoresis with immunofixation electrophoresis, serum free light chain analysis, and an abdominal fat pad aspirate and bone marrow biopsy.[1]
  1b. Diagnosis of systemic AL amyloidosis requires the presence of all of the following four criteria (International Myeloma Working Group):[2]
  - Presence of an amyloid-related systemic syndrome (e.g., renal, liver, heart, gastrointestinal tract, or peripheral nerve involvement).
  - Positive amyloid staining by Congo red in any tissue (e.g., fat aspirate, bone marrow, or organ biopsy).
  - Evidence that amyloid is light-chain-related established by direct examination of the amyloid using mass spectrometry-based proteomic analysis, or immunoelectron microscopy, and
  - Evidence of a monoclonal plasma cell proliferative disorder (serum or urine monoclonal protein, abnormal free light-chain ratio, or clonal plasma cells in the bone marrow)

  1c. The prognosis depends upon the stage of the disease. The Mayo 2012 staging system uses NT-proBNP ≥1,800 ng/L, cardiac troponin T ≥0.025 µg/L, and the difference between involved and uninvolved serum free light chains (dFLC) ≥18 mg/dL as risk factors.[3] There are four stages as follows:
  - Stage I—none elevated
  - Stage II—one elevated

- Stage III—two elevated
- Stage IV—three elevated

For patients classified as having stage I, II, III, or IV disease, median overall survival from diagnosis was 94, 40, 14, and 6 months, respectively.

1d. For patients classified as having stage I, II, III, or IV disease, median overall survival from diagnosis was 94, 40, 14, and 6 months, respectively.[3]

1e. Treatment includes induction therapy followed by stem cell transplant in fit patients. The preferred induction therapy varies and can include two, three, or four-drug regimens. The commonly used regimen is daratumumab plus cyclophosphamide, bortezomib, and dexamethasone (DaraCyBorD).[4]

Q2. A 35-year-old pregnant female with 7 months of gestation presents with bleeding from gums and fever for 7 days. She was found to have pancytopenia and her peripheral smear showed 40% atypical promyelocytes.

a. What is the diagnosis and how will you confirm it?
b. How will you treat this patient?
c. What is the risk to the fetus?

Ans:

2a. Bleeding manifestation with atypical promyelocytes on peripheral smear are suggestive of acute promyelocytic leukemia (APL). APL represents a medical emergency with a high rate of early mortality, often due to hemorrhage from a characteristic coagulopathy. It is strongly recommended to start treatment with a differentiation agent (e.g., tretinoin, also known as all-trans retinoic acid or ATRA) without delay as soon as the diagnosis is suspected based on cytologic and clinical criteria. If the diagnosis is not confirmed, ATRA can be discontinued and treatment changed to that used for other types of acute myeloid leukemia.

Reverse transcriptase polymerase chain reaction (RT-PCR) for promyelocytic leukemia retinoic acid receptor α (PML-RARA) is considered to be the current "gold standard" method for confirming the diagnosis of APL.[5]

2b. All-trans retinoic acid combined with arsenic trioxide (ATO) or anthracycline-based chemotherapy is the standard of care for APL. The combination of ATRA plus ATO yields excellent outcomes in low-risk APL and intermediate-risk APL. There is still relatively limited information on the comparative value of combination treatment with ATRA plus ATO in patients with high-risk APL.

APL with pregnancy: ATRA and chemotherapy are reasonably safe when given to patients with APL presenting during the second or third trimester of pregnancy.
ATO is only used after delivery. When ATO or chemotherapy are needed after delivery, breastfeeding is contraindicated.[6,7]

2c. Abortion rate significantly decreases as gestational age increases, with 88%, 30%, and 6% of pregnancies ending in abortion during the first, second, and third trimester, respectively.[8]

Q3. A 27-year-old female was diagnosed as a case of immune thrombocytopenia 2 years back and was treated with steroids for 4 weeks but was lost to follow-up after that. Now she presented with 10 weeks gestation and bleeding from gums. Her complete

blood count (CBC) revealed platelet count of 10,000/μL. Her white cell count was normal and there were no schistocytes.
a. What is your diagnosis?
b. Is it gestational thrombocytopenia or immune thrombocytopenia (ITP)? How will the treatment differ?
c. How will you manage this patient?
d. What will be your treatment approach if she does not respond to steroids?
e. What is the risk to fetus?

Ans:
3a. *Chronic ITP*
Immune thrombocytopenia (ITP) earlier called as idiopathic thrombocytopenic purpura, is an acquired immunological disorder caused by autoantibodies against platelet antigens. It is typically characterized by mucocutaneous bleeding and low platelet count on peripheral blood smear. It is the most common causes of thrombocytopenia in otherwise asymptomatic adults.
As per the time since diagnosis, ITP is classified as newly diagnosed, persistent, or chronic.[9]
- Newly diagnosed—up to 3 months since diagnosis.
- Persistent—3–12 months since diagnosis.
- Chronic—more than 12 months since diagnosis.

3b. It is ITP.
Gestational thrombocytopenia (GT) is also called as incidental thrombocytopenia of pregnancy. GT may occur during the first trimester, but it becomes more common as gestation progresses, with the highest frequency at the time of delivery, when the frequency is 5–10%.
While GT is a self-limited condition that requires no additional evaluation or treatment, for ITP immune suppressive therapy is must in patients with platelets <30,000/mm³ or bleeding or both.[10,11]

3c. Corticosteroid with or without intravenous immunoglobulin (IVIg)
The management of ITP during pregnancy is generally the same as ITP in a non-pregnant patient. The goal of therapy is to reduce the risk of bleeding, not to normalize the platelet count. Glucocorticoids or IVIg are given in individuals who are not bleeding only if the platelet count is below 30,000/mm³ or if a higher count is needed for an invasive procedure.[9]

3d. Splenectomy or azathioprine are treatment of choice in first trimester of pregnancy with steroid refractory ITP. Data on the safety of romiplostim and eltrombopag during pregnancy are limited.[12,13]

3e. Neonatal thrombocytopenia may result due to maternal ITP.
There is no strong correlation between maternal platelet count and neonatal platelet count in ITP. The risk factors for neonatal thrombocytopenia include a previous history of neonatal thrombocytopenia, prior splenectomy, severe thrombocytopenia (<50,000/mm³) at some point during the pregnancy, and possibly maternal platelet count <100,000/mm³ at the time of delivery. There is no evidence that ITP therapy for the mother raises the fetal platelet count.[14,15]

Q4. A 60-year-old diabetic male presented with nephrotic range proteinuria. He underwent renal biopsy which revealed proliferative glomerulonephritis with IgG kappa restriction. His bone marrow biopsy revealed 6% plasma cells and serum protein electrophoresis, immunofixation electrophoresis and free light chain assessment were normal. There were no lytic lesions, anemia or hypercalcemia.
   a. What is the diagnosis?
   b. How will you differentiate monoclonal gammopathy of renal significance (MGRS) from diabetic nephropathy?
   c. Does this patient require treatment? Why?
   d. How will you treat this patient?
   e. What is the prognosis of such patients?

Ans:
4a. Monoclonal gammopathy of renal significance [(MGRS)-proliferative glomerulonephritis with monoclonal immunoglobulin deposits (PGNMID)]:
- The MGRS is a group of disorders in which a monoclonal immunoglobulin secreted by a nonmalignant or premalignant B cell or plasma cell clone causes kidney damage. These disorders do not meet diagnostic criteria for multiple myeloma or a chronic lymphoproliferative disorder (CLPD).
- The MGRS-associated kidney diseases include lesions such as immunoglobulin-associated amyloidosis, the monoclonal immunoglobulin deposition diseases, light chain deposition disease, heavy chain deposition disease, and light and heavy chain deposition disease, PGNMID, C3 glomerulopathy with monoclonal gammopathy, light chain proximal tubulopathy, and several others.[16]

4b. Renal biopsy with immunohistochemistry (IHC) (showing monoclonal protein deposition): 70–80% of patients with PGNMID do not have a detectable circulating monoclonal gammopathy by serum and urine monoclonal protein testing and do not have detectable plasma cell or B-cell clones on bone marrow aspirate and biopsy. In these patients, the monoclonal protein is only found in the kidney, and the diagnosis of MGRS is established by kidney biopsy.[17]

4c. Treatment is indicated to save the kidney function.
There are several studies in patients with MGRS that have shown that kidney outcomes are closely associated with the hematologic response to chemotherapy. Therefore, once the kidney pathology is identified by kidney biopsy, it is preferred to treat with chemotherapy directed against the pathologic clone, with the primary goal of preserving kidney function.[18]

4d. Chemo-immunotherapy containing daratumumab, cyclophosphamide, and dexamethasone that does not require dose modification for kidney function is preferred, to limit the occurrence of adverse events (particularly cytopenias). Commonly used drugs are proteasome inhibitors (e.g., bortezomib, carfilzomib), monoclonal antibodies (e.g., rituximab, daratumumab), alkylating agents (e.g., cyclophosphamide, bendamustine, and melphalan), immunomodulatory drugs (e.g., thalidomide, lenalidomide, and pomalidomide), and glucocorticoids (e.g., prednisone, dexamethasone).[19]

4e. The prognosis of patients with MGRS is usually good [overall response rate (ORR) > 88%]. In a study, where 16 patients underwent treatment, the overall renal response rate was 88%, and 38% of patients experienced complete renal response (proteinuria reduction to under 0.5 g/24 hours) with initial treatment. All patients were end stage renal disease-free at last follow-up.[20]

Q5. A patient with metastatic carcinoma colon was admitted with breathlessness for 3 days. He was afebrile and his CBC revealed anemia and severe thrombocytopenia. His creatinine was 2.5 mg/dL. His peripheral blood smear revealed 3% schistocytes.
  a. What is your diagnosis?
  b. What are the secondary causes of thrombotic microangiopathy (TMA)?
  c. What is the role of therapeutic plasma exchange in cancer associated thrombotic microangiopathies?
  d. What is the prognosis of such patients?

Ans:
  5a. The most probable diagnosis is cancer associated TMA.
  Thrombotic microangiopathies are a group of disorders characterized by disseminated occlusive microvascular thrombosis, thrombocytopenia, and ischemic end-organ damage, most commonly in kidneys and brain. Most cases of cancer-associated TMA have been reported in patients with mucin-producing adenocarcinoma and in those with disseminated malignancies. A prospective study by Lohrmann et al., determined that 5.7% of patients with metastatic carcinoma have microangiopathic hemolytic anemia (MAHA).[20]
  5b. Malignancy, drugs, organ transplantation, sepsis, pregnancy (for preeclampsia and the hemolysis elevated liver enzymes low platelet count syndrome), and autoimmune diseases [systemic lupus erythematosus (SLE), antiphospholipid syndrome] are common causes of TMA.
  5c. There is no role of therapeutic plasma exchange in cancer associated TMA.
  Therapeutic plasma exchange is not effective in many of the causes of TMA seen in cancer patients, and where feasible, treatment of the underlying malignancy is important in controlling cancer-associated TMA driven by the disease.[21]

Q6. A 36-year-old male presented with fever, weight loss and generalized lymphadenopathy for 1 month duration. He had also noticed right testicular painless swelling for last 10 days. Lymph node biopsy revealed ABC type diffuse large B-cell lymphoma. His PET-CT scan and bone marrow biopsy were also done.
  a. Is CSF examination needed in this patient?
  b. How will you treat this patient?
  c. Will you consider orchiectomy or testicular irradiation in this case?
  d. How will you preserve the fertility of this patient?
  e. What is the prognosis of patients with testicular involvement?

Ans:

6a. Yes, cerebrospinal fluid (CSF) examination needed in this patient due to testicular involvement.

All patients of diffuse large B-cell lymphoma (DLBCL) should be assessed using the Central Nervous System International Prognostic Index (CNS IPI). Further evaluation should be performed for patients with neurologic abnormalities on clinical examination and for selected patients with higher risk for involvement of the neuraxis (stage III/IV disease, presence of B symptoms, retroperitoneal lymph node involvement, bone marrow involvement, involvement of > 1 extranodal site, elevated serum lactate dehydrogenase level, and low serum albumin concentration.

Age >60 years, aggressive or highly aggressive disease, high- or high-intermediate risk disease by the IPI, testicular involvement.[22]

6b. Six cycles of R-CHOP (rituximab, cyclophosphamide, doxorubicin, vincristine and prednisolone) chemotherapy with CNS prophylaxis intrathecal methotrexate (ITMTx), orchidectomy, and scrotal RT.

R-CHOP cures approximately 60% of patients with DLBCL, is associated with acceptable adverse effects, and has long been standard initial treatment for DLBCL.

Moreover, the index case has testicular involvement. Testicular involvement by DLBCL is associated with adverse prognosis, increased risk for CNS involvement, and requires distinct aspects of management. Apart from systemic chemotherapy, orchiectomy, CNS prophylaxis, and scrotal radiation therapy (25-30 Gy RT) is recommended.[23,24]

6c. Orchiectomy, and scrotal radiation therapy (25-30 Gy RT) are required in the index case. Unilateral orchiectomy is usually performed to obtain diagnostic tissue, but orchiectomy alone is not sufficient treatment, even with stage I disease because of the increased risk of CNS involvement and contralateral scrotal recurrence. RT alone is used only for patients who are not candidates for any chemotherapy. Doxorubicin-based regimens alone appear unable to cure most patients with lymphoma involving the testis, but CHOP with prophylactic intrathecal therapy and adjuvant scrotal radiotherapy appears promising.[25]

6d. Sperm cryopreservation should be advised to all such patients.

The extent of testicular injury due to radiation therapy is directly related to the dose of radiation delivered as well as the underlying cell type. The seminiferous tubules are more sensitive to radiation and as low as 0.1 Gy, RT results in temporary arrest of spermatogenesis and azoospermia has been reported at radiation doses of 0.65 Gy, with doses of 1 Gy, 2-3 Gy, and 4-6 Gy causing azoospermia lasting 9-18 months, 30 months, and 5 years to permanently, respectively. Leydig cells appear to be less susceptible to RT induced damage. Radiation doses as high as 20 Gy in prepubertal males and 30 Gy in postpubertal males are required to induce damage to Leydig cells, and thereby clinical hypogonadism.

Sperm cryopreservation is recommended for fertility preservation in postpubertal male patients undergoing RT to testis. It is achieved through semen collection prior to the initiation of RT or chemoradiation. Two to three samples are typically collected, due to frequently reduced semen quality in cancer patients.[26,27]

6e. It is associated with poor prognosis.

Testicular involvement by DLBCL is associated with adverse prognosis, increased risk for CNS involvement, and requires distinct aspects of management.[25]

Q7. A 6-year-old boy presented with swollen, painful left knee. He had prolonged bleeding following minor trauma since birth. His elder brother had died of intracranial hemorrhage.
   a. How will you evaluate the cause of bleeding in this child?
   b. How will you treat this child?
   c. Is there any cure for hemophilia?
   d. How will you differentiate hemophilia A form severe von Willebrand disease?
   e. How can hemophilia be prevented in further pregnancies?

Ans:
7a. This is a case of suspected hemophilia. The diagnostic evaluation typically begins with a thorough review of the patient's personal bleeding history and family history. Screening tests are then performed, and the diagnosis is confirmed with a specific clotting factor activity measurement(s) and/or genetic testing.
   Laboratory testing is similar for most of the patients with hemophilia. It starts with prothrombin time (PT), activated partial thromboplastin time (aPTT), and platelet count. If the aPTT is prolonged the mixing studies for the aPTT assay are performed. If mixing studies show correction, consistent with a factor deficiency rather than an inhibitor, then factor activity levels are measured.[28]

7b. Factor infusion and RICE (rest, ice compression, and elevation) should be started. Bleeding into a joint, as in the index case, is one of the most common manifestations of hemophilia. It is characterized by reduced range of motion associated with pain, palpable swelling, and warmth.
   Factor concentrates should be infused promptly at the first sign of joint bleeding. Other interventions to reduce bleeding, pain, and inflammation include avoidance of weight bearing on the affected extremity, application of ice packs, immobilization, and/or splinting (RICE).
   However, it is the regular prophylactic therapy (factor administration in the absence of bleeding), which is highly effective in reducing bleeding and long-term complications of bleeding (such as chronic arthropathy), is recommended in people with hemophilia. Emicizumab is a bispecific, FVIII-mimetic therapeutic antibody that has considerably reduced the annualized bleeding rates in congenital hemophiliacs with and without inhibitors with weekly or even 3–4-weekly subcutaneous treatment.[29,30]

7c. Yes, gene therapy can cure hemophilia.
   Gene therapy can cure hemophilia as infusion of the gene therapy construct (or treated cells) can provide the deficient factor. Efforts to establish gene therapy approaches for hemophilia are underway in various countries around the world. A small number of gene therapy constructs have been approved by the US Food and Drug Administration (FDA). However, aspects of this approach remain to be optimized and studied for longer durations, and clinician familiarity with the principles and logistics of gene therapy remains to be systematically addressed.[31]

7d. Platelet-dependent von Willebrand factor (vWF) activity, vWF antigen (vWF:Ag), and factor VIII binding assay differentiate hemophilia A from severe vWD.
   vWD types 2N and 3 usually have significantly low factor VIII levels and can share similar symptoms like hemophilia A. The differentiation is done by:

- *Bleeding severity:* In hemophilia A, bleeding can be severe and presents early in life, but bleeding may be mild and may present at an older age. In vWD type 2N, bleeding is variable but may be severe. In vWD type 3, bleeding is usually severe.
- *Type of bleeding:* In hemophilia A, bleeding occurs in joints and muscles. In vWD type 2N, bleeding can be mucocutaneous but also into joints and muscles. In vWD type 3, bleeding occurs in both mucocutaneous sites and joints and muscles.
- *Sex distribution:* Hemophilia A is X-linked recessive; males are generally more severely affected (female carriers may be affected). vWD types 2N and 3 are autosomal, hence, males and females both are equally affected.
- *Laboratory testing:* In hemophilia A, platelet-dependent vWF activity, vWF antigen (VWF:Ag), and factor VIII binding are normal. In vWD type 2N, platelet-dependent vWF activity and vWF:Ag can be normal, but binding of the patient's vWF to factor VIII is low. In vWD type 3, platelet-dependent vWF activity and VWF:Ag are undetectable or extremely low.[32]

7e. Genetic counseling and prenatal testing.

Ladies who are hemophilia carriers should receive preconception counseling about the genetic transmission and the various methods to determine the sex of the fetus and in case of a male fetus, whether he is affected with hemophilia. After preconception counseling, a couple decides they want to avoid the risk of having an affected child. If so, the possibilities of preimplantation genetic screening or antenatal genetic screening by chorionic villus sampling (weeks 10–14 of gestation) or amniocentesis (from week 15 of gestation) followed by (early) termination of pregnancy in case of an affected male fetus are there.[33]

Q8. A 56-year-old female presented with weakness and on evaluation was found to have anemia and thrombocytopenia. Her mean corpuscular volume (MCV) was 125 and peripheral smear did not reveal any atypical cells.
    a.   How will you evaluate this patient further?
    b.   What is the diagnostic test for megaloblastic anemia?
    c.   How is vitamin B12 deficiency treated?
    d.   How will you monitor the recovery of this patient?

Ans:

8a. A combination of history, physical examination, and laboratory evaluation are done to evaluate this case.

When an individual has suspected vitamin B12 or folate deficiency, the evaluation starts with history about previously diagnosed associated conditions, like celiac disease or inflammatory bowel disease; bariatric, gastric, or intestinal surgery; reduced dietary intake (e.g., vegan or vegetarian diet, lack of fresh vegetables); alcohol use (as an independent cause of macrocytic anemia and as a possible predictor of reduced dietary intake); and any symptoms, including subtle neurologic or psychiatric symptoms.

The physical examination is focused on dermatologic and gastrointestinal findings, including hepatosplenomegaly. Neurologic examination should also be conducted for signs of altered affect or mentation and/or findings associated with central or peripheral neuropathy (e.g., impaired sense of vibration, proprioception, or light touch, ataxia, and weakness).

Laboratory evaluation include, CBC and blood smear, serum vitamin B12 and folate levels, metabolite testing [methylmalonic acidemia (MMA) and homocysteine], and autoantibodies to intrinsic factor.[34]

8b. Megaloblastic anemia is diagnosed based on anemia (hemoglobin <12 g/dL for female and <13 g/dL for male), macrocytosis (MCV >100 fL or more so if MCV is >115 fL) and peripheral smear showing low reticulocytes and hypersegmented neutrophils.

Megaloblastic anemia is a form of macrocytic anemia in which nucleic acid metabolism is impaired, leading to reduced efficiency of cell division and nuclear-cytoplasmic dyssynchrony. Causes of megaloblastic anemia include deficiency of vitamin B12, folate, or copper, as well as a number of medications that interfere with DNA synthesis.[35]

8c. Injectable vitamin B12 1,000 µg intramuscular is administered daily for a week, followed by monthly maintenance.[36]

8d. Hemolysis markers start improving in 1–2 days, followed by reticulocytosis in 3–4 days. Anemia takes 1–2 weeks to start improving and 4–8 weeks to normalize. Disappearance of hypersegmented neutrophils takes 10–14 days. Leukopenia and thrombocytopenia resolves in 2–4 weeks. Improvement in neuropsychiatric features requires 3 months to a year.[37]

Q9. A 62-years-old female presented with pain and swelling of left lower limb of 10 days duration. Doppler ultrasound of the limb revealed left femoral and popliteal vein thrombosis.
   a. How will you evaluate this patient further? What is the role of thrombophilia work up?
   b. How will you initiate the treatment of this patient?
   c. How will you monitor this patient and how long will the anticoagulation continue?
   d. What are the indications for life long anticoagulation?

Ans:

9a. This is a newly diagnosed case of left lower limb (unprovoked, proximal) deep vein thrombosis (DVT): Compression ultrasonography (CUS) with Doppler is the diagnostic test of choice in patients with suspected DVT. The sensitivity and specificity of proximal CUS is greater than 95%. Once the diagnosis of DVT is established, the patient should undergo a thorough history and physical examination combined with review of diagnostic imaging studies and routine laboratory testing. This may reveal an acquired condition (e.g., major surgery) predisposing to the thrombotic event or provide clues to the presence of inherited thrombophilia (e.g., first-degree relatives with DVT at a young age).

It is recommended that routine testing for hypercoagulable disorders (inheritable thrombophilia and antiphospholipid syndrome) in unselected patients with a diagnosis of DVT is not warranted. This is because in most patients with DVT, the identification of an inheritable defect does not alter therapeutic anticoagulant management, and consequently it has not been associated with improved outcomes.[38]

9b. Newer oral anticoagulant (NOACs) are the preferred treatment for proximal DVT of lower limbs. The duration is for the 3 months. The alternative includes low-molecular-weight heparin (LMWH) (e.g., enoxaparin) overlapped with oral anticoagulation (e.g., warfarin).[39]

9c. Patients are monitored for the complications of both DVT and anticoagulation. Complications of DVT include extension of the thrombus, recurrence, embolization, and postthrombotic syndrome (PTS). It is monitored clinically for symptoms. Lower extremity compression ultrasound (CUS) following anticoagulant therapy is not routinely recommended on follow-up, unless the patient develops symptoms or signs of recurrent or persistent DVT. D-dimer can also be used to follow a patient with DVT.

Anticoagulation-related adverse effects (e.g., bleeding, thrombocytopenia) and for the development of conditions that affect the half-life of or contraindications for the anticoagulant used (e.g., kidney failure, pregnancy, and weight gain/loss) are also monitored.

9d. Indefinite anticoagulants is recommended in patients with DVT and active cancer or another persistent provoking factor (e.g., active inflammatory bowel disease), and in patients with a second unprovoked proximal DVT.[40]

Q10. A 26-year-old female with the history of systemic lupus erythematosus presented with sudden onset breathlessness, seizures, and decreased urine output. She was found to have pulmonary and renal artery embolism. Her magnetic resonance imaging (MRI) brain revealed middle cerebral artery territory infarct.
 a. **What is your diagnosis?**
 b. **What further investigations should be done in this patient?**
 c. **How can the mortality of this patient be reduced?**
 d. **What are the diagnostic criteria of catastrophic antiphospholipid antibody (APLA) syndrome?**

Ans:

10a. The diagnosis seems to be catastrophic antiphospholipid syndrome (CAPS).

The CAPS is a rare, life-threatening form of antiphospholipid syndrome (APS) characterized by severe thrombotic complications, usually microvascular as well as large-vessel thrombosis, affecting multiple organs, that develop simultaneously or over a short period of time.[41]

10b. The patient should be evaluated with CBC, blood smear, anticardiolipin (aCL) antibodies (IgG, IgM), anti-β-2 glycoprotein antibodies (IgG, IgM), lactate dehydrogenase (LDH), lupus anticoagulant (LA) assay, liver and kidney function test, and complement (C3, C4) levels are done in all cases.

Imaging [computed tomography (CT) scan or MRI] may be needed if large vessel occlusion is suspected or to evaluate neurologic findings. In selected cases, tissue biopsy may be helpful in cases of diagnostic uncertainty.[42]

10c. Treatment of CAPS is the combination of therapeutic plasma exchange, anticoagulation, corticosteroids, rituximab, and treatment of the condition that triggered CAPS.

Anticoagulation with unfractionated heparin has the most significant impact on the patient's prognosis. Heparin also appears to have anti-inflammatory and complement-inhibitory effects in CAPS. Corticosteroids are usually administered in intravenous pulses at doses of 0.5–1 mg/kg, followed by tapering to achieve a short treatment duration (typically 4–6 weeks). Rituximab may be used as an add-on therapy in patients with severe, refractory, or recurrent CAPS. Therapeutic plasma exchange is an established procedure in CAPS, especially for patients with microangiopathic features or renal involvement, despite a lack of evidence regarding prescription details, including frequency, choice of replacement fluid, timing, and number of sessions.[42]

10d. CAPS is defined as a condition characterized by multiple vascular occlusive events (defined as at least three distinct events), typically affecting small vessels, over a short period (defined as ≤7 days), confirmed by histopathology, and the persistent presence of aPL over 12 weeks, usually at high titers.[43]

REFERENCES

1. Gillmore JD, Wechalekar A, Bird J, Cavenagh J, Hawkins S, Kazmi M, et al. Guidelines on the diagnosis and investigation of AL amyloidosis. Br J Haematol. 2015;168(2):207-18.
2. Rajkumar SV, Dimopoulos MA, Palumbo A, Blade J, Merlini G, Mateos MV, et al. International Myeloma Working Group updated criteria for the diagnosis of multiple myeloma. Lancet Oncol. 2014;15(12):e538-48.
3. Kumar S, Dispenzieri A, Lacy MQ, Hayman SR, Buadi FK, Colby C, et al. Revised prognostic staging system for light chain amyloidosis incorporating cardiac biomarkers and serum free light chain measurements. J Clin Oncol. 2012;30(9):989-95.
4. Sanchorawala V, Boccadoro M, Gertz M, Hegenbart U, Kastritis E, Landau H, et al. Guidelines for high dose chemotherapy and stem cell transplantation for systemic AL amyloidosis: EHA-ISA working group guidelines. Amyloid. 2022;29(1):1-7.
5. Kakizuka A, Miller WH Jr, Umesono K, Warrell RP Jr, Frankel SR, Murty VV, et al. Chromosomal translocation t(15;17) in human acute promyelocytic leukemia fuses RAR alpha with a novel putative transcription factor, PML. Cell. 1991;66(4):663-74.
6. Lo-Coco F, Avvisati G, Vignetti M, Thiede C, Orlando SM, Iacobelli S, et al. Retinoic acid and arsenic trioxide for acute promyelocytic leukemia. N Engl J Med. 2013;369(2):111-21.
7. Culligan DJ, Merriman L, Kell J, Parker J, Jovanovic JV, Smith N, Grimwade D. The Management of Acute Promyelocytic Leukemia Presenting During Pregnancy. Clin Leuk. 2007;1:183-91.
8. Santolaria A, Perales A, Montesinos P, Sanz MA. Acute promyelocytic leukemia during pregnancy: A systematic review of the literature. Cancers (Basel). 2020;12(4):968.
9. Sandal R, Mishra K, Jandial A, Sahu KK, Siddiqui AD. Update on diagnosis and treatment of Immune thrombocytopenia. Expert Review of Clinical Pharmacology. 2021;14(5):553-68.
10. Aster RH. "Gestational" thrombocytopenia: a plea for conservative management. N Engl J Med. 1990;323(4):264-6.
11. Reese JA, Peck JD, Deschamps DR, McIntosh JJ, Knudtson EJ, Terrell DR, et al. Platelet Counts during Pregnancy. N Engl J Med. 2018;379(1):32-43.
12. Mishra K, Kumar S, Sandal R, Jandial A, Sahu KK, Singh K, et al. Safety and efficacy of splenectomy in immune thrombocytopenia. Am J Blood Res. 2021;11(4):361-72.
13. Patil AS, Dotters-Katz SK, Metjian AD, James AH, Swamy GK. Use of a thrombopoietin mimetic for chronic immune thrombocytopenic purpura in pregnancy. Obstet Gynecol. 2013;122(2 Pt 2):483-5.
14. Webert KE, Mittal R, Sigouin C, Heddle NM, Kelton JG. A retrospective 11-year analysis of obstetric patients with idiopathic thrombocytopenic purpura. Blood. 2003;102(13):4306-11.
15. Oyama S, Tomimatsu T, Kanagawa T, Kumasawa K, Tsutsui T, Kimura T. Reliable predictors of neonatal immune thrombocytopenia in pregnant women with idiopathic thrombocytopenic purpura. Am J Hematol. 2012;87(1):15-21.
16. Leung N, Bridoux F, Hutchison CA, Nasr SH, Cockwell P, Fermand JP, et al. Monoclonal gammopathy of renal significance: when MGUS is no longer undetermined or insignificant. Blood. 2012;120(22):4292-5.
17. Fish R, Pinney J, Jain P, Addison C, Jones C, Jayawardene S, et al. The incidence of major hemorrhagic complications after renal biopsies in patients with monoclonal gammopathies. Clin J Am Soc Nephrol. 2010;5(11):1977-80.

18. Cohen C, Royer B, Javaugue V, Szalat R, El Karoui K, Caulier A, et al. Bortezomib produces high hematological response rates with prolonged renal survival in monoclonal immunoglobulin deposition disease. Kidney Int. 2015;88(5):1135-43.
19. Gumber R, Cohen JB, Palmer MB, Kobrin SM, Vogl DT, Wasserstein AG, et al. A clone-directed approach may improve diagnosis and treatment of proliferative glomerulonephritis with monoclonal immunoglobulin deposits. Kidney Int. 2018;94(1):199-205.
20. Lohrmann HP, Adam W, Heymer B, Kubanek B. Microangiopathic hemolytic anemia in metastatic carcinoma: report of eight cases. Ann Intern Med. 1973;7:368-75.
21. Thomas MR, Scully M. How I treat microangiopathic hemolytic anemia in patients with cancer. Blood. 2021;137(10):1310-7.
22. Schmitz N, Zeynalova S, Nickelsen M, Kansara R, Villa D, Sehn LH, et al. CNS International Prognostic Index: A risk model for CNS relapse in patients with diffuse large B-cell lymphoma treated with R-CHOP. J Clin Oncol. 2016;34(26):3150-6.
23. Coiffier B, Lepage E, Briere J, Herbrecht R, Tilly H, Bouabdallah R, et al. CHOP chemotherapy plus rituximab compared with CHOP alone in elderly patients with diffuse large-B-cell lymphoma. N Engl J Med. 2002;346(4):235-42.
24. Vitolo U, Chiappella A, Ferreri AJ, Martelli M, Baldi I, Balzarotti M, et al. First-line treatment for primary testicular diffuse large B-cell lymphoma with rituximab-CHOP, CNS prophylaxis, and contralateral testis irradiation: final results of an international phase II trial. J Clin Oncol. 2011;29(20):2766-72.
25. Visco C, Medeiros LJ, Mesina OM, Rodriguez M, Hagemeister F, Mclaughlin P, et al. Non-Hodgkin's lymphoma affecting the testis: is it curable with doxorubicin-based therapy? Clin Lymphoma. 2001;2(1):40-6.
26. Pryzant RM, Meistrich ML, Wilson G, Brown B, McLaughlin P. Long-term reduction in sperm count after chemotherapy with and without radiation therapy for non-Hodgkin's lymphomas. J Clin Oncol. 1993;11(2):239-47.
27. Lee SJ, Schover LR, Partridge AH, Patrizio P, Wallace WH, Hagerty K, et al. American Society of Clinical Oncology recommendations on fertility preservation in cancer patients. J Clin Oncol. 2006;24(18):2917-31.
28. Lawn RM. The molecular genetics of hemophilia: blood clotting factors VIII and IX. Cell. 1985;42(2):405-6.
29. Simpson ML, Valentino LA. Management of joint bleeding in hemophilia. Expert Rev Hematol. 2012;5(4):459-68.
30. Oldenburg J. Optimal treatment strategies for hemophilia: achievements and limitations of current prophylactic regimens. Blood. 2015;125(13):2038-44.
31. Reiss UM, Mahlangu J, Ohmori T, Ozelo MC, Srivastava A, Zhang L. Haemophilia gene therapy-Update on new country initiatives. Haemophilia. 2022;28(Suppl 4):61-7.
32. Nichols WL, Hultin MB, James AH, Manco-Johnson MJ, Montgomery RR, Ortel TL, et al. von Willebrand disease (VWD): evidence-based diagnosis and management guidelines, the National Heart, Lung, and Blood Institute (NHLBI) Expert Panel report (USA). Haemophilia. 2008;14(2):171-232.
33. Leebeek FWG, Duvekot J, Kruip MJHA. How I manage pregnancy in carriers of hemophilia and patients with von Willebrand disease. Blood. 2020;136(19):2143-50.
34. Devalia V, Hamilton MS, Molloy AM; British Committee for Standards in Haematology. Guidelines for the diagnosis and treatment of cobalamin and folate disorders. Br J Haematol. 2014;166(4):496-513.
35. Torrez M, Chabot-Richards D, Babu D, Lockhart E, Foucar K. How I investigate acquired megaloblastic anemia. Int J Lab Hematol. 2022;44:236-47.
36. Green R. Vitamin B12 deficiency from the perspective of a practicing hematologist. Blood. 2017;129(19):2603-11.
37. Stabler SP. Clinical practice. Vitamin B12 deficiency. N Engl J Med. 2013;368(2):149-60.
38. Middeldorp S, van Hylckama Vlieg A. Does thrombophilia testing help in the clinical management of patients? Br J Haematol. 2008;143(3):321-35.
39. Ortel TL, Neumann I, Ageno W, Beyth R, Clark NP, Cuker A, et al. American Society of Hematology 2020 guidelines for management of venous thromboembolism: treatment of deep vein thrombosis and pulmonary embolism. Blood Adv. 2020;4(19):4693-738.
40. Kearon C, Kahn SR. Long-term treatment of venous thromboembolism. Blood. 2020;135(5):317-25.
41. Cervera R, Bucciarelli S, Plasín MA, Gómez-Puerta JA, Plaza J, Pons-Estel G, et al. Catastrophic antiphospholipid syndrome (CAPS): descriptive analysis of a series of 280 patients from the "CAPS Registry". J Autoimmun. 2009;32(3-4):240-5.

42. Legault K, Schunemann H, Hillis C, Yeung C, Akl EA, Carrier M, et al. McMaster RARE-Best practices clinical practice guideline on diagnosis and management of the catastrophic antiphospholipid syndrome. J Thromb Haemost. 2018;16(8):1656-64.
43. Jacobs L, Wauters N, Lablad Y, Morelle J, Taghavi M. Diagnosis and Management of Catastrophic Antiphospholipid Syndrome and the Potential Impact of the 2023 ACR/EULAR Antiphospholipid Syndrome Classification Criteria. Antibodies (Basel). 2024;13(1):21.

32 Interesting Cases in Hematology

Aditi Mittal

AMYLOIDOSIS

Q1. What is amyloidosis?

Ans: It is a rare condition defined by extracellular deposition of abnormal amyloid protein in various tissues and organs. Commonly affected organs include kidneys followed by heart, spleen, liver, adrenal, tongue, and brain.

Q2. What is amyloid?

Ans: Amyloid is an aberrant protein that has an alteration in its secondary structure and formed by ordinarily soluble proteins which misfolded and aggregate to form insoluble fibrils. Accumulation of amyloid outside of cells in organs leads to their impaired function.

Q3. What is the physical structure of amyloid?

Ans: *On electron microscopy*—it consists of nonbranching fibrils with diameter of 7.5–10 mm and indefinite length.
X-ray crystallography/infrared spectroscopy showed a cross β-pleated sheet conformation.

Q4. What are the three most common forms of amyloid?

Ans: AL (light-chain), AA (associated with chronic inflammation), and ATTR (transthyretin-related, hereditary or wild-type).

Q5. What are the staining characteristics of amyloid?

Ans: Following stains are used to confirm amyloid:[1]
- *Hematoxylin and Eosin (H&E):* Amyloid appears as amorphous, eosinophilic (pink) extracellular deposits **(Figs. 1A and B)**.
- *Congo red stain:* Most widely used stain for amyloid.
  - Under light microscopy: Amyloid appears as pink to red.
  - Under polarized light: Shows apple-green birefringence—a key diagnostic feature.
- *Methyl violet/crystal violet:* Metachromasia—rose-pink
- *Thioflavin T or S staining:* Fluorescent dyes used in research settings. Amyloid fluoresces bright green-yellow under ultraviolet (UV) or fluorescence microscopy.
- *Immunohistochemistry (IHC) and mass spectrometry:*
  - Used to type the specific amyloid protein (e.g., AL, AA, ATTR).

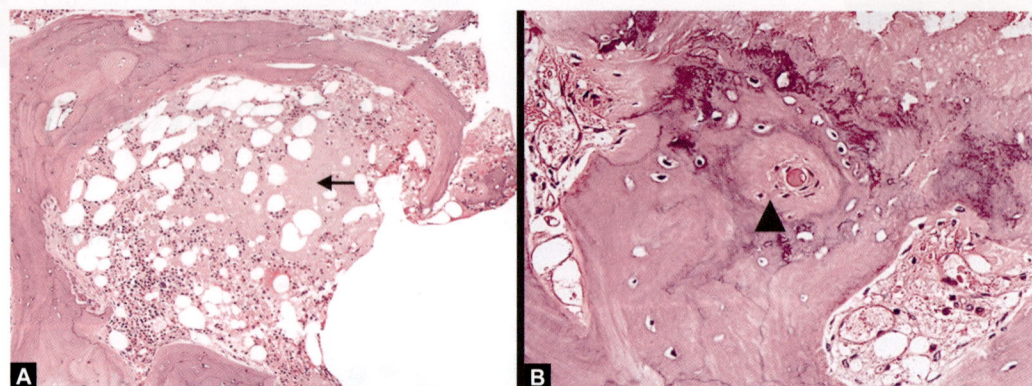

FIGS. 1A AND B: (A) Pink hyaline acellular homogeneous material suggesting amyloid deposit (arrow) in bone marrow biopsy (Hematoxylin and eosin; original magnification 100×). (B) Thickened blood vessel with widened tunica media and hyaline amorphous material suggestive of amyloid (arrowhead).

Q6. Describe the pattern of amyloid deposition in various organs?

Ans:
- *Kidney:* Most common type of systemic amyloidosis and most serious form of organ involvement.
  - The earliest pathological change seen in kidneys—thickening of glomerular basement membrane (GBM).
- *Heart:* Major organ involved in senile systemic amyloidosis.
  - The deposits start out as localized subendocardial collections and in the space between the heart's muscle fibers. Myocardial fiber pressure atrophy eventually results from the growth of these deposits.
- *Spleen:* Two patterns of deposition are seen:[1]
  i. Sago spleen—amyloid deposition in splenic follicles (white pulp).
  ii. Lardaceous spleen—amyloid deposit in splenic sinuses (red pulp).
- *Liver:* Amyloid gets deposited in space of disse.
- *Adrenal:* Deposition in zona glomerulosa.
- *Tongue:* Macroglossia
- *Brain:* In senile plaque of Alzheimer disease.[1]

Q7. Which amyloidosis is most commonly associated with plasma cell neoplasm?

Ans: AL amyloidosis

PLASMA CELL MYELOMA/MULTIPLE MYELOMA

Q8. What is plasma cell myeloma/multiple myeloma?

Ans: Plasma cell myeloma is multifocal neoplastic proliferation of plasma cells in bone marrow. Multiple myeloma is a combination of plasma cell myeloma usually associated with serum/urine monoclonal immunoglobulin (M-protein), and evidence of end-organ damage or diagnostic findings that suggest high risk of developing end-organ damage within 2 years.[2,3]

Q9. How does myeloma evolve?

Ans: All plasma cell myeloma evolve from monoclonal gammopathy of undetermined significance (MGUS) followed by smoldering myeloma.[2,3]
- Presence of <10% clonal plasma cells without evidence of M-protein and end-organ damage—defined as MGUS.
- Presence of 10% or more clonal plasma cells and M-protein in serum >30 g/L without evidence of end-organ damage—smoldering myeloma.
- Presence of all three features (>10% plasma cells, M-protein, and evidence of end-organ damage)—is defined as multiple myeloma.

Q10. What is the diagnostic criteria for myeloma?

Ans: *Essential:* Clonal bone marrow plasma cells ≥10% or biopsy-proven bony or extramedullary plasmacytoma and any one or more of the following myeloma—defining events:[2,3]

Evidence of end-organ damage that can be attributed to the underlying plasma cell proliferative disorder, specifically:
- *Hypercalcemia:* Serum calcium >0.25 mmol/L (>1 mg/dL) higher than the upper limit of normal or >2.75 mmol/L (>11 mg/dL).
- *Renal insufficiency:* Creatinine clearance <40 mL/min or serum creatinine >177 μmol/L (>2 mg/dL).
- *Anemia:* Hemoglobin value >2 g/dL below the lower limit of normal, or a hemoglobin value of <10 g/dL.
- *Bone lesions:* One or more osteolytic lesions on skeletal radiography, computed tomography (CT), or positron emission tomography (PET)-CT.

or
- Clonal bone marrow plasma cell percentage ≥60%.

or
- *Involved:* Uninvolved serum free light chain ratio ≥100 (involved free light chain level must be ≥100 mg/L).

or
- More than one focal lesion (≥5 mm in size) on magnetic resonance imaging (MRI) studies.

Q11. What does CRAB acronym stand for?

Ans: *C*alcium elevation, *R*enal failure, *A*nemia, *B*one lesions.

Q12. What is the most common presenting symptom of myeloma?

Ans: Bone pain especially in back and ribs. Lytic bone lesion is the most frequent multiple myeloma-associated end-organ damage.

Q13. What leads to pathologic fractures in myeloma?

Ans: Bone destruction is mediated by factors produced by neoplastic plasma cells such as macrophage inflammatory protein-1 alpha (MIP1α) (also called CCL3), a chemokine that promotes osteoclast development via a variety of pathways. Modulars of the Wnt pathway and other substances secreted by tumor cells inhibit osteoblast activity. The net result is a noticeable rise in bone resorption, which causes hypercalcemia and pathologic fractures.[1]

Q14. What are the peripheral blood and bone marrow findings in myeloma?

Ans:

Peripheral Blood Findings

- *Normocytic, normochromic anemia*: Common due to marrow infiltration and reduced erythropoiesis.
- *Rouleaux formation:* Red blood cells appear stacked like coins; caused by elevated serum globulins **(Fig. 2A)**.
- *Leukopenia and thrombocytopenia:* Seen in advanced disease due to marrow suppression.
- *Circulating plasma cells:* More than 5% circulating plasma cells in peripheral blood defined as plasma cell leukemia.
- *Elevated erythrocyte sedimentation rate (ESR):* Often markedly increased due to high levels of monoclonal protein.

Bone Marrow Findings (Figs. 2A to D)

- *Increased plasma cells*: ≥10% clonal plasma cells (can be up to 90% in severe cases).
- *Atypical/malignant plasma cells:* Eccentric nuclei, basophilic cytoplasm, perinuclear hof (clear zone), and prominent nucleoli.

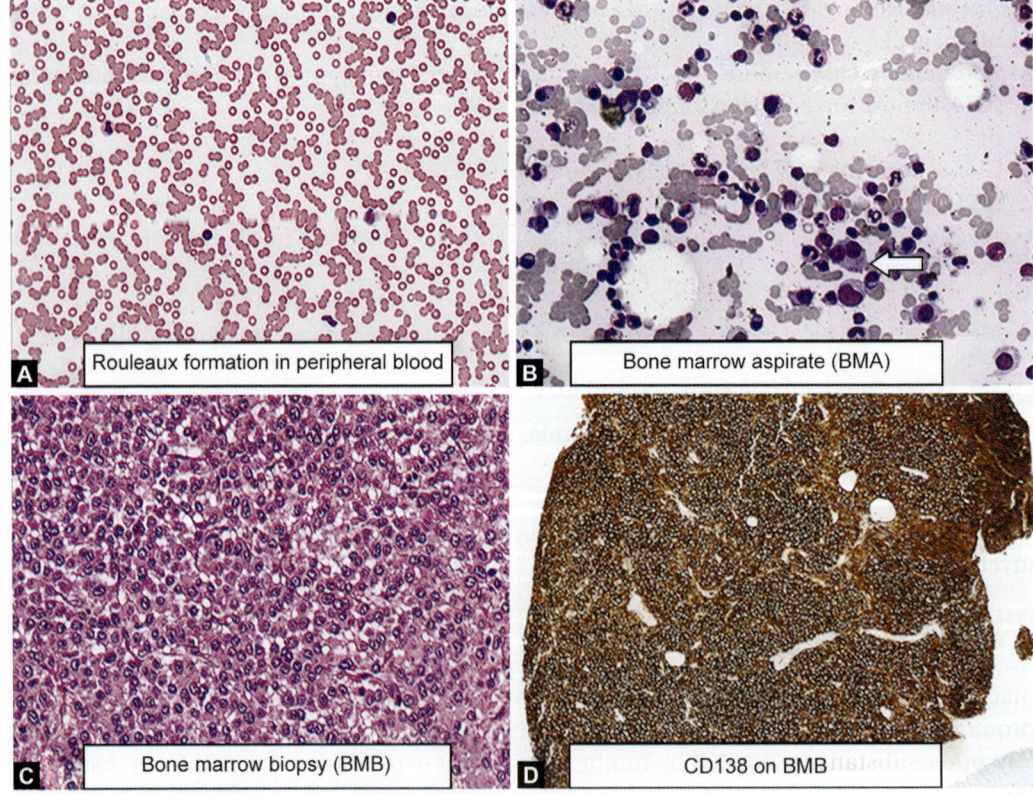

FIGS. 2A TO D: (A) Peripheral smear showing increased rouleaux formation (Giemsa; 200×). (B) Numerous plasma cells in BMA with few binucleated forms (arrow) (Wright Giemsa; 200×). (C) Bone marrow biopsy showing sheets of plasma cells (H&E; 400×). (D) CD138 positivity on sheets of plasma cells.

- *Suppressed normal hematopoietic elements*: Leading to anemia, leukopenia, and thrombocytopenia.
- *Multinucleated or binucleated plasma cells:* Indicative of dysplasia or aggressive disease.
- *Inclusions:*
    - *Russell bodies:* Large, eosinophilic cytoplasmic inclusions of immunoglobulin.
    - *Dutcher bodies:* Immunoglobulin inclusions appearing within or near the nucleus.
    - *Mott cells:* Plasma cells filled with multiple Russell bodies, giving a grape-like appearance.

Q15. What are the investigations that can be done in multiple myeloma?

Ans: Investigations include serum protein electrophoresis (SPEP), urine protein electrophoresis (UPEP), immunofixation electrophoresis (IFE), free light chain assay, skeletal survey, bone marrow examination, paraffin immunofluorescence, and renal function tests.

HEMOPHAGOCYTOSIS

The pathogenic process known as hemophagocytosis occurs when activated macrophages, also known as histiocytes, engulf and kill blood cells, including red, white, and platelets, in the bone marrow, spleen, liver, or lymph nodes. It is a defining feature of the uncommon but potentially fatal hyperinflammatory condition known as hemophagocytic lymphohistiocytosis (HLH) **(Figs. 3A and B)**.

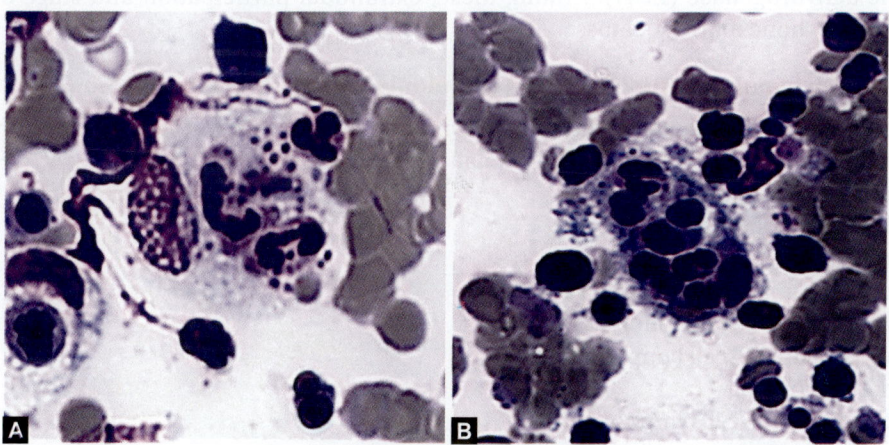

FIGS. 3A AND B: (A) Phagocytosis of neutrophil by histiocyte. (B) Erythrophagocytosis.

Types of Hemophagocytic Lymphohistiocytosis

- *Primary (Familial):* Due to genetic mutations (e.g., *PRF1, UNC13D*)
- *Secondary:* Due to infections [(*especially Epstein-Barr virus (EBV)*], *malignancies* (e.g., lymphomas), *autoimmune diseases* [e.g., systemic lupus erythematosus (SLE)], or certain *drugs*.

Q16. What are the characteristic bone marrow findings in HLH?

Ans: Activated histiocytes engulfing red blood cells (RBCs), white blood cells (WBCs), and platelets.

Q17. What are the HLH-2004 diagnostic criteria?

Ans: Fever, splenomegaly, cytopenias, hyperferritinemia, hypertriglyceridemia, low fibrinogen, hemophagocytosis, elevated sCD25/decreased natural killer (NK) activity (five of eight required).

Q18. What is the role of IHC in hemophagocytosis?

Ans: Identifies histiocytes using CD68 immunostain.

Q19. What is the treatment of HLH?

Ans: Immunosuppressive therapy (dexamethasone, etoposide), treatment of underlying cause (e.g., infection, autoimmune disease) and stem cell transplantation in familial HLH.

MARROW INFILTRATION BY LYMPHOMA

Q20. What is the significance of bone marrow infiltration in lymphoma patients?

Ans: Bone marrow infiltration by lymphoma is crucial for accurate staging, prognosis, and treatment planning. The marrow involvement often indicates advanced disease (stage IV) and may impact therapeutic decisions. The prognosis of patients depends on the determination of their bone marrow status. The five clinical factors that make up the International Prognostic Index (IPI) are age, performance status (PS), stage, extranodal involvement, and serum levels of lactic dehydrogenase (LDH). Among these, extranodal participation and stage can be influenced by bone marrow status.

Q21. Which lymphoma subtypes most commonly infiltrate the bone marrow?

Ans: The incidence of marrow infiltration by lymphoma are as follows (in descending order).
- Chronic lymphocytic leukemia (CLL)/small lymphocytic lymphoma (SLL)
- Mantle cell lymphoma (MCL)
- Follicular lymphoma (FL)
- Marginal zone lymphoma (MZL)
- Lymphoplasmacytic lymphoma (LPL)
- Diffuse large B-cell lymphoma (DLBCL)
- T-cell rich large B-cell lymphoma
- Burkitt lymphoma
- Hepatosplenic T-cell lymphoma

Q22. What are the common histological patterns of bone marrow infiltration by lymphoma (Figs. 4A to F)?

Ans:
- *Focal, random:* Discrete, randomly located infiltrates [e.g., SLL, MCL, splenic marginal zone lymphoma (SMZL)].
- *Paratrabecular:* Infiltrate aligned along trabeculae (classically in FL).
- *Interstitial:* Scattered neoplastic cells in marrow interstitium without effacement. Seen in CLL/SLL.
- *Diffuse*: Complete effacement of marrow. Common in *aggressive B-cell lymphomas*.
- *Intrasinusoidal:* Neoplastic cells within marrow sinusoids. Seen in hepatosplenic T-cell lymphoma (*HSTL*), *SMZL, intravascular large B-cell lymphoma (IVLBCL)*.

CHAPTER 32: Interesting Cases in Hematology

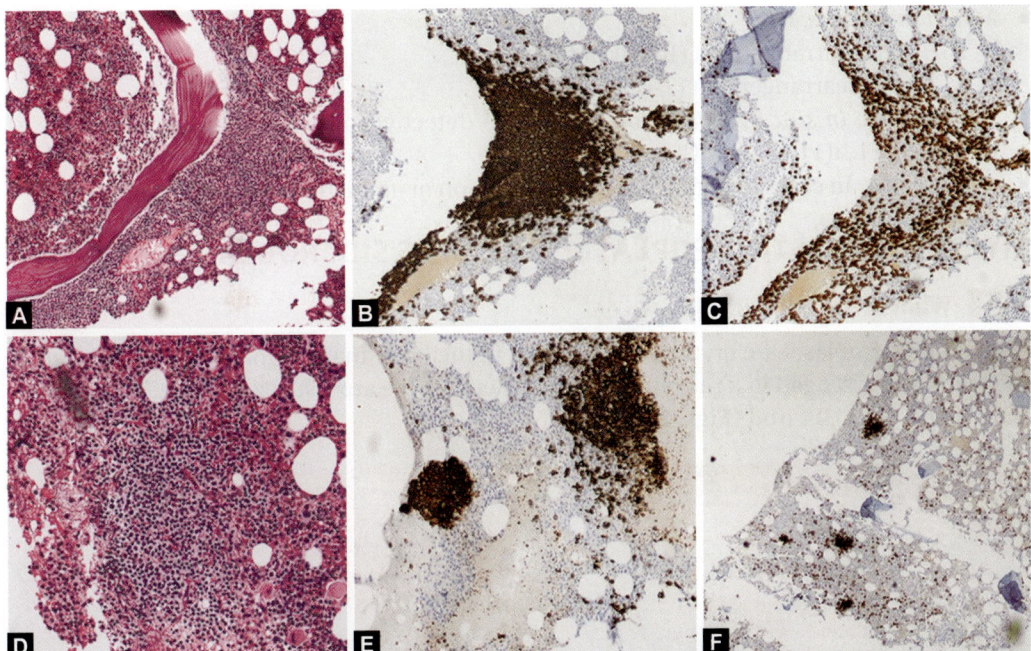

FIGS. 4A TO F: (A) Case of follicular lymphoma showing paratrabecular infiltration of marrow (H&E; 100×). (B) Strong CD20 positivity in the paratrabecular aggregate (100×). (C) Cuffing of the same paratrabecular aggregate by CD3 positive T-cells (100×). (D) Nodular lymphoid aggregate (H&E; 200×). (E) CD20 immunostain showing nodular as well as paratrabecular aggregate (100×). (F) Focal and interstitial marrow involvement by lymphoma in splenic marginal zone lymphoma (SMZL) (CD20; 40×).

Q23. Correlate the marrow infiltration patterns with immunophenotyping profiles.

Ans: Correlation of the marrow infiltration patterns with immunophenotyping profiles are given in **Table 1**.

TABLE 1: Correlation of the marrow infiltration patterns with immunophenotyping profiles.

Pattern	Typical lymphomas	Immunophenotype
Focal, random	SLL, MCL, SMZL	CD20+, CD5+ (MCL), Cyclin D1+ (MCL), CD23+ (SLL)
Paratrabecular	Follicular lymphoma	CD10+, BCL2+, BCL6+
Interstitial	CLL/SLL	CD5+, CD23+, CD20 dim
Diffuse	DLBCL, Burkitt	CD20+, Ki-67 high (Burkitt >90%)
Intrasinusoidal	HSTL, IVLBCL, SMZL	CD3+, TCRγδ+ (HSTL); CD20+, CD79a+ (IVLBCL)

(CLL: chronic lymphocytic leukemia; DLBCL: diffuse large B-cell lymphoma; HSTL: hepatosplenic T-cell lymphoma; IVLBCL: intravascular large B-cell lymphoma; MCL: mantle cell lymphoma; SMZL: splenic marginal zone lymphoma; SLL: small lymphocytic lymphoma; TCRγδ: T-cell receptors gamma delta)

Q24. What additional investigations aid diagnosis in marrow-involved lymphoma?

Ans:
- *Flow cytometry:* Identifies clonal B-cell/T-cell populations.

- *Molecular studies:*
  - IGH gene rearrangement (B-cell clonality)
  - TCR gene rearrangement (T-cell clonality)
- *Fluorescence in situ hybridization (FISH):* To detect chromosomal translocations [e.g., t(14;18) in FL, t(11;14) in MCL].
- *Cytogenetics:* In cases of high-grade transformation or ambiguous morphology.

MYELODYSPLASTIC NEOPLASM WITH RING SIDEROBLASTS

Q25. What are ring sideroblasts?

Ans: Ring sideroblasts are erythroid precursors in the bone marrow that contain *iron-loaded mitochondria* arranged in a ring around the nucleus. These are visualized using *Prussian blue stain* (Perls' stain) for iron **(Figs. 5A and B)**.

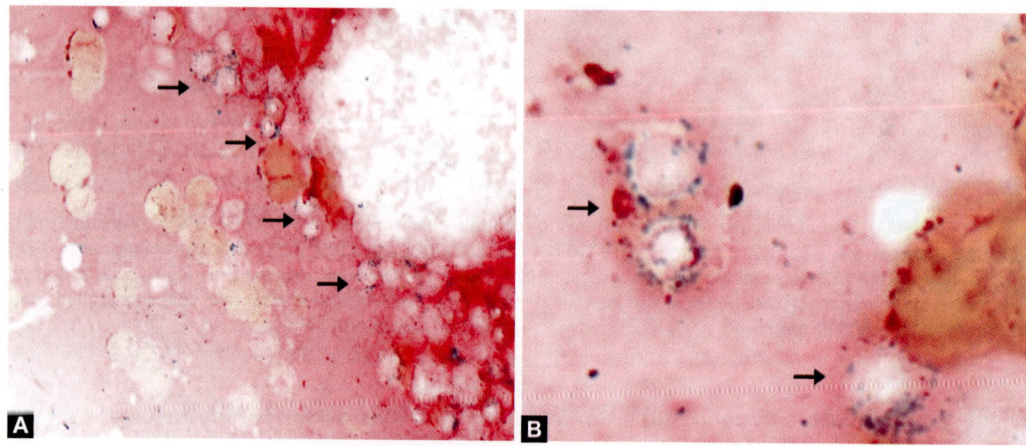

FIGS. 5A AND B: More than 15% of ring sideroblasts (arrow) in a diagnosed case of MDS with low blasts and *SF3B1* mutation in a 75-year-old male [Prussian blue stain; (A) 100×; (B) 400×].

Q26. How do ring sideroblasts differ from sideroblasts?

Ans: *Sideroblasts* are normal erythroid precursors with iron granules. *Ring sideroblasts* are pathologic, with *five or more iron granules* encircling at least *one-third of the nucleus* in a perinuclear distribution.

Q27. What are common causes of ring sideroblasts?

Ans:

Inherited

- X-linked sideroblastic anemia (*ALAS2* mutation)
- Autosomal recessive (*SLC25A38, GLRX5* mutations)

Acquired

- Myelodysplastic neoplasm (MDS)
- Drugs (chloramphenicol, isoniazid, linezolid)

- Alcohol
- Copper deficiency
- Lead poisoning
- Vitamin B6 deficiency

Q28. **Which mutation is commonly associated with the increased number of ring sideroblasts in myelodysplastic syndrome?**

Ans: *SF3B1* mutation.

Q29. **What is the role of the *SF3B1* mutation in ring sideroblasts?**

Ans: *SF3B1*, a splicing factor gene, is mutated in *70–90%* of MDS cases with ring sideroblasts. Heterozygous mutations in *SF3B1*, which codes for a fundamental part of the U2 small nuclear ribonucleoprotein (snRNP) spliceosome that is essential for RNA splicing, leads to *aberrant splicing of mitochondrial genes*, resulting in *iron-laden mitochondria*. It is associated with *indolent course* and *favorable prognosis*.[3]

BONE MARROW METASTASIS (FIGS. 6A TO F)

Q30. **What is bone marrow metastasis?**

Ans: Bone marrow metastasis is the infiltration of bone marrow by malignant cells from a nonhematologic primary tumor, such as carcinomas or sarcomas.

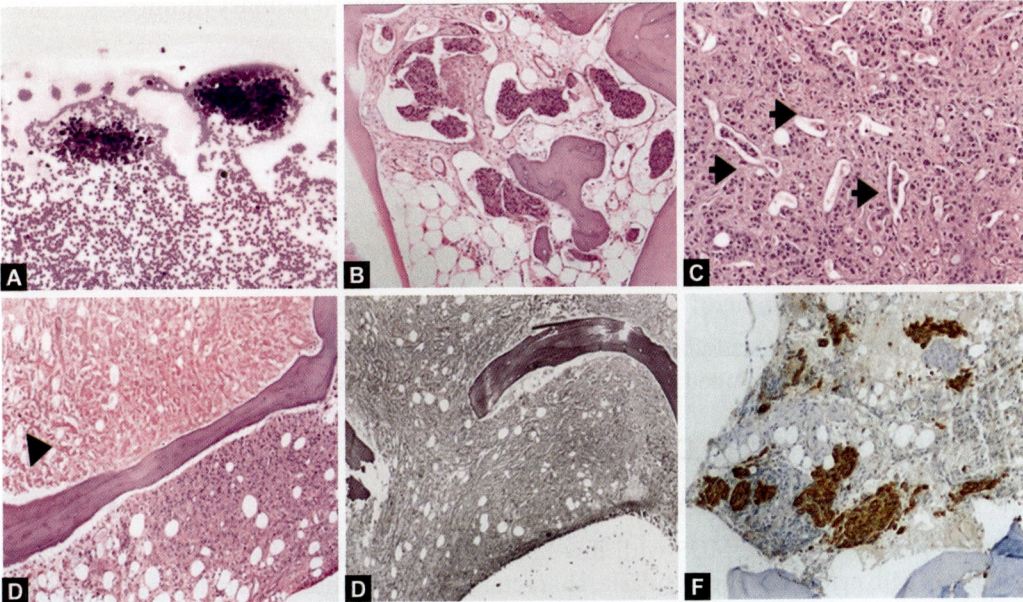

FIGS. 6A TO F: (A to C) A case of 45-year-old female with carcinoma breast. (A) Tumor cells lying in tight clusters in bone marrow aspirate suggesting nonhematopoietic origin. (B) A bone marrow biopsy with infiltration by metastatic tumor cells lying in nests and clusters in a known case (H&E; 100×). (C) Sheets of tumor cells in the same case with intrasinusoidal infiltration (arrows) (H&E; 100×). (D to F) A case of 55-year-old male with prostatic adenocarcinoma. (D) A bone marrow biopsy infiltrated by metastatic tumor cells lying in sheets along with area of necrosis (arrowhead) (H&E; 100×). (E) Desmoplasia in bone biopsy as evidenced by reticulin stain (reticulin; 100×). (F) Tumor deposits as highlighted by Pan-cytokeratin immunostains (Pan-Ck; 100×).

Q31. Which adult cancers most commonly metastasize to the bone marrow?

Ans: Common adult cancers include breast carcinoma, prostate carcinoma, lung carcinoma, and gastrointestinal cancers.

Q32. Which pediatric tumors commonly show bone marrow metastasis?

Ans: Neuroblastoma, Ewing's sarcoma, and rhabdomyosarcoma are the most frequent tumors that metastasize to bone marrow.

Q33. What are typical peripheral blood findings in marrow metastasis?

Ans: A leukoerythroblastic blood picture, including nucleated red blood cells, immature granulocytes, and anemia, is commonly seen.

Q34. What are the bone marrow biopsy findings in metastatic infiltration?

Ans: Bone marrow biopsy shows clusters, sheets, or nests of malignant cells, often with fibrosis (desmoplasia) and suppression of normal hematopoietic elements.

Q35. What is the role of IHC in diagnosing bone marrow metastasis?

Ans: IHC helps to identify the tissue of origin using specific markers, distinguishing metastatic carcinoma from primary hematologic malignancies.

Q36. Name some common IHC markers and their associated primary tumors.

Ans:
- *Cytokeratin*—general epithelial marker
- *Thyroid transcription factor-1 (TTF-1)*—lung adenocarcinoma
- *Prostate-specific antigen (PSA)*—prostate carcinoma
- *S100*—melanoma
- *Synaptophysin/chromogranin*—neuroendocrine tumors
- *CD99*—Ewing's sarcoma

Q37. How does bone marrow metastasis affect prognosis and treatment?

Ans: Bone marrow metastasis usually indicates advanced disease and poor prognosis, and it influences staging and the need for systemic therapy (e.g., chemotherapy, targeted therapy).

MYELODYSPLASTIC NEOPLASM WITH DEL (5Q)

Q38. What is MDS with 5q deletion?

Ans: As per latest WHO, MDS with low blasts and 5q deletion (MDS-5q) is a myeloid neoplasm with cytopenia and dysplasia, characterized by chromosome 5q deletion occurring in isolation or with one additional cytogenetic abnormality other than monosomy 7 or 7q deletion **(Figs. 7 and 8)**.[3]

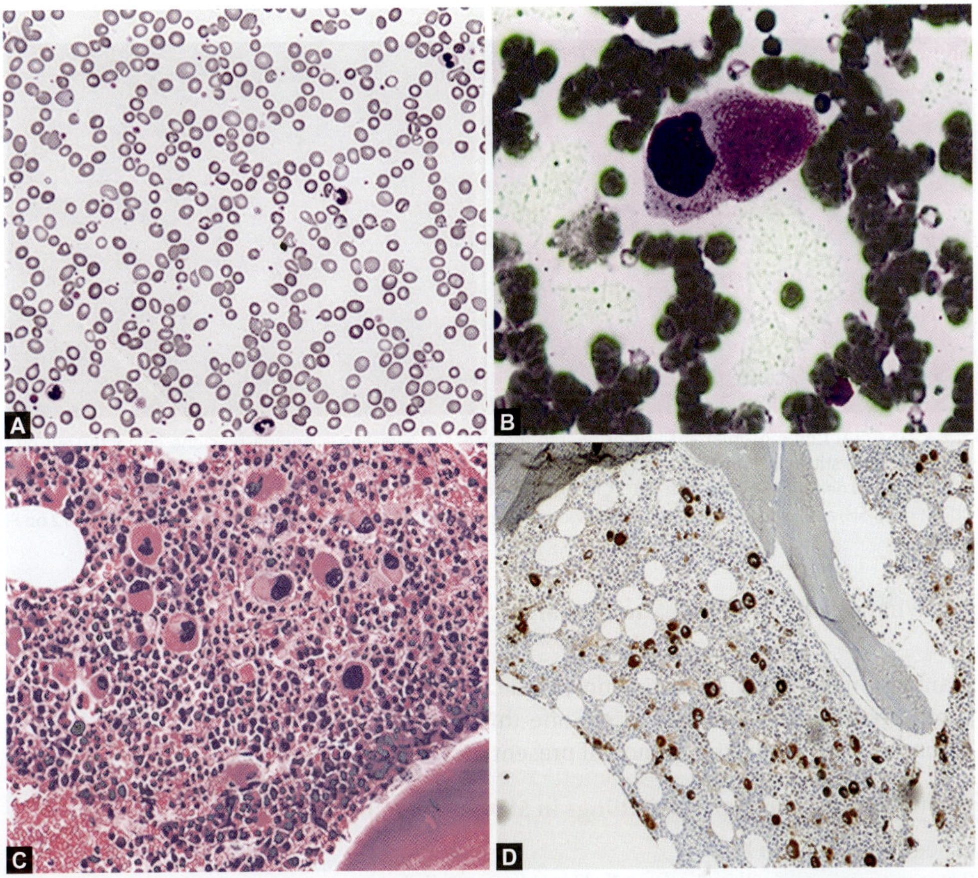

FIGS. 7A TO D: (A) Dimorphic anemia on peripheral blood (Giemsa; 200x) in a 60-year-old male presented with transfusion dependent anemia for 8 months. (B) Bone marrow aspirate showing presence of monolobated megakaryocytes. (C) Bone marrow biopsy showing monolobated megakaryocytes in a hypercellular marrow. (D) Megakaryocytes got highlighted by CD61 immunostain.

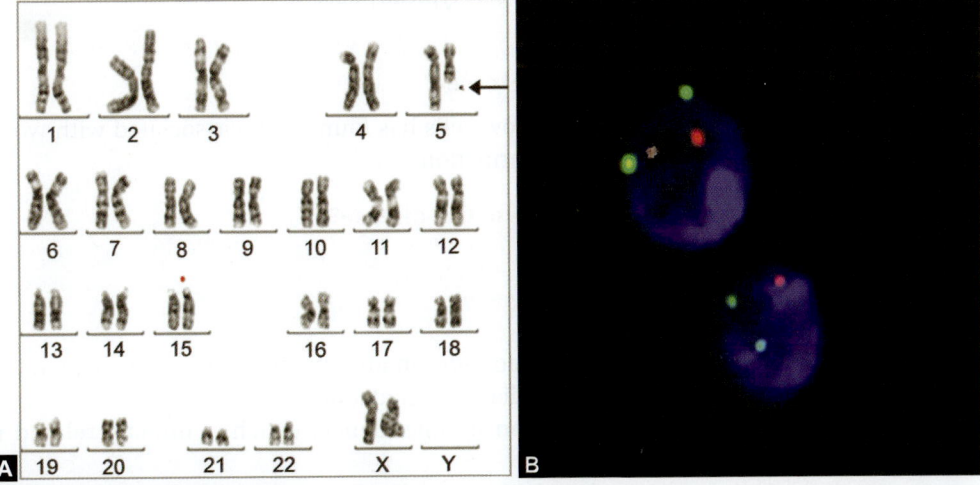

FIGS. 8A TO C: *Continued*

Continued

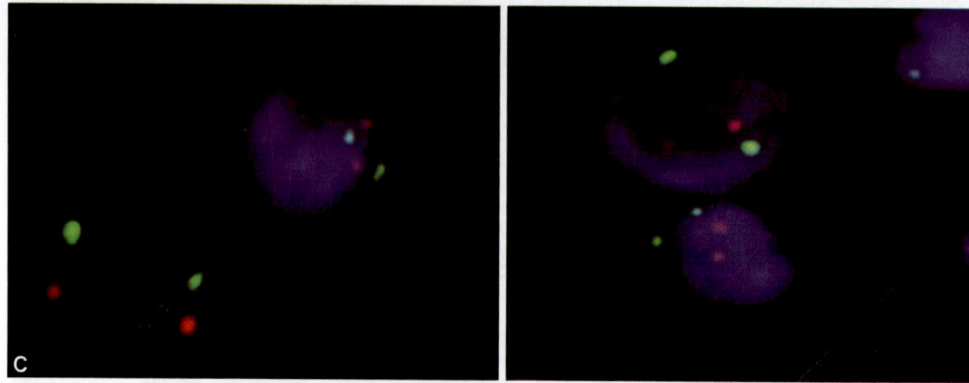

FIGS. 8A TO C: (A) Chromosomal analysis of twenty metaphases revealing a neoplastic clone characterized by the presence of an interstitial deletion of the long arm of chromosome 5 (arrow) in eighteen metaphases analyzed. Karyotype [ISCN 2020]: 46,XX,del(5)(q13q33)[18]/46,XX[2]. (B) Only one orange light indicating deletion 5q31 on fluorescence in situ hybridization (FISH) analysis. (C) Two orange and two green lights indicating normal patterns for 7q31 and 20q12 on FISH analysis.

Q39. What are the clinical features of MDS-5q?

Ans:
- Transfusion dependent anemia, mostly macrocytic.
- Thrombocytosis (>4.5 Lakh/mm^3) in one-third cases.
- Thrombocytopenia is uncommon, if present indicates advanced disease.

Q40. What are bone marrow findings in MDS-5q deletion?

Ans: See **Figures 7A to D**.
- Bone marrow—usually normocellular or hypercellular.
- Erythroid hypoplasia is the most common.
- Megakaryocytes—increased, usually nonlobulated or hypolobated.
- Dyserythropoiesis and dysgranulopoiesis—less common.
- Ring sideroblasts can be seen. Marrow fibrosis typically absent.
- Blasts <5% of all nucleated cells.

Q41. What is the role of p53 in MDS-5q del cases?

Ans: Strong p53 expression in >1% of marrow cells has found to be associated with worse prognosis and higher risk of leukemic transformation.

Q42. What is the treatment and prognosis of this disease?

Ans:

Treatment
- Patients with MDS-5q benefit from lenalidomide, an immunomodulatory medication that targets casein kinase 1A for ubiquitin-mediated degradation.
- Two-thirds of patients attain transfusion independence, which is directly related to suppressing the aberrant clone.

Prognosis

- In the Revised International Prognostic Scoring System (IPSS-R), the majority of patients are classified as low-risk or intermediate-1-risk, and the defining cytogenetic parameters for MDS-5q fall into the "good" prognostic cytogenetic grouping.[2]
- Poor prognosis is linked to male sex, advanced age, transfusion need, low platelet count, and low absolute neutrophil count.[2]
- Up to 18% of individuals have a TP53 mutation at diagnosis, which is linked to a worse response to lenalidomide and a higher chance of developing acute myeloid leukemia (AML).[2]
- TP53, RUNX1, and TET2 mutations have been found in patients who had AML transition.
- Additionally, *SF3B1* mutations may indicate worse outcomes in MDS-5q.[2]

REED–STERNBERG CELLS

Q43. What are Reed–Sternberg (RS) cells?

Ans: Reed–Sternberg cells are large, abnormal, binucleated or multinucleated cells with prominent eosinophilic nucleoli, classically described as having an "owl's eye" appearance. They are diagnostic hallmark cells of classical Hodgkin lymphoma (CHL).

Q44. What is the origin of RS cells?

Ans: Reed–Sternberg cells originate from germinal center B cells that do not exhibit their typical B-cell phenotype. Despite B-cell origin, they often lose expression of B-cell markers (e.g., CD20). RS cells exhibit crippled immunoglobulin gene rearrangements and constitutive NF-κB activation, promoting survival.

Q45. What is the immunophenotype of classical RS cells?

Ans: The immunophenotype of classical RS cells are given in **Table 2**.

TABLE 2: The immunophenotype of classical RS cells.

Marker expression in classical Hodgkin's lymphoma	Reed–Sternberg (RS) cells
CD30	Strongly positive (membranous/Golgi)
CD15	Positive in ~75% (Golgi + membranous)
CD20	Usually negative or weak
CD45 (LCA)	Negative
PAX5	Weakly positive (dim nuclear)
EBER	Often positive (especially mixed cellularity subtype)

Note: The dim expression of *PAX5* helps distinguish RS cells from other large B-cell neoplasms.

Q46. What are the different morphological variants of RS cells?

Ans: Morphological variants of RS cells are given in **Table 3** and **Figures 9A and B**.

TABLE 3: Morphological variants of Reed–Sternberg (RS) cells.		
Variant description	Description	Subtype
Classic RS cell (See **Fig. 9A**)	Binucleate with eosinophilic nucleoli ("owl eyes")	All classical Hodgkin lymphoma (CHL) subtypes
Hodgkin cell (See **Fig. 9B**)	Identical to classic RS cell except that they have single large round nucleus with a large eosinophilic inclusion like nucleus	CHL
Lacunar cell	RS variant with clear space ("lacunae") around nucleus	Nodular sclerosis CHL
Mummified cell	Shrunken, pyknotic RS cell	Nodular sclerosis
Anaplastic/pleomorphic	Irregular, bizarre cells	Lymphocyte-depleted CHL
Popcorn cell	Polylobated nucleus with small nucleoli	Nodular lymphocyte predominant HL (NLPHL) (NOT true RS cell)

Note: Popcorn cells are lymphocyte-predominant (LP) cells, CD20+, CD30–, and not considered RS cells.

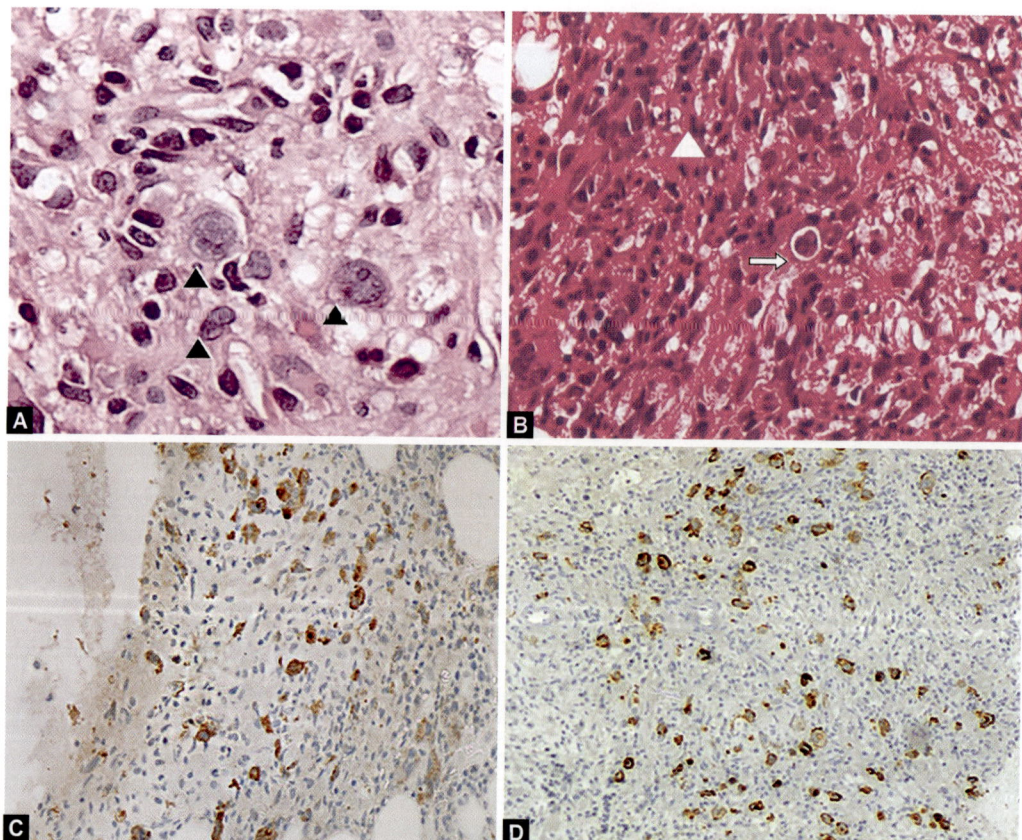

FIGS. 9A TO D: (A) Classical Reed–Sternberg (RS) cells (arrowhead) having bilobed nucleus with prominent eosinophilic nuclei "Owl-eye appearance" [Bone marrow biopsy (BMB); H&E; 200×]. (B) Bone marrow biopsy involvement by Hodgkin cells (arrow) in a fibrotic background with occasional collection of epithelioid histiocytes forming ill formed granuloma (arrowhead) (H&E; 200×). (C) Epstein–Barr virus (EBV) immunostain positivity on Hodgkin and Reed–Sternberg cells (EBV; 100×). (D) CD30 membranous positivity on RS cells (CD30; 100×).

CHAPTER 32: Interesting Cases in Hematology

Q47. How do RS cells differ in classical HL and nodular lymphocyte predominant HL (NLPHL)?

Ans: Differences of RS cells in CHL and NLPHL are given in **Table 4**.

TABLE 4: Differences of Reed–Sternberg (RS) cells in classical Hodgkin lymphoma (CHL) and nodular lymphocyte predominant HL (NLPHL).

Feature	CHL	NLPHL
RS cell type	Classic RS	Lymphocyte-predominant (LP) cell ("Popcorn cell")
CD30 (See **Fig. 9D**)	Positive	Negative
CD15	Often positive	Negative
CD20	Weak/negative	Positive
CD45	Negative	Positive
Epstein–Barr virus (EBV) association (See **Fig. 9C**)	Often positive (especially mixed cellularity type)	Rare
PD-L1 expression	Upregulated	Not expressed

Q48. What is the diagnostic role of RS cells?

Ans: It is essential for diagnosing CHL.
- Must be seen in an appropriate reactive background (mixed inflammatory infiltrate: Eosinophils, plasma cells, and histiocytes).
- Confirmed by immunophenotyping and EBV studies [EBER/latent membrane protein 1 (LMP1)] if needed.

Q49. What is the role of PD-L1 in RS cells?

Ans:
- RS cells often show 9p24.1 amplification, leading to overexpression of PD-L1 and PD-L2, allowing immune evasion.
- Checkpoint inhibitors (e.g., nivolumab) target this mechanism and are used in relapsed/refractory CHL.
- In over 40% of cases, strong expression of PD-L1 IHC is seen in majority of Hodgkin and Reed–Sternberg (HRS) cells.

Q50. How do RS cells escape the immune system?

Ans:
- Hodgkin and Reed–Sternberg cells release various chemokines (e.g., CCL17/TARC, CCL5), cytokines [Interleukin (IL)-5, IL-7, IL-13], and growth factors (e.g., FGF2, M-CSF) that attract and modulate CD4+ helper/regulatory T cells, eosinophils, macrophages, mast cells, fibroblasts, and stromal cells. Rather than being reactive, this cellular environment supports HRS cell survival, angiogenesis, and immune evasion.[1]
- Immune escape is facilitated by CD4+ T-cell rosettes around HRS cells, polarization toward regulatory T cells, differentiation of monocytes into M2 macrophages, and secretion of suppressive cytokines such as IL-10 and transforming growth factor-beta (TGF-β). A critical mechanism involves HRS cell expression of PD-L1 and PD-L2, which engage PD-1 on T cells—an interaction now targeted by checkpoint inhibitors.[1]

- In EBV-positive cases, HRS cells exhibit type II latency, expressing EBERs, EBNA1, LMP1, and LMP2A. LMP1 mimics CD40 signaling, while LMP2A substitutes for B-cell receptor activity, together providing essential survival signals for malignant B cells.

Q51. What is the typical histopathological background of RS cells in CHL?

Ans:
- Mixed inflammatory milieu, including eosinophils, plasma cells, lymphocytes (mostly T cells), macrophages, and fibrosis (especially in nodular sclerosis type).
- Background varies by subtype and helps classify CHL.

Q52. What are mimickers of RS cells?

Ans: Immunoblasts
RS-like cells can also be seen in:
- Peripheral T-cell lymphoma (PTCL) not otherwise specified (NOS) and anaplastic large cell lymphoma.
- EBV+ DLBCL
- T-cell/histiocyte-rich large B-cell lymphoma (THRLBCL)
- EBV+ mucocutaneous ulcer
- Immune deficiency/dysregulation–associated lymphoproliferative disorders (IDD-LPDs)
- Low grade B-cell lymphomas with immunoblastic proliferations
- Infectious mononucleosis

Use of IHC panel (CD15, CD30, CD20, ALK, and CD45) is crucial to avoid misdiagnosis.

GRANULOMA

Q53. What is a granuloma?

Ans: Granulomas are localized clusters of active macrophages (epithelioid cells) that are frequently encircled by lymphocytes and occasionally contain multinucleated giant cells. They are created in reaction to a prolonged irritant, such as an autoimmune trigger, infection, or foreign material.

Q54. What are the types of granulomas?

Ans:
- *Caseating granulomas*—central necrosis [e.g., tuberculosis (TB)] **(See Figs. 10A to D)**
- *Noncaseating granulomas*—no necrosis (e.g., sarcoidosis, Crohn's disease).
- *Suppurative granulomas*—with central neutrophilic abscess (e.g., cat scratch disease).
- *Foreign body granulomas*—response to inert materials.
- *Immune granulomas*—due to persistent antigen (e.g., fungi, TB).

Q55. Name three infectious causes of granuloma.

Ans: *Mycobacterium tuberculosis, Histoplasma capsulatum,* and *Schistosoma species.*

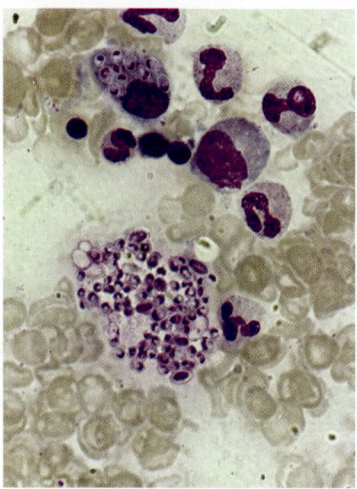

FIG. 1: Histoplasmosis.
Courtesy: Dr Aastha Gupta.

Q56. Enumerate causes of noninfectious granulomas.

Ans:
- Sarcoidosis
- Crohn's disease
- Chronic beryllium disease
- Wegener's granulomatosis (GPA)
- Drug-induced (e.g., methotrexate, allopurinol)

Q57. Describe the cellular components and pathogenesis of granuloma formation.

Ans:
- *Macrophages* become *epithelioid cells* and sometimes fuse into *giant cells.*
- Driven by *Th1-type immune response*, especially *interferon (IFN)-γ, TNF-α,* and *IL-12.*[1]
- Persistent antigenic stimulus → sustained macrophage activation → granuloma formation.

Q58. How are immune granulomas different from foreign body granulomas?

Ans: Differences between immune granulomas and foreign body granulomas are given in **Table 5**.

TABLE 5: Differences between immune granulomas and foreign body granulomas.

Feature	Immune granulomas	Foreign body granulomas
Etiology	Persistent immune stimulus [e.g., tuberculosis (TB), fungi]	Inert material (e.g., sutures, silica)
T-cell involvement	Present (Th1-mediated)	Absent or minimal
Necrosis	May be caseating	Rare
Surrounding cells	Lymphocytes, plasma cells	Few inflammatory cells

Q59. What are the morphological differences between TB and sarcoid granulomas?

Ans: The morphological differences between TB and sarcoid granulomas are given in **Table 6**.

TABLE 6: Morphological differences between tuberculosis (TB) and sarcoid granulomas.

Feature	Tuberculous granuloma	Sarcoid granuloma
Necrosis	Caseating	Noncaseating
Giant cells	Langhans-type	Asteroid/Schwann or foreign-body type
Organisms	Acid-fast bacilli (Ziehl–Neelsen)	None seen
Fibrosis	Minimal early, later present	Prominent

Q60. What is the role of special stains and ancillary studies in diagnosing granulomas in tissue?

Ans:
- *Ziehl–Neelsen (ZN) stain*—Mycobacteria
- *Grocott's methenamine silver (GMS) and periodic acid-schiff (PAS) stains*—Fungi
- *Polarization*—Foreign materials (e.g., talc)
- *Polymerase chain reaction (PCR)*—Mycobacterial DNA
- *Culture*—Always advised in marrow granulomas for specific etiology.

Q61. Write the diagnostic approach to a granuloma seen on bone marrow biopsy.

Ans: Stepwise approach:
- *Clinical context*—immunosuppression, fever, hepatosplenomegaly, and travel history.
- *Histology*—caseating versus noncaseating.
- *Special stains*—ZN, PAS, and GMS.
- *Molecular testing*—TB PCR, fungal PCR.
- *Cultures*—mycobacterial, fungal, and blood.
- *Serological/autoimmune tests*—angiotensin-converting enzyme (ACE) levels, antineutrophil cytoplasmic antibody (ANCA), and serum calcium.
- *Exclude* HLH, lymphoma, and drugs.

Q62. What are Langhans giant cells (See Figs. 10A to D)?

Ans: They are multinucleated giant cells formed by fusion of macrophages, with peripherally arranged nuclei in a horseshoe pattern, typically seen in tuberculous granulomas.

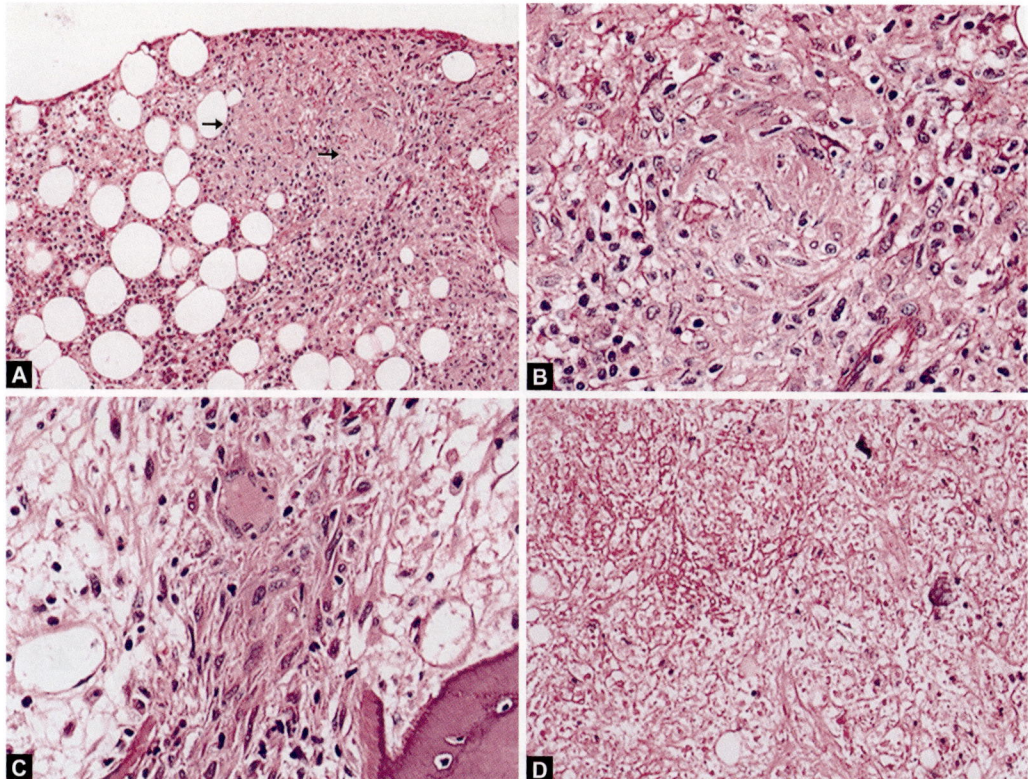

FIGS. 10A TO D: Bone marrow biopsy findings of a case of 18-year-old male presented with unexplained weight loss and pyrexia of unknown origin since 1 month. He came positive for *Mycobacterium tuberculosis* and confirmed by marrow culture and Ziehl–Neelsen (ZN) stain for acid-fast bacilli. (A) Epithelioid cell granulomas in bone marrow biopsy (BMB; H&E; 200×). (B) Caseating epithelioid cell granuloma surrounded by lymphocytes (BMB; H&E; 400×). (C) Langhans giant cells (BMB; H&E; 400×). (D) Caseous necrosis in focal area of the same biopsy (BMB; H&E; 100×).

OSTEITIS FIBROSA CYSTICA

Q63. What is osteitis fibrosa cystica (OFC)?

Ans: Osteitis fibrosa cystica is a skeletal complication of advanced hyperparathyroidism, characterized by increased bone resorption, marrow fibrosis, cyst formation, and presence of brown tumors.

Q64. Which condition most commonly causes OFC?

Ans:
- Primary hyperparathyroidism (e.g., parathyroid adenoma).
- Secondary hyperparathyroidism due to chronic kidney disease (CKD).

Q65. What is the pathophysiology of OFC?

Ans:
- Excess parathyroid hormone (PTH) stimulates osteoclast-mediated bone resorption.
- Leads to trabecular thinning, marrow fibrosis, and formation of cystic spaces.
- Accumulation of hemosiderin-laden macrophages forms "brown tumors."

Q66. Discuss the bone histopathology of OFC.

Ans: See **Figures 11A to F**.
- Increased osteoclastic resorption of cortical and trabecular bone.
- Peritrabecular marrow fibrosis.
- Replacement of marrow by fibrovascular tissue.
- Formation of cyst-like spaces and hemorrhage.
- Presence of multinucleated giant cells (especially in brown tumors).

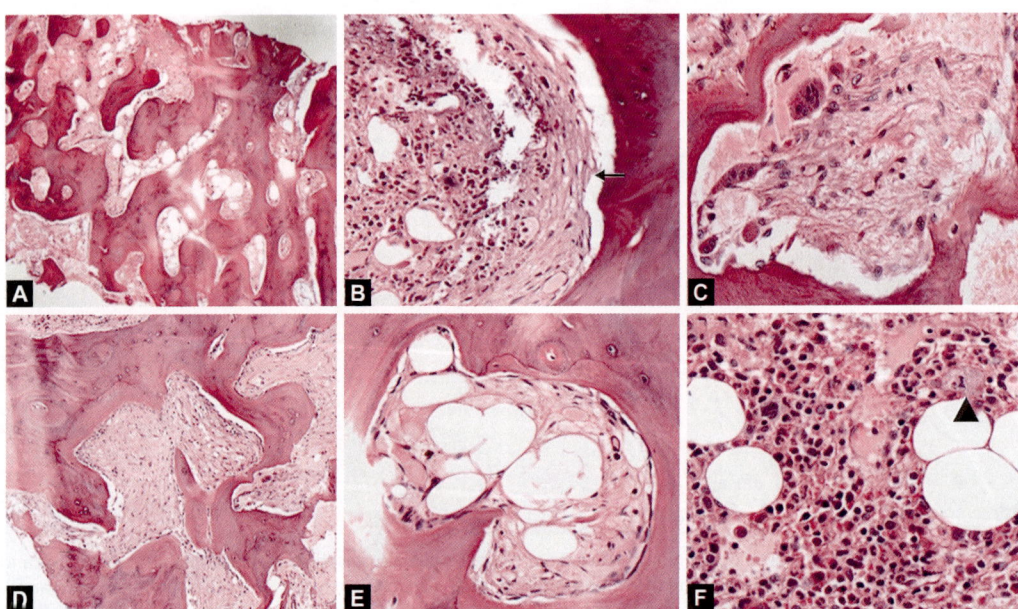

FIGS. 11A TO F: Bone marrow biopsy findings of a 66-year-old male with chronic kidney disease (CKD) stage-5 and high parathyroid (PTH) levels—suggestive of osteitis fibrosa cystica. (A) Bone marrow biopsy (BMB) showing a disorganized marrow architecture with extensive marrow remodeling and thickened bony trabeculae and replacement by fibrocollagenous tissue (H&E; 40×). (B) Peritrabecular fine fibrosis (arrow; H&E; 200×). (C) Increased osteoclastic activity with cystic dilatation of marrow space replaced by fibrous band (H&E; 400×). (D) Replacement of marrow spaces by fibrous tissue (H&E; 200×). (E) Increased osteoblastic activity with osteoblastic rimming of trabeculae (H&E; 400×). (F) Focal preserved area of trilineage hematopoiesis in the same biopsy with reduced erythroid cells, disproportionate to anemia, few histiocytes (arrowhead), and dysplastic megakaryocyte (thick arrow) (H&E; 400×).

Q67. Differentiate between primary and secondary hyperparathyroidism in the context of OFC.

Ans: Differences between primary and secondary hyperparathyroidism are given in **Table 7**.

TABLE 7: Differences between primary and secondary hyperparathyroidism.

Feature	Primary hyperparathyroidism (HPT)	Secondary HPT (CKD)
Cause	Parathyroid adenoma/hyperplasia	CKD → hypocalcemia ← ↑PTH
Calcium	↑ (Hypercalcemia)	↓ or normal
Phosphate	↓	↑ (due to CKD)
PTH	↑↑	↑
OFC occurrence	More common in late-stage	Common with long-standing CKD

(CKD: chronic kidney disease; OFC: osteitis fibrosa cystica; PTH: parathyroid hormone)

Q68. What is the significance of OFC in bone marrow biopsy reports?

Ans:
- Bone marrow biopsy may reveal fibrosis, cystic changes, and giant cells.
- In CKD patients, it helps differentiate between anemia due to myelofibrosis versus marrow fibrosis from secondary hyperparathyroidism.
- Important to correlate with PTH levels and renal function.

REFERENCES

1. Kumar V, Abbas AK, Aster JC, Debnath J, Das A. Robbins & Cotran Pathologic Basis of Disease, 11th edition. Philadelphia, PA: Elsevier; 2025.
2. Means Jr. RJ, Rodgers GP, Glader B, Arber DA, Appelbaum FR, Dispenzieri A, et al. Wintrobe's Clinical Hematology, 15th edition. Philadelphia, PA: Wolters Kluwer; 2024.
3. World Health Organization. WHO Classification of Tumours: Haematolymphoid Tumours, 5th edition, volume 1. Lyon, France: International Agency for Research on Cancer (IARC); 2022.

Index

Page numbers followed by *b* refer to box, *f* refer to figure, *fc* refer to flowchart, and *t* refer to table.

A

ABO
  incompatibility 284
  Rh grouping cards 271*f*
Absolute eosinophil count 33, 33*t*
Absolute neutrophil count 8, 10
Acid phosphatase reaction 130
Acid-fast bacilli 329*f*
Acoustic-assisted flow cytometry 136
Acquired immune deficiencies 27
Activated partial thromboplastin time 63-65, 67-69, 68*t*, 69*t*, 304
  clinical use of 68
Activated protein C 112
  resistance 65
Acute lung injury, transfusion related 275
Acute lymphoblastic leukemia 153, 196
Acute megakaryoblastic leukemia 215, 217
  characteristics features of 217
Acute myeloid leukemia 129, 152, 172, 175, 215, 216, 218
  morphological classification of 215
  risk of 206
  subtypes of 221
Acute myelomonocytic leukemia 215

Acute promyelocytic leukemia 221, 222, 222*f*, 224, 226, 227, 299
  clinical of 221
  genetics features of 221
  low risk 225
  molecular monitoring of 223
  morphological of 221
  treatment of 227
  variants of 223
Acute thrombotic episodes 65
Adaptive immune system 114
Adenocarcinoma, prostatic 319*f*
Adenosine diphosphate receptor blockers 76
Adhesion defects 19
Advanced mass spectrometry techniques 248
Afibrinogenemia 71
Air embolism 275
Air-dried smears 125
Albinism 23
Albumin 237
Alcoholism 43, 51
Alder–Reilly anomaly 16, 16*t*
Alkaline extraction 159
Allergic reaction 275, 276
  severe 276
Allogeneic stem cell transplant 49, 290, 291, 296
  role of 121, 227
Alloimmunization 275, 291
Allopurinol 327
All-trans retinoic acid 221
  therapy 224

Alpha-naphthyl butyrate esterase 129
Alpha-thalassemia 43, 58, 59
Alphoid repetitive probes 163
Altered light chain metabolism 264
Alzheimer disease, senile plaque of 312
Amyloid 241, 298, 311
  deposition, pattern of 312
  laser capture microdissection of 241
  physical structure of 311
  primary 241
  related systemic syndrome 298
  staining characteristics of 311
Amyloidosis 241, 311, 312
  primary 241
  secondary 241
Anaphylactic reactions 275
Anaplastic large cell lymphomas 203, 203*t*, 234
  characteristics features of 203
Anaplastic lymphoma kinase 203
Ancillary studies 328
Anemia 51, 284, 301, 330*f*
  aplastic 49, 50, 124, 208
  causes of 49
  congenital dyserythropoietic 50
  dimorphic 321*f*
  hemolytic 46, 51

Index

megaloblastic 59, 306
microcytic 58
normochromic 314
sideroblastic 43, 51
Angioimmunoblastic T-cell lymphoma, features of 202
Anisocytosis 142
Annual joint bleed rate 102
Anti-β2-glycoprotein-1 antibodies 111
Antibody 141, 283
  deficiencies 115
  panel testing 283
  production 291
  reduction 289
  screen 283
  selection 143
  testing 292
  titration 141
Anticardiolipin antibodies 111
Anticoagulants 1, 64, 83
  therapy 65
Antigen variation 282
Antiglobulin crossmatch 270
Antinuclear antibody 47
  test 47
Antiphospholipid syndrome 65, 67
Antithrombin 111
Apheresis 288, 290
Arsenic trioxide 221, 299
Aspirin 103
Asplenia 24
Autoimmune diseases 26, 137, 140
Autoimmune disorders 26, 109
Autoimmune lymphoproliferative syndrome 118
Autoimmunity 21
Autologous chimeric antigen receptor-cell therapy 294
Automated hemoglobin electrophoresis systems 60
Autosomal dominant 89, 115, 176
Autosomal recessive 89, 115, 176
Azathioprine 300

B

Babesia 6
Bactericidal assay 23
B-acute lymphoblastic leukemia 130
Banding, steps of 149
Basophilia 36
  causes of 36, 36t
B-cell 183f, 188
  aplasia 295
  lymphoma 164, 182-184, 184t, 192, 302
  malignancies 172
  rich lymphoid proliferation 183
Bence Jones protein 247, 253
  test 247
Bendamustine 301
Beryllium disease, chronic 327
Beta-globulins 238
Beta-thalassemia 53
  lab diagnosis of 53
  major 42
  trait 54f, 59
Bethesda assay 102, 108
Bioassay 73
Biomarker 31
Biopsy 205
Bleeding
  acquired causes of 103
  disorder 98
    screening of 68
  episode 97
  manifestation 95, 299
  mucocutaneous 300
  severe 78
  types of 85
Blood
  bank 285
    procedures 282
  cells 30, 30t
  components 274, 286
  group 269, 273, 291
    antigen removal 289
    crossmatch 289
    incompatibility 284
    techniques of 269
    typing 289
  sample 1, 63
  smear 2
    examination serves 2
    limitations of 6
  transfusion
    noninfectious complications of 274
    reactions 274
  vessel, thickened 312f
Bloom syndrome 117
B-lymphoblastic lymphoma 130
Bone
  biopsy 319f
  lesions 313
Bone marrow 120, 188, 289, 315, 316, 320, 322
  aspirate 5f, 124, 125, 125f, 127, 205, 319f, 321f
  biopsy 125, 266, 292, 301, 302, 312f, 314f, 319f, 320, 321f, 324f, 328, 329f, 330f, 331
    immunohistochemical staining of 131
    indications for 124
    reports 331
  disorders 11, 137
  evaluation 126
  examination 124
    indications of 124, 127
  failure syndromes 50, 175t
  findings 49, 188, 189, 205, 314, 322
  hypercellularity 220
  impact 291
  infiltration 316
    significance of 316
  metastasis 319, 320
  samples 146
  smear 30f
  specimen 147f
  transplantation 109
  trephine biopsy 130
    sections 130
Bortezomib 301
Brain 312
  magnetic resonance imaging of 307

Break-apart probes 163
Breast
  carcinoma 319f, 320
    implant-associated anaplastic large cell lymphomas 203
Breathlessness 302
  sudden onset 307
Bridging therapy 296
Brown tumors 329, 330
Bruton's tyrosine kinase deficiency 116, 191
Buffers 144
Burkitt lymphoma 28, 188, 189, 316

C

Calcium elevation 313
Cancer
  cells 294
  research 141
  surveillance 27
Capillary electrophoresis systems 60
Cardiac surgery 80
Cardiac toxicity 226
Cardiopulmonary bypass liver disease 76
Carfilzomib 301
Catastrophic antiphospholipid syndrome 307
  treatment of 307
Cell
  atypical clustering of 180
  collection 122
  cycle analysis 140
  made up of 114
  of origin 190, 191, 200, 229
  sorting 136
  type 30
  viability 141
Central nervous system 211
  international prognostic index 303
Centrifugation 280
Centroblasts 185
Cerebrospinal fluid 303
Cetyltrimethylammonium bromide extraction 159

Chediak–Higashi syndrome 23, 117, 118
  pathophysiology of 23t
Chemiluminescence 252
  assay 82, 250
  immunoassays 252
Chemoimmunotherapy 301
Chemotaxis
  assay 22
  defects 19
Chemotherapy 38, 109, 226
Chimeric antigen receptor T-cell 294, 295
  exhaustion of 296
  therapy 294, 296
    complications of 295
    side effects of 294
Chromogenic assay 72, 108
  procedure 72
Chromogenic enzyme-linked immunoassays activity assay 108
Chromogranin 320
Chromosomal microarray 146, 147
Chromosome
  analysis 151
  deletion of 154
  tetrasomy of 154f
  trisomies of 154f
Chronic kidney disease 260, 329, 330, 330f
Chronic lymphocytic leukemia 3f, 150, 164, 188, 190, 316, 317
  flow cytometry analysis of 195f
Chronic lymphoproliferative disorders 188, 190, 191, 197, 198, 301
  subtyping of 188t
Chronic myeloid leukemia 154, 155b, 211, 212
  microscopic features of 210
Chronic myelomonocytic leukemia 211, 218
Chronic neutrophilic leukemia 212

Ciclosporin-based immunosuppressive therapy 49
Circadian rhythm 65
Cisplatin 109
Clonal cytopenia 207
Clonal hematopoiesis 207
Clonal plasma cells 298
Clopidogrel 109
Clotting disorder 96
Clotting factor
  deficiencies 76
  level 97
Coagulation disorders 95, 95t, 100
  pathophysiology of 96
Coagulation parameters 64t, 65t
Codeine 99
Codocytes 40
Collagen 76
  binding assays 108
Collection procedure 287
Column agglutination test 269
Common phagocytic disorders 19
Complete blood count 53, 78, 87, 193, 299
  basics of 45
Concizumab 101
Congo red stain 298, 311
Conventional cytogenetic 146, 151, 222
  studies, method of 148b
Coombs test, direct 271, 292
Copy number variations 147
Cord 290
Core binding factor 216
Coronavirus disease-2019 66
Cortical bone 330
Cortical expansion, nodular pattern of 181t
Corticosteroid 300
Crohn's disease 327
Cross-linked fibrin, degradation of 113
Cryoprecipitate 100, 279
Crystal violet 311

Cyanotic congenital heart disease 103
Cyclic neutropenia 12, 13
Cyclooxygenase-2 inhibitors 76
Cyclophosphamide 109, 301, 303
Cyclosporine 109
Cyst formation 329
Cytochemical analysis 222
Cytochemistry 127
Cytogenetics 146, 148*t*, 151
  abnormalities 153, 156
  evaluation 150
  role of 151-154, 156
  techniques 147*t*
  types of 146
Cytokeratin 320
Cytokine release syndrome 224, 294
Cytomorphology 200, 201
Cytopenia 205, 239, 316
Cytoplasmic
  abnormalities 14
  alterations 205
  hairy projections 193*f*

D

Daratumumab 301
D-dimer
  measurement 113
  role of 112
Deep vein thrombosis 111, 306
  assessment of 112
Defective molecule 20
Defensive immune system 114
Degranulation
  assay 23
  defects 20
Delayed hemolytic transfusion reaction 275, 278
Dental extraction 63
Deoxyribonucleic acid 50, 294
  analysis 57
  based assay 73
  extraction method, silica column-based 159
  isolation of 158
Dermatologic disorders 99
Desensitization protocols 289

Dexamethasone 301, 316
Diabetes mellitus 99
Diamond–Blackfan anemia 176
Diffuse large B-cell lymphoma 28, 186, 189, 190, 191, 303, 316, 317
DiGeorge syndrome 116
Dihydrorhodamine
  flow cytometry 22
  test 21
Dimethyl sulfoxide 279
Direct antiglobulin test 272*f*
Direct oral anticoagulant 83
Direct tubular toxicity 259
Disseminated intravascular coagulation 224
Dodecyl sulfate detergent 158
Döhle bodies 18, 19
  etiology of 19*t*
Donor
  assessment 288
  lymphocyte 288
    harvest, indications for 288
    infusion, types of 288
  matching 121
  red blood cells unit
    selection 270
    testing 270
Downey cells 27
Doxorubicin 303
Dry marrow 124
Dual-color fusion probes 163
Dutcher bodies 315
Dyserythropoiesis 322
Dysfibrinogenemia 71
Dyskeratosis 175
Dysplasia 205, 208, 211, 214
Dysplastic megakaryocyte 330*f*
Dyspnea, transfusion associated 275

E

Echocardiography 298
Electronics system 134
Electrophoresis 262
Elevated erythrocyte sedimentation rate 314
Elution studies 283
Emapalumab 295

Emicizumab 101
  mechanism of action of 101
Endocrine disorders 11
Endocrinopathy 36, 240
Enzyme immunoassay, types of 47
Enzyme-linked immunosorbent assay 47, 70, 82, 113, 248, 286
Eosin-5-maleimide binding test 41
Eosinophil 36*f*
Eosinophilia 33*t*, 34, 36*f*
  causes of 32, 33*t*
  degree of 33, 33*t*
  mild 32
  moderate 32
  severe 32
Epigenetic, role of 207
Epinephrine 76
Epithelioid cell 327
  granuloma 329*f*
Epstein–Barr virus 27, 28, 324*f*
  infection 184
  latent 229
  role of 230
Erythroblasts, mitochondria of 44
Erythrocyte sedimentation rate 46
  significance of 47
Erythroid
  cells 330*f*
  hypoplasia 322
Erythrophagocytosis 315*f*
Escherichia coli 12, 109
Essential thrombocythemia 213
Esterases, nonspecific 128
Ethylenediaminetetraacetic acid 1, 63, 64
Etoposide 316
European Leukemia Network 223
Ewing's sarcoma 320
Excision biopsy 179
Expanded marginal zone cells, monomorphic appearance of 184
Extranodal tumorous infiltrate 148

Index

F

Failure to thrive 142
Fanconi anemia 50, 175
Febrile nonhemolytic
 transfusion reaction 275, 276
Fetal hemoglobin 43
 persistence of 43, 59
Fever 302
 prolonged 124
 recurrent 13
Fibrinogen 70
 assay
  clinical use of 70
  uses of 70*f*
 estimation 70
 levels 70
Fibroblasts 214
Fibrocollagenous tissue 330*f*
Fibrosis 260
Fibrotic marrow 124
Fibrovascular tissue 330
Fitusiran 101
Flame cells 28
Florid reactive lymphoid
 hyperplasia 184, 184*t*
Flow cytometer, calibration of 141
Flow cytometric
 analysis 119
 immunophenotypic testing 141
 profile, characteristics of 189, 190*fc*
Flow cytometry 22, 23, 32, 119, 134, 136, 138, 138*t*, 143, 194*f*-196*f*
 advantages of 134
 limitations of 135
 principle of 135
 role of 184
 significance of 206
Fluidics system 134, 135
Fluorescence
 activated cell sorting 136
 calibration 141
 detection 135
 minus one controls 144
 resonance energy transfer
  assay 108

Fluorescence in situ
 hybridization 127, 146, 147, 151, 162, 205, 206, 212, 222, 318
 advantages of 166
 analysis 322*f*
  interphase 147*f*, 153*f*, 157*f*
 basic principle of 162
 limitations of 166
 technique 166
 testing 162
Fluorochrome selection 143, 144
Follicular hyperplasia 185*f*
Follicular lymphoma 179, 184, 184*t*, 185, 185*f*, 188, 189, 191, 316, 317*f*
Food and Drug Administration 171
Foreign body granulomas 326-328, 328*t*
Fractures, pathologic 313
Free light chains 247, 248, 252, 262
 abnormal serum 261
 assays 249
 concentration 254, 255
 diagnostic role of 264
 normal renal clearance of 262
 prognostic role of 264
 ratio, abnormal 298
 role of 264
Fresh frozen plasma 100, 279
 features of 100*t*
Functional flow cytometry 136
Fungi 328

G

Gamma globulins 238
Gastrointestinal bleeding,
 chronic 51
Gaucher cells 241
Gemcitabine 109
Genes 12, 175, 176
 deletions 58
 modification 122
 panel 174
 therapy 120, 122, 304
  role of 122

Genetics 12, 35, 36
 abnormalities 151*t*, 215
 alterations 229
 analysis 120, 222
 counseling 305
 defect 20, 122
 inheritance 17
 mutations 21, 224
 testing 22, 53, 120, 242
  role of 92
Genome-wide association
 studies 161
Genomic stability, master
 regulator of 208
Germline mutation 174, 175
 recognition of 172
Germline predisposition
 syndromes 172
Giant platelets 18
Giemsa stain 34*f*
Globulin patterns 237
Glomerular basement
 membrane, thickening of 312
Glomerulonephritis,
 proliferative 301
Glucocorticoids 301
Good-quality trephine biopsy
 specimen 49
Graft manipulation techniques 289
Graft-versus-host disease 140, 275, 291
Granular lymphocyte leukemia 197, 198
Granuloma 326, 328
 causes of 327
 formation 21
 pathogenesis of 327
 noncaseating 326
 noninfectious 327
 suppurative 326
 tuberculous 328
 types of 326
Granulomatous disease,
 chronic 21, 116
Granulomatous slack skin 200
Green-blue granules,
 perinuclear ring of 44
Grocott's methenamine silver 328

H

Hairy cell leukemia 127, 132, 172, 188-192
  flow cytometry analysis of 194f
  variant 132
Hallmark cell 234
Harvest procedures 148
Harvesting donor lymphocytes 288
Heart 312
  muscle fibers 312
Heat
  precipitation test 248
  solubility 247
Heinz body 40, 43
Hematocrit, high 65
Hematological diseases 171, 174, 239
Hematological disorders 137, 162
Hematological malignancies 140, 163, 172, 217
Hematology 159, 311
Hematolymphoid malignancies 196
Hemato-oncology 159
Hematopoietic stem cell transplantation 120, 227, 273
Hemoglobin 4
  E disease 58
  electrophoresis 43, 53, 55
  fast-moving 40
  fractions 54
  high-performance liquid chromatography 55f
  S 56
  variants 54
Hemoglobinopathy 46, 59, 60
Hemoglobinuria, paroxysmal nocturnal 50, 112
Hemolysis 64
Hemolytic disease 283
Hemolytic transfusion reaction, acute 275
Hemophagocytic lymphohistiocytosis 28, 295
  treatment of 316
  types of 315

Hemophagocytosis 315, 316
Hemophilia 85, 95-99, 102-104
  A 72-74, 74t, 100
    inheritance of 72
    mild-moderate 73
  acquired 97, 98t, 99
  B 100
  carriers 305
  clinical history of 96
  complications of 101
  inherited 97, 98t
  seldom, moderate 100
  severity of 97t
  treatment of 101, 101t
  types of 95
Hemorrhage, intracranial 304
Hemosiderin-laden macrophages, accumulation of 329
Hemostasis 63
  period of 96
Heparin contamination 64, 66
Heparin-induced thrombocytopenia 80, 81, 83
  pathogenesis of 80
Hepatic disorders 103
Hepatic dysfunction 51
Hepatitis B virus 160
Hepatosplenic T-cell lymphoma 204, 204t, 317
Hepatosplenomegaly 284
Heterozygosity, loss of 147
Heyde syndrome 93
High reticulocyte index, causes of 46
High-molecular weight 89
  multimers 75, 78
High-performance liquid chromatography 53, 55, 212
  systems 60
  role of 54
Histopathology 266
Histoplasmosis 327f
Hodgkin's cells 229, 324f, 325
  classical 179
Hodgkin's disease 33
Hodgkin's lymphoma 28, 137, 182, 183, 229, 234
  classical 229, 323, 325, 325f
  histopathology of 230

  immunophenotype of 231
  interfollicular 179
  nodular lymphocyte predominant 325, 325t, 235
  pathogenesis of 230
  pathophysiology of 230
  subtypes of 231
Human cytomegalovirus 160
Human immunodeficiency virus 101, 106, 160
Human leukocyte antigen matching 289
Hybrid capture 287
Hydrops fetalis 284
Hypercalcemia 301
Hypercellular marrow 321f
Hypereosinophilia 34
  clinical subtypes of 35t
Hypereosinophilic syndrome 34
Hyperferritinemia 316
Hypergammaglobulinemia 263
Hyper-immunoglobulins
  E syndrome 116
  M syndrome 117
    autosomal recessive 117
Hyperparathyroidism
  primary 329, 330, 330t
  secondary 329, 330, 330t
Hyperplasia, megakaryocytic 220
Hypertriglyceridemia 316
Hyperviscosity 239
Hypocellular myelodysplastic syndrome 49
Hypochromia 142
Hypofibrinogenemia 71
Hypoplastic myelodysplastic syndrome 49, 131
Hypothyroidism 93

I

Idiopathic thrombocytopenic purpura 300
Imaging flow cytometry 136
Immature B cell 130
  malignancies 130t
Immature T cell malignancies 131t

Immune
  cell attack 291
  defects 118*t*
  dysregulation, diseases of 115
  effector cell-associated neurotoxicity syndrome 295
  function tests 120
  granulomas 326, 327, 328, 328*t*
  hemolytic anemia 27
  reaction 275, 291
  response 27
  system 114, 325
    replacement of 121
  thrombocytopenia 27, 173, 299, 300
Immunity, inborn errors of 114, 116, 117, 122
Immunoassay 73
  platforms 250, 251
Immunoblasts 235
Immunodeficiency 116
  diseases 114
  disorders 140
  severe combined 116, 121, 122
  syndromes 115
Immunoelectron microscopy 241
Immunofixation electrophoresis 239, 248, 301, 315
Immunofluorescence
  indirect 47
  microscopy 266
Immunoglobulins 28, 167
  G 80, 252
    normal serum half-lives of 252
  increased production of 263
  intravenous 285
  replacement therapy 120
  surface 190
Immunohistochemistry 41, 49, 132*t*, 138, 138*t*, 184, 311
  interpretation of 132
  markers 183*t*186
  role of 316

Immunomodulation, transfusion related 275
Immunomodulatory drugs 301
Immunophenotype 317, 323, 323*t*
Immunophenotypic abnormalities, typical 200
Immunosuppressive therapy 316
Immunoturbidimetry 248
Impaired fibrinolysis 224
Inclusions, types of 28
Infections 11, 24, 66, 103, 137
  monitoring 140
  severe 12
  viral 26, 137, 140, 286
Infectious diseases 160
Inflammation 21, 260
Inflammatory bowel disease 99
Inheritance, pattern of 77, 78
Inherited bone marrow failure 49
  syndromes 176
    management of 175
Inherited platelet disorders 173
Insoluble amyloid proteins 241
Intensive care unit 65
Intermittent flow apheresis machines 288
International Myeloma Working Group 240, 298
International Normalized Ratio 227
International Society on Thrombosis and Haemostasis Bleeding Assessment Tool 96
Iron 318
  deficiency anemia 42, 54
  loaded mitochondria 318
  overload 275
  staining 128, 129
Irritable bowel syndrome 42

J

Janus kinase 229
Jaundice 284
Job syndrome 115, 116
Joint bleeding, episodes of 73
Jordan anomaly 18

K

Karyotyping 146, 147
Kernicterus 284
Kidney
  biopsy 266
  disease, chronic 260, 329, 330, 330*f*
Killing defects 20
Kostmann's syndrome 12

L

Lactic dehydrogenase, serum levels of 316
Langerhans cell histiocytosis 218
Langhans giant cells 328, 329*f*
Lardaceous spleen 312
Large cell lymphoma 182, 183, 316
  intravascular 317
  refractory diffuse 296
Large granular lymphocytes 25, 26*t*
  role of 27
  types of 26, 26*t*
Laser light source 135
Latent membrane protein 230
Latex agglutination assays 113
Left ventricular ejection fraction 298
Leishman stain 25, 36*f*
Lenalidomide 301
Leukemia 98, 137, 192
  acute 124, 125*f*
    basophilic 215
    erythroid 215, 216
    monocytic 215
  juvenile myelomonocytic 219
Leukemoid reaction 31
  evaluation of 31*t*
Leukocyte
  adhesion
    defects 20
    deficiency 20, 20*t*, 115, 116
  alkaline phosphatase score 31, 129
Leukopenia 27, 314

Light chain
  deposition disease 239, 253, 265
  immunohistochemistry 244
    role of 245
  myeloma 247
  only multiple myeloma 252
Light microscopy 311
Light transmission aggregometry 77
Limb, Doppler ultrasound of 306
Liver
  disease 64
    alcoholic 51
  dysfunction 67
Low reticulocyte index, causes of 46
Low-grade indolent lymphomas 184
Lung carcinoma 320
Lupus anticoagulant 65, 111
Lupus test 66
Lymph node 180*t*, 186*f*
  architecture of 179
  biopsy 302
  evaluation of 179
  follicle 182*f*, 183*f*
  immunohistochemical evaluation of 182
  immunohistochemistry of 186
  reactive 182*f*
  retroperitoneal 179
  sinuses 180*t*
  sinusoidal architecture 180
  vascular architecture 180
Lymphadenopathy, generalized 302
Lymphocyte 25, 235, 329*f*
  preponderance of 193*f*
  reactive 25*f*
  subset analysis 119
  trafficking 180
  types of 25*t*
Lymphocytosis 27
  atypical 27
  causes of 23, 24*t*
Lymphoid
  cells 186*f*
  leukemias, precursor 173
  neoplasms 127, 172

Lymphoma 124, 137, 150, 183, 191, 316, 317*f*
  diagnosis 179, 181*t*, 184
  evaluation 179, 180
  subgroups of 182
  type 183
  typical 317
Lymphomatoid papulosis 200
Lymphomatous conditions 180, 181
Lymphopenia 119
Lymphoplasmacytic lymphoma 188-191, 316
Lymphoproliferative
  disease 197, 239
  disorders 24, 28, 188
Lysosomal abnormalities 23

M

Macroglossia 312
Macrophage 327
  inflammatory protein-1 alpha 313
Malignancy 109, 302
  risk of 13
Malignant disorders 137
Malignant plasma cells 29, 29*t*, 314
Malmo protocol 100, 101
Mansonella 6
Mantle cell lymphoma 190, 191, 316, 317
Marginal zone
  expansion 184
  lymphoma 184, 188-191, 316
Marrow
  aplasia 27, 124
  infiltration 316
    patterns, correlation of 317*t*
  involved lymphoma 317
  metastasis 320
  paratrabecular infiltration of 317*f*
  replacement of 330
Marstacimab 101
Mass spectrometry 60, 248, 250, 251, 311
Mature B cell 130, 225
  malignancies 130*t*
  neoplasms 188
Mature lymphocytes 3*f*, 193*f*

Mature T cell
  malignancies 131*t*
  neoplasms 197
May–Hegglin anomaly 18, 18*t*
Mean corpuscular volume 4, 45, 106, 305
Megakaryocytes 322
  atypia 214
  morphological characteristics of 213
Megakaryocytic markers 217
Melphalan 301
Menorrhagia 96
Mental retardation syndrome 59
Metalloproteinase 107
Metastasis 124
Metastatic
  carcinoma colon 302
  infiltration 320
  tumor cells 319*f*
Methotrexate 327
Methyl violet 311
Microangiopathy, thrombotic 41
Microarray 151
Microcytic hypochromic red blood cells 42*f*
Microcytosis 142
Microenvironment, role of 230
Microfluidic flow cytometry 136
Microplate test 209
Minimal residual disease 167, 176
Misfolded monoclonal proteins 239
Mitochondrial poisoning 43
Mitomycin 109
Mixed-phenotype acute leukemia 217
Molecular
  assays, limitations of 161
  cytogenetics 146
  genetics 203
  markers 196
Monitoring disease progression 254, 254
Monoclonal antibodies 301
Monoclonal band, significance of 239
Monoclonal free light chains 259, 265

Monoclonal gammopathy 243, 301
Monoclonal immunoglobulin deposits 301
Monoclonal plasma cell disorder 240
 proliferative disorder, evaluation of 298
Monoclonal production 254
Monoclonal protein 238, 239, 266
 deletion of 253
Monocytopenia 37
 causes of 38t
Monocytosis 37
Monomorphic epitheliotropic intestinal T-cell lymphoma 202
Mononucleosis, infectious 27, 326
Monosomal karyotype 152
Monosomy 154
Monospecific direct antiglobulin test 272, 273f
Morphine 99
Morphology, role of 180
Mortality rate 225
Mosaicism 73
Mott cells 315
Mucopolysaccharidosis
 diagnosis of 17t
 types of 16t
Mucosa-associated lymphoid tissue 184
Multicolor flow cytometry 136
Multiparametric analysis 134
Multiple factor deficiency 69
Multiple myeloma 5f, 137, 150, 156, 156t, 239, 254, 257, 312, 315
 oncogene 232
 risk stratification of 156
Multiplex ligation-dependent probe amplification 73
Mutation 151
Mycobacteria 328
Mycobacterium tuberculosis 329f
Mycosis fungoides 200
Myelodysplasia 124
Myelodysplastic disorders 132

Myelodysplastic neoplasm 150, 161, 151f, 205, 318, 320
 pathognomonic of 206
 pathophysiology of 207
 treatment of 207
Myelodysplastic syndrome 137, 151, 172, 164, 205, 319, 320
 cytogenetic-based risk classifications of 206
 diagnosis of 206
 management of 175
Myelofibrosis 124, 155, 213
Myeloid 127
 antigens 296
 lineage 217
 malignancies 131t, 215
 neoplasms 172
Myeloma 239, 255, 313, 314
 diagnosis of 244
 evaluation 124
 symptom of 313
Myeloperoxidase 128, 216
Myeloproliferative disorders 132, 154
Myeloproliferative neoplasm 37, 112, 172, 210, 219
 overlap syndromes 172
Myelosuppression 226

N

Naphthol 129
National Cancer Institute 171
Natural killer cell 197, 198
Neoplastic disorders 38
Neoplastic follicles 185f
Nephelometers 250
Nephrotic range proteinuria 301
Nephrotoxicity, mechanisms of 259
Neural cell adhesion molecule 245
Neuroblastoma 320
Neutralizing antibodies 108
Neutropenia 10, 11, 119
 causes of 8, 8t, 10, 10t
 classification of 10t
 congenital 10, 12
 drug-induced 11
 immune-associated 10

 mild 10
 moderate 10
 postinfectious 11
 severe 10
 congenital 12, 12t
Neutrophilia 10f
 factitious 8
 primary 8
 reactive 9
 secondary 9
Neutrophils 13, 14t, 18t
 function
 assessment of 22t
 defects 19, 19t, 22
 hereditary hypersegmentation of 17
 hypersegmentation of 17
 morphologic features of 18t
 phagocytosis of 315f
Newborn screening methods 59
Next-generation sequencing 170, 171, 175t
 limitations of 176
 role of 50
Nitroblue tetrazolium test 21, 22
Nodal T-follicular helper 234
Nodular lymphoid 317f
Nonchemotherapy approaches 226
Nonfactor therapies 101
Nonhematological disorders 138
Non-Hodgkin lymphoma 130, 131, 137, 186f, 203
Nonimmune chronic idiopathic neutropenia 11
Nonimmune hematologic disorders 10
Nonimmune hemolysis 275
Non-neutralizing antibodies 108
Nonsense mutations 53
Nonsteroidal anti-inflammatory agents 103
Nuclear abnormalities 14
Nucleic acid
 isolation of 158
 testing 286
Nutritional deficiencies 11, 51

O

Oncogenic potential mutations, conal hematopoiesis of 207
One stage clotting assay 71, 71*t*
Optical filters 135
Optical genome mapping 146
Optics system 134
Orchiectomy 303
Organic extraction 158
Organomegaly 240
Osteitis fibrosa cystica 329, 330, 330*f*
  bone histopathology of 330
  pathophysiology of 329
  significance of 331
Osteoblastic activity 330*f*
Owl-eye appearance 324*f*
Oxidative burst
  defects 20
  test 22

P

Packed cell volume 45
Pagetoid reticulosis 200
Pain 306
  management of 99
Pancytopenia 299
Panel optimization 144
Paracetamol 99
Paraffin embedded tissue 170
Para-nitro aniline 98
Parathyroid
  adenoma 329
  hormone 330
    stimulates 329
Passenger lymphocyte syndrome 274, 292
Pelger–Huët anomaly 14, 15, 15*t*
  diagnosis of 15*t*
  differential diagnosis of 15*t*
Perinephric fluid collections 240
Perinuclear clearing 231
Periodic acid-Schiff 126
  reaction 128
  stains 328

Peripheral blood 33*t*, 148, 314, 321*f*
  findings 314
  typical 320
  low magnification microscopic picture of 193*f*
  smear 1, 2*f*, 3*f*, 5*f*, 6*f*, 7, 10*f*, 26, 31, 34*f*, 36*f*, 40, 42*f*, 45, 52*f*, 53, 65, 78, 107*f*, 188, 189, 302, 314*f*
  stem cell 287, 289
Peripheral nerve involvement 298
Peripheral smear 6
  examination 6
Peripheral T-cell lymphoma 204
  characteristics of 203
Peritrabecular marrow fibrosis 330
Perls' reaction 128, 129
Perls' stain 43, 318
Phagocyte function tests 120
Phagocytic disorders 19
Phagocytosis
  assay 22
  defects 19
Phenol-chloroform method 159
Phenytoin 65
Philadelphia chromosome 155*f*
Phosphate-buffered saline 185
Plasma
  exchange 289
  normal pooled 75
Plasma cell 5, 28, 30*f*, 127, 235, 241, 301, 314, 314*f*, 326
  atypical 314
  binucleated 315
  disorders 172, 247
    monitoring of 253
  immunophenotype of 29
  morphology of 28, 28*t*
  multifocal neoplastic proliferation of 312
  myeloma 164, 312
  reactive 29
Plasmacytoid lymphocytes 28
Plasmapheresis 280

Plasmic score 106
Plasmodium 6
  vivax schizont 6*f*
Platelet 18*t*, 91, 95
  activation assays 82
  contamination 66
  count 65, 304
  disorders 95, 95*t*
  function
    assay 76, 76*f*
    defects, acquired 76
    disorder 76
  washing 82
Plump high-endothelial venules vascular hyalinization 180
POEMS syndrome 240
Poikilocytosis 142
Point-of-care devices 60
Polarization 328
Polyadenylation signal mutations 53
Polychromasia 43
Polychromatophilic cells 41
Polyclonal
  expansion 264
  gammopathies 237
  gaussian curve 168
  production 254
Polycythemia vera 213
Polymerase chain reaction 12, 73, 158
  quantitative 154
  single-cell 229
  techniques, role of 159
Polyneuropathy 240
Polyvinyl sulfonate 82
Pomalidomide 301
Popliteal vein thrombosis 306
Positive Prussian blue 129
Postharvest care 287
Post-thrombotic syndrome 307
Post-transplantation lymphoproliferative disorder 28
  immunotherapy 288
Prednisone 301
Pregnancy 109
Primary cutaneous anaplastic large cell lymphomas 203

Index

Primary immunodeficiency
　disease 20, 114, 121
　disorder 21, 114
Procoagulant substances,
　release of 224
Proinflammatory cytokines,
　release of 225
Prolonged prothrombin time
　69t
　causes of 67t
Prominent nucleoli 192
Promoter region mutations 53
Promyelocytes, atypical 299
Prostate
　carcinoma 320
　specific antigen 320
Protein
　C deficiency 112
　electrophoresis, major
　　importance of 237
　fractions 239
　typing 242
Proteinuria 260, 298
　diagnosis of 253
Prothrombin gene mutation
　111
Prothrombin time 63-65, 67,
　304
　clinical use of 67
Prussian blue stain 44, 128, 129,
　318, 318f
Pseudomonas aeruginosa 12
Pseudo-Pelger-Huët anomaly
　15
Pure red cell aplasia,
　pathophysiology of 291
Pyogenic infections, recurrent
　23
Pyrexia of unknown origin 329f

Q

Quality control 285
　frequency of 160
Quality metrics 174
Quantitative analysis 140, 248,
　251
Quantitative immunoglobulins
　120
Quinidine 109

R

Random donor platelets 280
Rapid screening tests 82
Reactive oxygen species 21
Recurrent cerebral vein
　thrombosis episodes 65
Red blood cell 2f, 40, 289
　agglutination 5f
　contamination 289
　distribution width 45
　engraftment 290
Reed-Sternberg cells 179, 229,
　231, 323-325, 324f, 324t,
　325f
　classical 323, 323t, 324f
　diagnostic role of 325
　mimickers of 326
　origin of 323
Refractile bodies 241
Refractory multiple myeloma
　296
Reinfusion 122
Renal amyloidosis 243
　histological features of 242
Renal artery embolism 307
Renal biopsy 301
Renal disease 103
Renal dysfunction 264
Renal failure 313
Renal hemodynamics 259
Renal impairment 262
　impact of 262
Renal significance, monoclonal
　gammopathy of 243, 301
Respiratory diseases 99
Reticulocyte 41
　count 43
　　significance of 41
　index 46
　production index 46
Retinoic acid
　receptor alpha 221
　syndrome 224
Reverse transcriptase
　polymerase chain reaction
　222, 299
Revised International Prognostic
　Scoring System 152
Rh incompatibility 284

Rhabdomyosarcoma 320
Ribonucleic acid, isolation of
　158, 159
Ring sideroblasts 44, 205, 206,
　318, 319, 322
　causes of 318
Ristocetin-induced platelet
　agglutination 75, 78, 88
　procedure 77
Rituximab 301, 303
Romanowsky stains 7
Rouleaux formation 5f, 6f, 314,
　314f
Russell bodies 315

S

Sago spleen 312
Salting-out method 159
Sarcoid granulomas 328, 328t
Sarcoidosis 327
Schistocytes 107f, 299, 302
Schnitzler syndrome 240
Scleromyxedema 240
Seizures 65, 307
Sensitivity 50, 239
　high 250, 251
Sepsis 30, 30t, 31t, 98
Serum amyloid levels 242
Serum free light chain 254, 256,
　257, 262, 263
　analysis, limitations of 258
　assays 248, 250t
　measurements 257
　rapid response assessment,
　　mechanisms of 262
　short half-life of 259
　tests 266
Serum immunofixation
　electrophoresis 238, 239t
Serum protein electrophoresis
　237, 237t, 238, 239, 239t,
　266, 301, 315
Sézary syndrome 197, 200
　cell of origin of 200
Shwachman-Diamond
　syndrome 12, 176
Sickle cell
　anemia 46
　disease 43
　　severity of 43
　trait 56f

Sickle solubility test 57
Sideroblast 318
Silica-based methods 158
Siltuximab 295
Single nucleotide
   polymorphism 161
Skin bleed, types of 95
Small B-cell lymphoma 182,
   183, 183t
Small lymphocytic lymphoma
   188, 190, 191, 316, 317
Sodium dodecyl sulfate-
   polyacrylamide gel
   electrophoresis 108
Soft tissue bleeding 74
Solitary plasmacytoma 239, 261
Somatic mutation 174
Sparse population 230
Sperm cryopreservation 303
Spherocytosis, hereditary 51
Spiculated red cells, types of 40
Splenectomy 300
Splenic marginal zone
   lymphoma 132, 190, 191,
   192t, 317
Splenomegaly 316
Splice site mutations 53
Standard donor lymphocyte
   infusion 288
Standard flow cytometry 136
Staphylococcus aureus 12
Stem cell 279, 287, 289
   products 289
   transplant 120, 273
      recipient 289
Stress 24
   cytogenetics 50
Swelling 306
Synaptophysin 320
Systemic inflammatory
   response syndrome 295
Systemic lupus erythematosus
   109, 302, 307

T

T-acute lymphoblastic leukemia
   131
Target cells 40

Tartrate-resistant acid
   phosphatase reaction 130
T-cell 183f, 316
   acute lymphoblastic
      leukemia
      diagnosis of 196f
      precursor 196
   chronic lymphoproliferative
      disorders 197
   function tests 120
   large granular lymphocytic
      leukemia 197-199
      features of 199
   leukemia 197-199
   lineage 198
   lymphoid lymphomas,
      primary cutaneous 200
   lymphoma 164, 182, 183,
      196, 197
      adult 197, 198
      cutaneous 200t
      enteropathy-associated
         202
      intestinal 202
   neoplasms 172
   prolymphocytic leukemia
      197-199
   receptor
      gamma delta 317
      gene rearrangements 167
   therapy 294
      adoptive 288
Telomere biology disorders 175
Thalassemia 40, 53, 54
   carriers 173
Thalidomide 301
Thioflavin 311
Thrombin time 64, 65
Thrombocytopenia 18, 87, 305,
   307, 314, 322
   causes of 80
   gestational 300
   heparin-induced 80, 81, 83
   neonatal 300
   severe 302
Thrombocytosis 322
Thrombophilia 111
   hereditary 111
   inherited 111

Thrombotic disorders,
   screening of 68
Thrombotic thrombocytopenic
   purpura 106
   diagnosis of 107, 108
   pathophysiology of 106
   primary 106
   secondary 106
Thyroid transcription factor-1
   320
Ticlopidine 109
Time-of-flight flow cytometry
   136
T-lymphoblastic
   lymphoma 131
   proliferation, indolent 196
T-lymphoid neoplasms 196
Tocilizumab 295
Toluidine blue stain 130
Tongue 312
Total body irradiation 109
Toxic granules 19
Trabecular bone 330
Tramadol 99
Tranexamic acid 227
Tranfusion transmitted
   infection 101
Transforming growth factor-
   beta 230
Transfusion
   associated circulatory
      overload 275-277
   medicine 282
   basics of 269
Transient abnormal
   myelopoiesis 217
Transplantation 140
Transretinoic acid 225
Traumatic venipuncture 64
Trephine sections 127
Tru-cut biopsy 179
Trypanosoma 6
Tube test 269
Tuberculosis 328t
Tubular dysfunction 260
Tumor
   antigen 295
   cells 295, 319f
      sequencing of 170

media 312f
microdissection 170f
pediatric 320
staging 124
Turbidimeters 250
Two stage clotting assays 71, 71t
Tyrosine kinase mutation 212

U

Ulcers, aphthous 13
Ultralarge immune complexes 81
Unbalanced clonal abnormalities 152
Unfractionated heparin therapy 67
Upshaw–Schulman syndrome 106
Uremia 76
Urine
  concentrations 253
  detection 247
  levels 254
  monoclonal immunoglobulin 312
  protein 298
  protein electrophoresis 242, 248, 315
  role of 252, 253
  sample collection 248
  tests 260, 266
Utrecht protocol 101

V

Vaccine development 141

Venipuncture 1
Venous thromboembolism 111
Versatility 251
Vesicular trafficking, congenital disorders of 11
Viral infections 26, 137, 140, 286
  treatment of 288
Virus-associated hemophagocytic syndrome 27
Vitamin
  B12 42, 306
  K
    antagonist therapy 67
    deficiency 67
von Willebrand antigen 97
von Willebrand collagen binding activity 75, 78
von Willebrand disease 74t, 77, 77t, 78, 85-87, 89, 89t, 90, 91, 97, 98
  assays 74t
  diagnosis of 74, 75fc, 86, 93
  evaluation of 92
  second-line tests for 88
  subtypes 77t
von Willebrand factor 74, 75, 78, 81, 89, 106
  activity
    levels 91
    platelet-dependent 304
    ratio of 92
  antigen 75, 78, 86, 92
    assay 90
    levels 91
  propeptide 75
von Willebrand syndrome 93
  acquired 93

W

Waldenström's macroglobulinemia 172, 239
Warning signs 115, 115t
Wegener's granulomatosis 327
Weight loss 329f
Westergren method 46
Western blotting 108
White blood cell 3, 8
  count 27, 30
Whole-exome sequencing 173, 174
Whole-genome sequencing 173, 174
Wilson disease protein gene 43
Wintrobe method 46
Wiskott–Aldrich syndrome 12, 116, 122
World Health Organization 127
Wright-Giemsa stain 125
Wuchereria bancrofti, microfilaria of 34f

X

X-linked agammaglobulinemia 116
X-linked recessive 74, 176
  disorders 95
XmnI polymorphism 58

Z

Zeta sediment ratio 46
Ziehl–Neelsen stain 328, 329f